Sexually Transmitted Infections and AIDS in the Tropics

Edited by
O.P. Arya and C.A. Hart

Department of Medical Microbiology and Genitourinary Medicine
University of Liverpool, Liverpool, UK

CABI *Publishing*

CABI *Publishing* – a division of CAB INTERNATIONAL

CABI *Publishing*
CAB INTERNATIONAL
Wallingford
Oxon OX10 8DE
UK

Tel: +44 (0)1491 832111
Fax: +44 (0)1491 833508
Email: cabi@cabi.org

CABI *Publishing*
10E 40th Street
Suite 3203
New York, NY 10016
USA

Tel: +1 212 481 7018
Fax: +1 212 686 7993
Email: cabi-nao@cabi.org

A catalogue record for this book is available from the British Library, London, UK

Library of Congress Cataloging-in-Publication Data
Sexually transmitted infections and AIDS in the tropics / edited by
O.P. Arya and C.A. Hart.
p. cm.
Includes bibliographical references and index.
ISBN 0–85199–262–5 (alk. paper)
1. Sexually transmitted diseases– –Tropics. 2. AIDS (Disease)– –Tropics. 3. Tropical medicine. I. Hart, C.A. (Charles Anthony)
[DNLM: 1. Acquired Immunodeficiency Syndrome– –epidemiology.
2. Acquired Immunodeficiency Syndrome– –prevention & control.
3. Sexually Transmitted Diseases– –epidemiology. 4. Tropical Climate. WC 503 S518 1998]
RC200.1.S495 1998
616.95´1´00913– –dc21
DNLM/DLC
for Library of Congress 98–23327
CIP

ISBN 0 85199 262 5

Typeset in 10pt Souvenir by Solidus (Bristol) Limited
Printed and bound in the UK by Biddles Ltd, Guildford and King's Lynn

CONTENTS

The colour plate section can be found after the index

CONTRIBUTORS

A.B. Alawattegama, *Department of Genitourinary Medicine, Royal Liverpool University Hospital, Prescot Street, Liverpool L7 8XP, UK.*

O.P. Arya, *Department of Medical Microbiology and Genitourinary Medicine, University of Liverpool, Duncan Building, Daulby Street, Liverpool L69 3GA, UK.*

H.D.L. Birley, *Department of Medical Microbiology and Genitourinary Medicine, University of Liverpool, Duncan Building, Daulby Street, Liverpool L69 3GA, UK.*

V. Chandeying, *Department of Obstetrics and Gynaecology, Faculty of Medicine, Prince of Songkla University, Hat Yai 90112, Thailand.*

J.B.S. Coulter, *Liverpool School of Tropical Medicine, Pembroke Place, Liverpool L3 5QA, UK.*

C.A. Hart, *Department of Medical Microbiology and Genitourinary Medicine, University of Liverpool, Duncan Building, Daulby Street, Liverpool L69 3GA, UK.*

J. Kayita, *Department of Paediatrics and Child Health, Makerere University Medical School, PO Box 7072, Kampala, Uganda.*

K. Keersmaekers, *Department of Epidemiology and Community Medicine, University of Antwerp, Universiteitsplein 1, B-2610 Antwerp, Belgium.*

A.S. Latif, *Department of Medicine, University of Zimbabwe, PO Box A178, Avondale, Harare, Zimbabwe.*

A. Meheus, *Department of Epidemiology and Community Medicine, University of Antwerp, Universiteitsplein 1, B-2610 Antwerp, Belgium.*

A.O. Osoba, *Division of Microbiology, King Khalid National Guard Hospital, PO Box 9515, Jeddah 21423, Saudi Arabia.*

P. Phanuphak, *Department of Medicine, Faculty of Medicine, Chulalongkorn University, Rama IV Road, Bangkok 10330, Thailand.*

J. Richens, *Department of Sexually Transmitted Disease, University College London Medical School, Mortimer Market Centre, Mortimer Market, London WC1E 6AU, UK.*

T.F. Schulz, *Department of Medical Microbiology and Genitourinary Medicine, Duncan Building, University of Liverpool, Liverpool L69 3GA, UK.*

D.M. Serwadda, *Institute of Public Health, Makerere University Medical School, PO Box 7072, Kampala, Uganda.*

A. Sivayathorn, *Department of Dermatology, Faculty of Medicine, Siriraj Hospital, Mahidol University, Prannok Road, Bangkok 10700, Thailand.*

G.B. Wyatt, *Liverpool School of Tropical Medicine, Pembroke Place, Liverpool L3 5QA, UK.*

PREFACE

Sexually transmitted infections (STI) are a major public health problem both in their own right and because of their link with HIV infection. This has elevated their control to an absolute priority throughout the world. In developing countries, which account for approximately 75% of the easily curable STI, as estimated by the WHO, and where sexually transmitted HIV infection has reached epidemic proportions, the need is even more acute. Here AIDS is claiming hundreds of thousands of lives, and will continue to do so for the foreseeable future. In addition, because of inadequate resources, the sequelae of STI (e.g. infertility and some cancers) contribute greatly to ill health in the tropics. The inevitable consequences are social and economic upheaval in societies in developing countries. Whereas a change in sexual behaviour is the most important preventive measure, the appropriate management of STI is equally important for the prevention and control of these infections, including AIDS.

Despite its limitations, the 'syndromic' or problem-oriented approach will continue to play a significant role in STI/HIV control in many tropical countries lacking resources. These approaches are, therefore, well covered in the book. At the same time, efforts must continue to be made to strengthen the infrastructure and improve and expand appropriate diagnostic and treatment facilities at the primary health care level. As Professor Phanuphak makes clear in his chapter, tropical countries are at varying stages of economic development. Consequently, some countries can better afford to provide more appropriate and effective intervention strategies and support components for STI and HIV control.

This book, written by acknowledged experts working in, or with experience of, the tropical countries, provides authoritative, clear, concise and up-to-date knowledge and understanding on all aspects of STI. It should be useful for all those involved in the appropriate management and control of STI, HIV and AIDS in various settings, ranging from peripheral and rural urban health centres to the large hospitals of the tropical countries at various stages of development. We envisage that this book will also be helpful in training health care professionals in the various aspects of STI, HIV and AIDS in these countries.

The book is divided into three sections. Part I includes epidemiology and other basic considerations, Part II describes clinical and management aspects, and Part III covers some special topics and control aspects including problem-oriented approaches. Although the book is multi-authored, we have attempted to ensure a uniform style, avoiding duplication wherever possible, except for the chapters on problem-oriented approaches which are meant to stand on their own. Extensive bibliography has been avoided except for the chapter on epidemiology. Most other chapters provide a short list of further reading at the end.

Acknowledgements

OPA is grateful to Churchill Livingstone, the publisher of *Tropical Venereology*, 2nd edition, 1988 (by O.P. Arya, A.O. Osoba and F.J. Bennett) for clearance to develop this book, and for permission to reproduce several illustrations.

We wish to thank Mrs Heather Stefaniak, Mrs Linda Jones and Mrs Marilyn Forster for typing the manuscript with patience and care, Mr Noel Blundell for his help in collating the final version, and our publishers, CAB INTERNATIONAL, for their support and understanding.

O.P. Arya and C.A. Hart
Liverpool, 1998

Whilst every effort has been made to check the drug dosages, some errors may have occurred or the drug regimen(s) may subsequently have been revised. In addition, due to space constraints, the various contraindications and side effects have been omitted. Readers are, therefore, urged to consult their national formularies and/or the drug manufacturers' literature before prescribing the drugs mentioned in this book.

ABBREVIATIONS

AHU	arginine, hypoxanthine, uracil
AIC	AIDS Information Centre
AIDS	acquired immune deficiency syndrome
APC	antigen-presenting cells
BCG	bacille Calmette-Guérin
BV	bacterial vaginosis
CFT	complement fixation test
CIN	cervical intraepithelial neoplasia
CMRNG	chromosomally mediated penicillin-resistant *N. gonorrhoeae*
CMV	cytomegalovirus
CRP	C-reactive protein
CRPV	cottontail rabbit papillomavirus
CSF	cerebrospinal fluid
CTL	cytotoxic T lymphocytes
d4T	stavudine
DALYs	disability-adjusted life years
ddC	zalcitabine
ddI	didanosine
DEAFF	direct early antigen fluorescent foci
DEC	diethylcarbamazine
ECG	electrocardiogram
ELISA	enzyme-linked immunosorbent assay
EM	electron microscopy
EPI	extended programme of immunization
ESR	erythrocyte sedimentation rate
FP	family planning
FTA-ABS	fluorescent treponemal antibody absorption test
GPA	gel protein agglutination
GPI	general paralysis of the insane
GUD	genital ulcer disease
H(X)V	hepatitis (X) virus
HBcAg	hepatitis B core antigen
HBeAg	hepatitis B e-antigen
HBsAg	hepatitis B surface antigen
HIV	human immunodeficiency virus
HPV	human papillomavirus
HSV	herpes simplex virus
IEC	information, education, communication
IFAT	immunofluorescent antigen test
Ig	immunoglobulin
IL	interleukin
IUCD	intrauterine contraceptive device
IVDU	intravenous drug users
JH	Jarisch–Herxheimer
KS	Kaposi's sarcoma
KSHV	Kaposi's sarcoma-related herpesvirus

LCR	ligase chain reaction
LE	leukocyte esterase
LED	leukocyte esterase dip-stick test
LGV	lymphogranuloma venereum
LOS	lipo-oligosaccharide
LPA	latex particle agglutination
LSA	lichen sclerosus et atrophicus
MCH	maternal and child health
MCV	molluscum contagiosum virus
MHC	major histocompatibility complex
MIC	minimum inhibitory concentration
MIF	microimmunofluorescence
MOMP	major outer membrane protein
NGO	non-governmental organization
NGU	non-gonococcal urethritis
OMS	Organisations Mondiale de la Santé
Opa	opacity protein
ORF	open-reading frame
ORS	oral rehydration solution
PAHO	Pan-American Health Organization
PAS	Periodic acid–Schiff
PBMC	peripheral blood mononuclear cells
PCP	*Pneumocystis carinii* pneumonia
PCR	polymerase chain reaction
PDGF	platelet-derived growth factor
PEP	post-exposure prophylaxis
PGU	postgonococcal urethritis
PHC	primary health care
PI	prevention indicator
PID	pelvic inflammatory disease
PMN	polymorphonuclear leukocytes
PPE	pruritic papular eruption
PPLO	pleuropneumonia-like organism
PPNG	penicillinase-producing *N. gonorrhoeae*
Rb	retinoblastoma
RIA	radioimmunoassay
RPR	rapid plasma reagin
RT	reverse transcriptase
SIV	simian immunodeficiency virus
STI	sexually transmitted infection(s)
TASO	The AIDS Support Organization
3TC	lamivudine
T_H	T-helper
TPHA	*T. pallidum* haemagglutination assay
TRNG	tetracycline-resistant *N. gonorrhoeae*
UNAIDS	United Nations Programme on HIV/AIDS
VDRL	Venereal Disease Reference Laboratory
VLP	virus-like particle
VZV	varicella zoster virus
WHO	World Health Organization
ZDV	zidovudine

PART I
Epidemiology and Basic Considerations

CHAPTER 1
Epidemiology of sexually transmitted infections and AIDS in developing countries

K. Keersmaekers and A. Meheus
Department of Epidemiology and Community Medicine, University of Antwerp, Antwerp, Belgium

Public health importance and socioeconomic impact of STI in developing countries

The magnitude of the STI problem

Infections by a number of viruses, bacteria, fungi, protozoa or arthropods are transmitted primarily through heterosexual or homosexual contact. These sexually transmitted infections (STI) can result in a wide variety of clinical conditions (Table 1.1). This chapter will focus on those that have a high impact from a public health point of view.

STI rank among the most frequent infectious diseases (De Schrijver and Meheus, 1990). The World Health Organization (WHO) (1995a) estimated the incidence of four selected curable sexually transmitted diseases – gonorrhoea, syphilis, chlamydial infection and trichomoniasis – among adults aged 15–49 at 333 million cases for the whole of 1995 (Fig. 1.1). Of these, the vast majority occurred in the developing world: 45% in South and Southeast Asia, 20% in sub-Saharan Africa and 11% in Latin America and the Caribbean (Table 1.2) (WHO, 1995a).

Epidemiological monitoring in developing countries is not an easy task, and data on STI have to be interpreted with great caution. The aforementioned WHO figures are estimates based on a heterogeneous variety of data collected through official reporting systems and isolated studies, which means that quality and the degree to which they can be generalized vary considerably. Prevalence data from many countries can be found, usually from point prevalence studies conducted in selected populations. These data are not representative of the population as a whole, and an additional weakness of prevalence figures is that they are influenced not only by the magnitude of the STI epidemics, but also by the quality of STI treatment services provided for curable STI.

Data on STI incidence from most developing countries are scarce and

Table 1.1. Conditions associated with sexually transmitted infections (Goeman *et al.*, 1991).

Pathogen	Clinical condition
Bacteria	
Neisseria gonorrhoeae	Urethritis, epididymitis, orchitis, urethral stricture, infertility (in men)
	Cervicitis, endometritis, amnionitis, premature rupture of membranes (PROM), PID and sequelae, bartholinitis, perihepatitis (in women)
	Proctitis, pharyngitis (in both sexes)
	Conjunctivitis in the newborn
Chlamydia trachomatis	Urethritis, epididymitis, orchitis, urethral stricture, infertility (in men)
	Cervicitis, endometritis, amnionitis, PROM, PID and sequelae, bartholinitis, perihepatitis (in women)
	Proctitis, pharyngitis, Reiter syndrome (in both sexes)
	Conjunctivitis and pneumonia in the newborn
Treponema pallidum	Syphilis, pregnancy wastage and prematurity, congenital syphilis
Haemophilus ducreyi	Chancroid
Calymmatobacterium granulomatis	Donovanosis
Mycoplasma hominis	PID
Mycoplasma genitalium	Urethritis (?), PID (?)
Ureaplasma urealyticum	Urethritis (?), epididymitis (?), PID (?)
Viruses	
HSV-1 and HSV-2 (HHV-1 and HHV-2)	Genital and orolabial herpes, meningitis, encephalitis, neonatal herpes, pregnancy wastage, preterm birth
Hepatitis B virus	Acute and chronic hepatitis, liver cirrhosis, hepatocellular carcinoma
Cytomegalovirus (HHV-5)	Congenital infection
Human papillomavirus	Condylomata acuminata, carcinoma of the cervix
Molluscum contagiosum virus	Molluscum contagiosum
HTLV-1	Leukaemia
HIV-1 and HIV-2	AIDS
Protozoa	
Trichomonas vaginalis	Vaginitis, urethritis
Entamoeba histolytica	Amoebiasis
Giardia lamblia	Giardiasis
Parasites	
Phthirus pubis	Pubic lice infestation
Sarcoptes scabiei	Scabies

usually not very reliable. Consultation rates for STI and associated clinical conditions, although likely to be biased by sociocultural differences in health care-seeking behaviour, have often been used to estimate the magnitude of the STI problem in countries and to determine trends over time. STI rank among

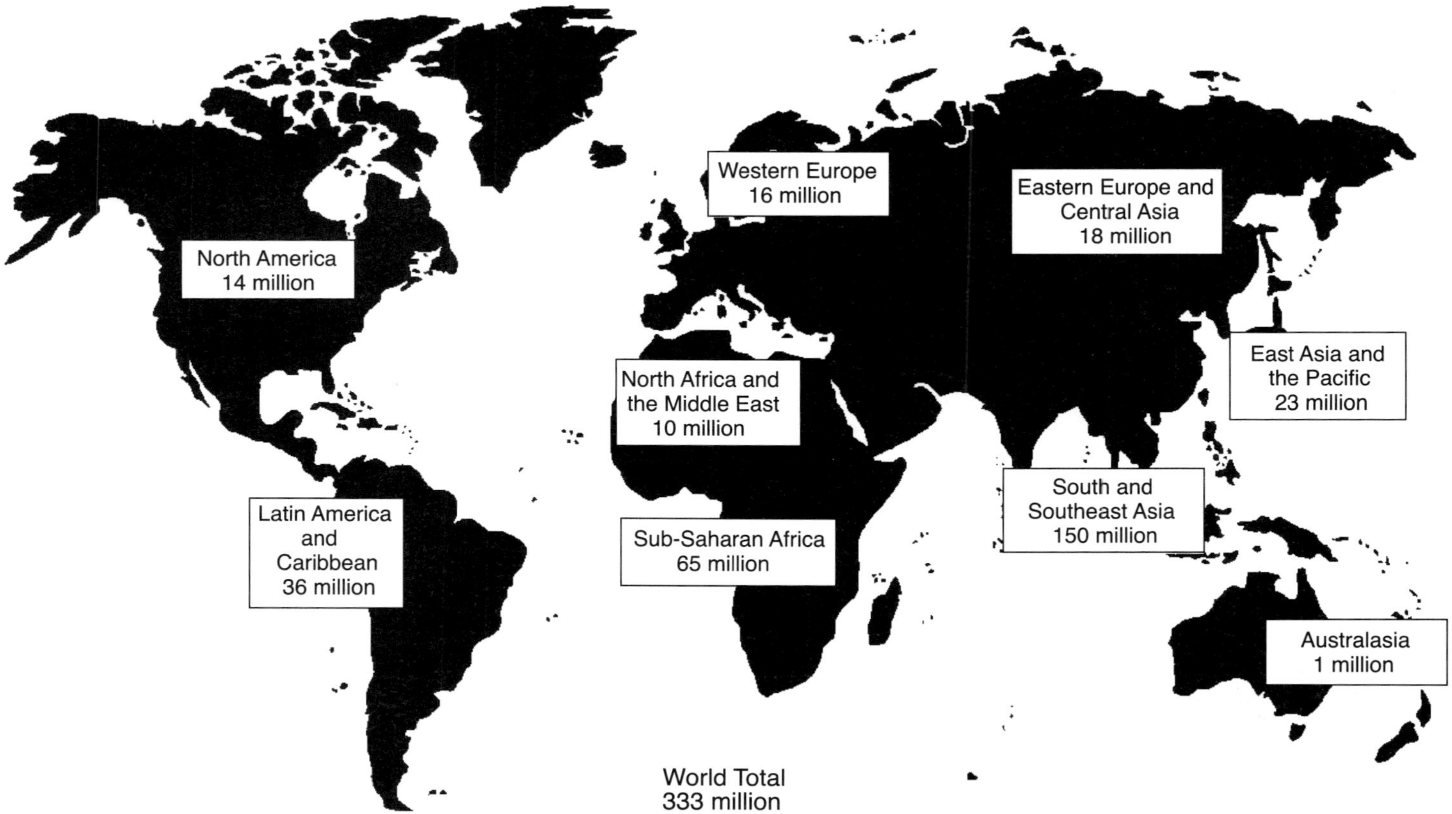

Fig. 1.1. Incidence of four curable STI (WHO, 1995a).

Table 1.2. Estimated new cases of four curable STI in 1995, in thousands (WHO, 1995a).

Region	Syphilis	Gonorrhoea	Chlamydia	Trichomoniasis
North America	140	1,800	4,000	8,000
Latin America and Caribbean	1,300	7,100	10,000	18,000
Western Europe	200	1,200	5,000	10,000
Eastern Europe and Central Asia	100	2,300	5,000	10,000
East Asia and Pacific	330	3,000	6,200	13,000
South and Southeast Asia	5,800	29,000	40,000	75,000
Australasia	10	130	300	1,000
North Africa and Middle East	620	1,500	2,900	4,600
Sub-Saharan Africa	3,500	16,000	15,000	30,000
Global total	12,000	62,030	88,400	169,600

the five most predominant reasons for health service consultations in most African countries, even more so when age-specific consultation rates are used for the most sexually active age groups between 15 and 44 years old (Meheus *et al.*, 1990). This type of proxy for incidence rates has to be interpreted cautiously, as factors such as inconsistency of the reporting system or changes in accessibility of health care facilities can be important determinants. This was illustrated in Kenya and Zimbabwe, which have a relatively well-functioning reporting system: the introduction of a fee for health care services in 1989 and 1992, respectively, resulted in a decline of reported STI cases, whereas the actual incidence of STI can be expected to have increased because of delayed treatment of infected individuals (Moses *et al.*, 1992).

Prevalence studies or official reports from sub-Saharan countries with a still well-functioning health care system show that STI remain alarmingly high. For instance, Zimbabwe reports 1 million STI cases a year for a total population of only 10 million inhabitants (Piot and Laga, 1994), and the situation is likely to be similar in most of Central, East and Southern Africa.

Socioeconomic impact of STI/HIV infection

It has become increasingly clear over the past two decades that STI, and in particular acquired immunodeficiency syndrome (AIDS), have a major impact on societies in developing countries. This is a result of both the magnitude of the STI epidemic and its impact on an individual's health and productivity. STI can undermine the economic development of low-income countries through increased morbidity and mortality in the younger sexually active age groups, as they tend to have more frequent changes of sexual partners (Brunham and Ronald, 1991). In the typical broad-based pyramidal age structure of most developing countries, which results from high birth rates and low life expectancies, the younger age groups comprise a much higher proportion of the population as a whole than in industrialized countries.

It has been estimated that AIDS and other STI combined account annually for almost 15% of the global burden of disease in adults between 15 and 44 years of age. Classical STI are the second most major cause of a healthy life lost in adults in developing countries; in the male population, human immunodeficiency virus (HIV) infection ranks number one; in women, classical STI are preceded only by obstetric problems (World Bank, 1993).

Besides the direct morbidity they cause and the ensuing loss of economic productivity, complications and long-term sequelae of STI are equally important. Furthermore, sexually transmitted agents have been identified as causal factors of cancers, both genital and extragenital. The role of human papillomavirus (HPV) in the development of cervical, vulvovaginal, anal and penile cancer, and of hepatitis B virus (HBV) infection in hepatocellular carcinoma is discussed elsewhere in the book.

Infertility, which commonly complicates pelvic inflammatory disease (PID), can strongly affect the social position of women in traditional societies. Involuntarily childless women become socially isolated as marriages are often broken. As a result, some end up in prostitution to secure some income (Meheus, 1992).

HIV is predominantly sexually transmitted, and WHO (1993) estimates that 75% of HIV infections result from sexual contact. Thus, HIV-related morbidity and mortality strongly affect young people, the population segment which contributes most to the countries' economy and development. Consequently, the epidemic has a strong negative economic impact on households, enterprises and entire countries (World Bank, 1997).

Although the number of children dying as a result of HIV transmission from mother to newborn is considerable, it is assumed that around 70% of children born from seropositive mothers do not become infected. This has resulted in an explosive increase in the number of orphans in regions that are highly affected by the AIDS epidemic; the total number of AIDS orphans (infants and children under 15 years of age who lost their mother or both parents due to AIDS) was estimated to be 8.2 million by December 1997 and this figure will almost double by the year 2000 (UNAIDS/WHO, 1997a). These children are often forced to discontinue their school education for financial reasons or to take over the care of the family, which jeopardizes their own future and the development potential of the country.

High numbers of AIDS cases also create a direct economic burden by considerably increasing health care expenditure. For instance, 30–70% of hospital beds in some African countries are occupied by patients with HIV-related conditions.

Although AIDS treatment options in most developing countries do not include expensive antiviral treatment but remain limited to palliative measures, such as pain alleviation and treatment of some opportunistic infections in immune-depressed individuals, the World Bank (1993) estimates that developing countries spent about US$340 million on care for AIDS cases in 1992. It is obvious that in a health care system which was already heavily under strain, less resources will be available for care of other health problems as the number of AIDS cases increases. Thus, data from Nairobi (Kenya) indicate that the increased need to care for HIV/AIDS patients has squeezed out some HIV-negative people who otherwise would have received care (World Bank, 1997).

Immune depression caused by HIV infection leads to reactivation of latent infections such as *Mycobacterium tuberculosis*; this explains the emergence of a new tuberculosis (TB) epidemic in populations with high HIV prevalence. On a global scale, tuberculosis is still the number one killing infectious disease, causing 3 million deaths each year, 75% of which are in Asia or Africa (Murray *et al.*, 1990; De Cock *et al.*, 1992; Narain *et al.*, 1992). Tuberculosis control in the AIDS era is complicated further because AIDS patients cannot be treated safely with traditionally used, cheap drug combinations and because of the development of single and multiple drug-resistant tuberculosis strains, the latter most likely accelerated by HIV coinfection (Carpels *et al.*, 1995; Van Gorkom and Kibuga, 1996).

Demographic impact of STI/HIV infection

The concept that STI epidemics can be important determinants of population dynamics is a relatively new one. In general, diseases can reduce population growth through three mechanisms: they can cause death prior to reproduction, affect reproductive competitiveness or reduce fertility in men or women.

Among sexually transmitted diseases, a distinction needs to be made between HIV infection, which mainly will influence demography by causing premature deaths (high number of years of potential life lost), and some conventional STI, which are rarely fatal but will have an impact through pregnancy complications and infertility (Brunham and Embree, 1992). Up to 30% of women in some African countries remain involuntarily childless, and up to two-thirds of these result from tubal infertility (Belsey, 1976). However, patterns of infertility differ considerably between Africa and other parts of the developing world. Secondary type infertility was much more common among African women, and a history of STI was found in 9% of the women, compared with 1% in Asia, Latin America and the eastern Mediterranean (Cates *et al.*, 1985). Ectopic pregnancies frequently have a fatal outcome when treatment facilities are limited, and are 6–10 times more common in women with a history of PID (Meheus, 1992). Spontaneous abortion can be the result of infection with a number of pathogens, including *Treponema pallidum,* herpes simplex virus (HSV) and, possibly, *Chlamydia trachomatis* (Bergström, 1990).

The AIDS epidemic has an effect on countries' population growth by increasing mortality, particularly in young adults. In sub-Saharan Africa, this could result in a reduction of population growth rates from an average 3% to less than 2% by the year 2000. A combination of relatively high HIV endemicity and low population growth independent of HIV will result in a much higher reduction and even negative population growth, as is expected to occur in certain countries in Asia. In high endemic countries, AIDS has reversed the successes of child survival initiatives and life expectancy is being reduced: in Botswana, for instance, life expectancy rose from 43 years in 1955 to 61 years in 1990, and with 25–30% of the adult population infected with HIV, life expectancy might drop back to levels seen in the late 1960s (UNAIDS/WHO, 1997b; Fig. 1.2).

Impact of STI on mother and child health and reproduction

Many STI potentially can complicate pregnancies or influence the health of mother or newborn. These include infections by bacteria such as *T. pallidum, Neisseria gonorrhoeae, C. trachomatis, Mycoplasma hominis, Ureaplasma urealyticum* and group B streptococci, as well as viruses, i.e. HSV, HPV, cytomegalovirus (CMV) and HIV. They are preventable causes of infertility, ectopic pregnancy, postpartum upper genital tract infections, cervical cancer, fetal wastage, low birth weight, infant blindness, neonatal pneumonia and mental retardation.

Whereas the assumed baseline infertility rate (i.e. not resulting from infection or trauma) is approximately 3–7%, up to 30% of couples in parts of sub-Saharan Africa remain involuntarily childless, and infertility in 50–80% of these couples is assumed to result from STI (Wasserheit and Holmes, 1992). Ectopic pregnancies are more common in the developing countries and have a much higher fatality, as medical facilities are often substandard.

Approximately 99% of all maternal deaths are assumed to occur in developing countries, very often resulting from sepsis following a pathologic pregnancy or delivery, or from a clandestine abortion in the presence of a genital infection (Bergström, 1990).

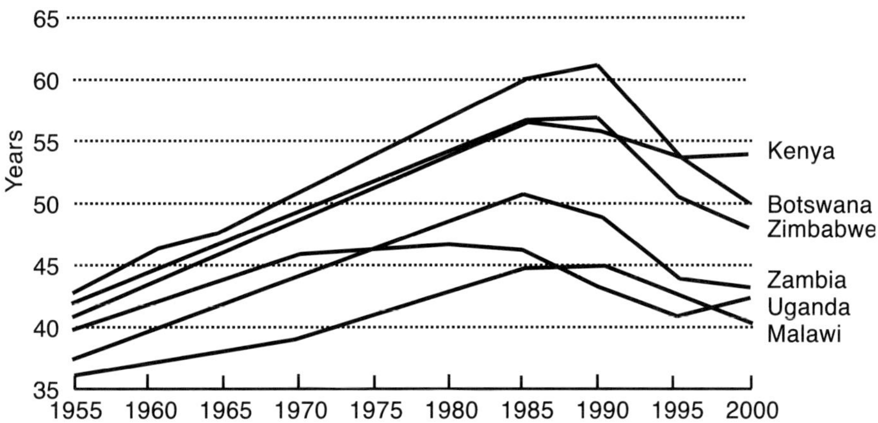

Fig. 1.2. Projected life expectancy at birth in selected sub-Saharan countries. Source: UNAIDS/WHO (1997a).

Characteristics of STI epidemiology in the 1980s and 1990s

Importance of demographic, political and socioeconomic factors in STI epidemiology

The demography of developing countries is characterized by a number of factors which favour the development of STI epidemics (Brunham and Embree, 1992). As a result of high birth rates and low life expectancy, the younger age groups make up a larger proportion of the population than in developed countries. Consequently, the age groups with the highest rate of sex partner change, young adults, are more predominant.

Rapid urbanization results in selective migration of the economically active population into the cities. Between 1965 and 1988, the proportion of people living in cities doubled in sub-Saharan Africa from 14% to 28% (Brunham and Embree, 1992). In these cities, the 20–45 year age groups are more predominant than in rural areas, and this is particularly true for young adult males. This results in an increase in commercial and non-commercial casual sex, and spread of STI.

Prostitutes are a core group in STI acquisition and transmission because of their high rates of partner change, and they can contribute considerably to the spread of STI in the general population via their clients. Due to poverty, prostitution can lead to a further increase in risk behaviour through either an increase in the number of sex partners or low use of condoms due to the low bargaining power of the women. This might explain the differences seen in STI prevalence between different social classes of commercial sex workers. For instance, in Nairobi, Kenya, the prevalence of gonorrhoea was 64.8% in 'low class' commercial sex workers compared with 22.5% in their 'high class' colleagues, and syphilis rates were 53 and 37% respectively (D'Costa *et al.*, 1985).

Poverty not only has an impact on prostitution and migration, the poor and deteriorating economic situation in many developing countries, and increasing expenditure on the military, also lead governments to spend less on health care and prevention programmes, and health care becomes less affordable to the patients.

Classical STI as determinants of the HIV pandemic

Much of the attention accorded to STI nowadays results from the important role they have in determining the dynamics of the HIV pandemic. STI and HIV may mutually influence each other: STI by facilitating HIV transmission and HIV by changing the natural history, clinical picture, diagnosis and treatment response of the 'classical' STI (Wasserheit, 1989; Laga *et al.*, 1994, 1995) (see also Chapter 11.4). A randomized intervention trial conducted from 1991 to 1994 in 12 communities in the Mwanza region, Tanzania, reportedly resulted in reduction of HIV incidence by 42% following improved STI case management (Grosskurth *et al.*, 1995). All this has thrown new light on the importance of STI control, which has not long been a priority for health policy makers, even in countries where STI are very common.

Increased importance of antibiotic resistance

The rapidly changing antimicrobial susceptibility of two organisms, *N. gonorrhoeae* and *Haemophilus ducreyi*, has created an important problem for STI treatment and control worldwide, but has a much higher impact in developing countries. Because of the widespread resistance, the older and usually cheaper antibiotics, such as penicillins and tetracyclines, have lost their usefulness in treatment of gonorrhoea.

Neisseria gonorrhoeae

Penicillin-resistant *N. gonorrhoeae* is an example of antibiotic resistance in which both chromosomal- and plasmid-mediated mechanisms are involved. Today, the prevalence of penicillinase-producing *N. gonorrhoeae* (PPNG) with plasmid-mediated resistance, which were first isolated in 1975 in the Far East and West Africa, is very high in Africa and Southeast Asia. By 1981, 30 and 42% of *N. gonorrhoeae* isolates, respectively in Bangkok and Singapore, were penicillinase-producing, but this seems to be stabilizing in most parts of the Far East to around 35% of isolates (Lind, 1990; Laga, 1994). In China, 4.3% of strains are PPNG (Ye, 1994). Figure 1.3 summarizes the PPNG prevalence among isolates from different countries in the early 1990s and clearly highlights the different situation in the developing world as opposed to some industrialized countries (Laga, 1994).

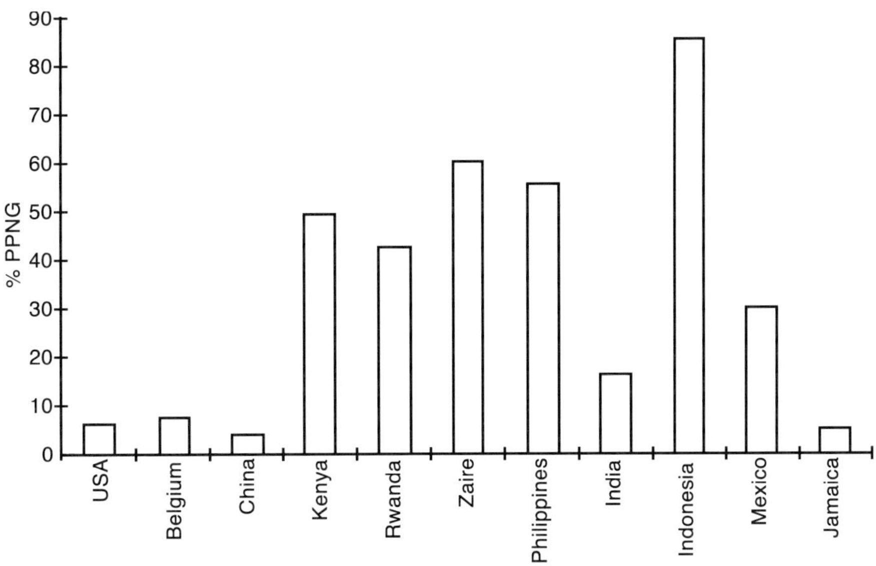

Fig. 1.3. PPNG proportions of *Neisseria gonorrhoeae* isolates in different countries (Laga, 1994).

Also, the importance of chromosomally mediated penicillin-resistant *N. gonorrhoeae* (CMRNG) strains has been increasing, as was seen in a longitudinal study in Senegal, where the percentage of non-PPNG strains with decreased susceptibility to penicillin rose from 12% in 1982 to 31% in 1986.

As is the case for penicillin, both chromosomal- and plasmid-mediated resistance to tetracycline have been identified in gonococci. One of the highest prevalence rates (98%) for tetracycline-resistant *N. gonorrhoeae* (TRNG) was reported in Indonesian prostitutes (Joesoef *et al.*, 1994). Plasmid-mediated tetracycline resistance of *N. gonorrhoeae* is spreading rapidly in many African countries, as was clearly demonstrated in a cohort of prostitutes in Kinshasa, Zaire, where the prevalence of TRNG rose from 11% to 45% over a period of 2.5 years (Van Dyck *et al.*, 1992, 1995). High prevalences of TRNG have also been documented in Singapore, Malaysia and Vietnam (Tapsall, 1995).

Furthermore, resistance of gonococci to many newer antibiotics has been reported, e.g. to quinolones in Thailand, Japan and Rwanda, and increasing levels of resistance to spectinomycin, ceftriaxone and cefotaxime have been reported from a number of regions (Ye, 1994).

Haemophilus ducreyi

Plasmid-mediated resistance of *H. ducreyi* is well documented and has been described for sulphonamides, aminoglycosides, tetracyclines, chloramphenicol and β-lactam antibiotics. Occurrence of multiple resistance plasmids in a single strain was not unusual (Trees and Morse, 1995). The epidemiology and mechanisms of chromosomal-mediated antibiotic resistance in *H. ducreyi* is much less documented. Nevertheless, resistance to penicillin, trimethoprim, ciprofloxacin and ofloxacin has been observed in *H. ducreyi* strains that lack resistance plasmids, suggesting chromosomally mediated resistance.

Regional epidemiology of viral STI

HIV/AIDS

When reference is made to HIV in the coming text, HIV-1 is intended, unless HIV-2 is mentioned explicitly.

Infections with HIV-2 mainly occur in some West African countries and in Angola and Mozambique. Elsewhere in the world, HIV infections are nearly always due to HIV-1. Figure 1.4 summarizes HIV-2 seroprevalence rates in low-risk urban populations on the African continent (Marlink, 1994).

It is assumed that the infectivity of HIV-2 is much lower than that of HIV-1, which could explain why HIV-2 infection usually occurs at a later age and is rare in young children.

Current size of the AIDS pandemic

By 20 November 1997, a total of 1,736,958 cumulative AIDS cases worldwide had been reported to WHO (UNAIDS/WHO, 1997a, b). However, the vast majority of AIDS cases, particularly in developing countries, are still not

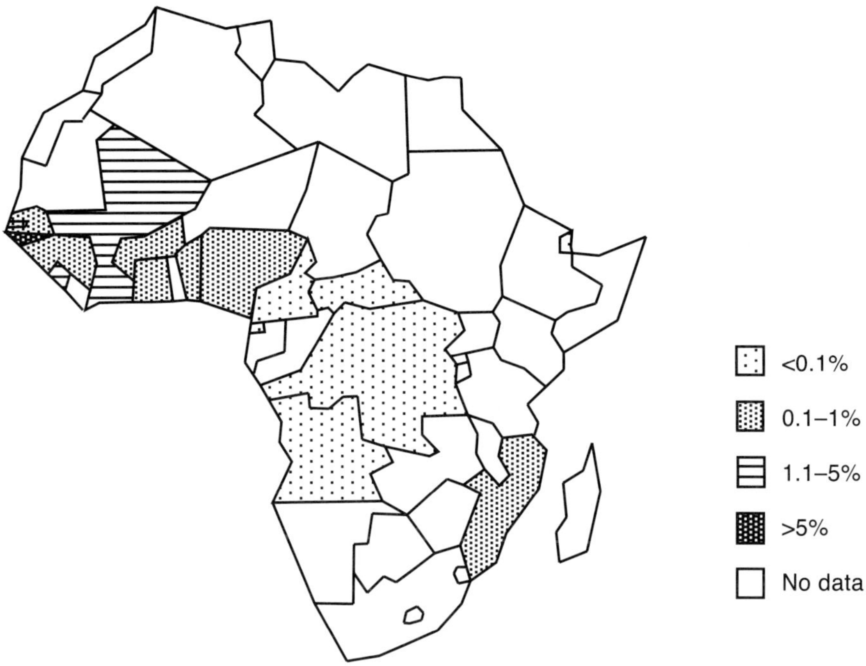

Fig. 1.4. HIV-2 seroprevalence among urban adults in Africa, reports from 1989 to 1992 (Marlink, 1994).

diagnosed or escape the WHO surveillance set-up, which strongly limits the usefulness of these figures to describe the ongoing AIDS pandemic. The absence of reliable data is due to the highly varying facilities in different countries to diagnose AIDS cases and the lack of homogeneity in the countries' AIDS surveillance programmes. For instance, the implementation of sentinel HIV seroprevalence activities varies considerably even between different countries in one region (Mertens *et al.*, 1994). Based on country prevalence data and taking into account the factors of underdiagnosis, incomplete reporting and reporting delay, WHO estimates that 12.9 million cumulative adult and paediatric AIDS cases had occurred worldwide by late 1997, with more than 90% in the developing world (UNAIDS/WHO, 1997a); 11.7 million of them had died from AIDS. Approximately 2.3 million (one-fifth of cases) died during 1997. Overall, reported cases represent only 15% of the estimated total number of AIDS cases that have occurred.

The United Nations Programme on HIV/AIDS (UNAIDS) and WHO have developed a global surveillance system. The last estimate (November 1997) yields a figure of 30.6 million people living with HIV/AIDS in the world (Fig. 1.5), of whom 5.8 million were newly infected during 1997, including 590,000 children. The HIV/AIDS pandemic is still evolving rapidly; there are major regional differences in the levels of HIV prevalence in adults and in the ways in which the virus spreads in the different areas of the world (Table 1.3).

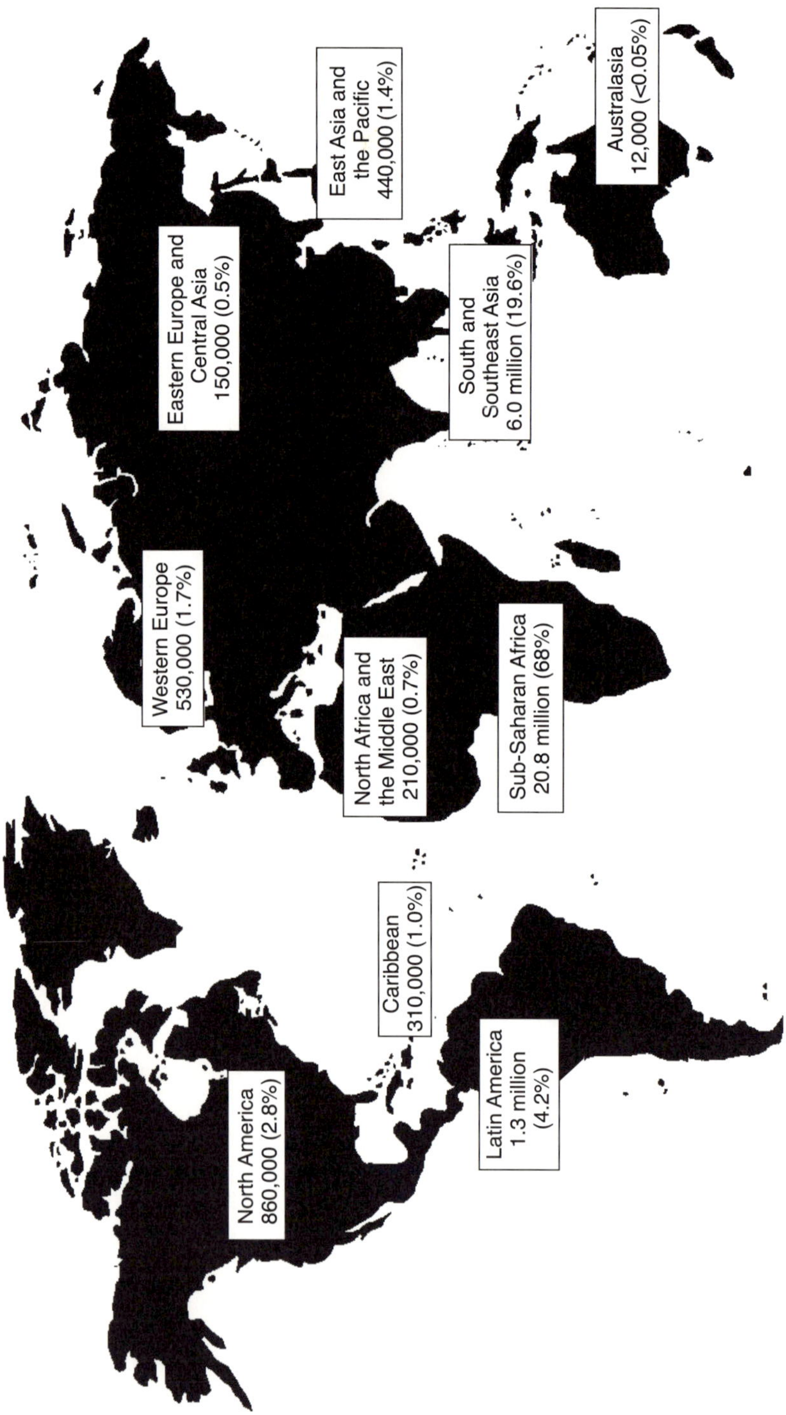

Fig. 1.5. Estimated number and geographical distribution of people living with HIV/AIDS: end 1997 (estimated total 30.6 million). The figures have been rounded up. (Adapted from: UNAIDS/WHO, 1997a.)

Table 1.3. Regional HIV/AIDS statistics and features, December 1997 (UNAIDS/WHO, 1997a).

Region	Epidemic started	Adults and children living with HIV/AIDS	Adult prevalence rate[a](%)	Cumulative no. of orphans[b]	Percentage of women	Main mode(s) of transmission[c] for those living with HIV/AIDS
Sub-Saharan Africa	Late 1970s – early 1980s	20.8 million	7.4	7.8 million	50	Hetero
North Africa, Middle East	Late 1980s	210,000	0.13	14,200	20	IDU, hetero
South and South-east Asia	Late 1980s	6.0 million	0.6	220,000	25	Hetero
East Asia, Pacific	Late 1980s	440,000	0.05	1,900	11	IDU, hetero, MSM
Latin America	Late 1970s – early 1980s	1.3 million	0.5	91,000	19	MSM, IDU, hetero
Caribbean	Late 1970s – early 1980s	310,000	1.9	48,000	33	Hetero, MSM
Eastern Europe and Central Asia	Early 1990s	150,000	0.07	30	25	IDU, MSM
Western Europe	Late 1970s – early 1980s	530,000	0.3	8,700	20	IDU, MSM
North America	Late 1970s – early 1980s	860,000	0.6	70,000	20	MSM, IDU, hetero
Australia and New Zealand	Late 1970s – early 1980s	12,000	0.1	300	5	MSM, IDU
Total		30.6 million	1.0%	8.2 million	41%	

[a]The proportion of adults living with HIV/AIDS in the adult population (15–49 years of age).
[b]Orphans are defined as HIV-negative children who lost their mother or both parents to AIDS when they were under age 15.
[c]MSM (men who have sex with men), IDU (injecting drug users), hetero (heterosexual transmission).

Africa

It is estimated that 68% of the world's 30.6 million people living with HIV/AIDS at the end of 1997, and 80% of the estimated 12.9 million AIDS cases that had developed by the end of 1997, had occurred in sub-Saharan Africa. It is assumed further that the number of new infections during the year 1996 was close to 3.8 million (UNAIDS/WHO, 1997a,b). Nevertheless, there are considerable regional differences in HIV prevalence within and between different countries and it is important to realize that the epidemic in Africa is still moving fast. While it has been said that the situation is stabilizing in certain parts of East and Central Africa, the epidemic is still advancing rapidly in Southern and Western Africa.

CENTRAL, EAST AND SOUTHERN AFRICA. The first AIDS cases in Africa were seen in East and Central Africa, and the epidemic is now firmly established among the general population of both these regions, with prevalence rates of HIV-1 infection in several urban areas of ≥20%. Here, infected women outnumber men (Serwadda *et al.*, 1994). This phenomenon is now also seen in several southern African countries, with 50% of reported AIDS cases being women in Swaziland, 52% in South Africa and 56% in Lesotho (UNAIDS/WHO, 1997c).

Apart from differences between countries, within-country variations have been reported to be considerable. As a rule, prevalence rates have been consistently higher in urban areas compared with rural regions. For instance, in Burundi, the HIV-1 infection rate in 1989 in the adult general population was 20 times higher in the capital (15.4%) than in rural areas of the country, a situation very similar to neighbouring Rwanda, with 17.8 and 1.8% of the urban and rural population HIV seropositive in 1986 (Bugingo *et al.*, 1988). As the epidemic becomes more strongly rooted in the general population, these differences tend to disappear, as was seen in Uganda, where rural and urban prevalence rates became nearly equal in the early 1990s (Sewankambo *et al.*, 1994).

Uganda is arguably the country that has suffered most from the AIDS pandemic, but now things seem to be changing for the better. At three different surveillance sites, a 20% decrease of infection levels was seen between 1996 and 1997, to between 5 and 9%. Particularly in younger age groups, infection rates are dropping, following intensive education campaigns leading to later sexual initiation, fewer partners and more condom use. As a result, life expectancy there recently started to rise again, unlike the picture in other countries in the area, such as Kenya, Zambia and even more so Zimbabwe, Malawi and Botswana, where AIDS as the leading cause of death in adults is expected to continue cutting life expectancy (UNAIDS/WHO, 1997a).

The epidemic seems to have affected Ethiopia later than the other countries of East Africa, and prevalence rates are still lower. The situation here has also experienced rapid changes, as was indicated by a rise in HIV prevalence among prostitutes from 18.5% in 1988 to 29.2% in 1989 (Serwadda *et al.*, 1994). HIV-1 seroprevalence also rose in blood donors, from 12.0% in

1994 to 16.7% in 1995 (Rahlenbeck *et al.*, 1997). Today, the number of reported AIDS cases has reached a total of 21,569 in a population of nearly 50 million (UNAIDS/WHO, 1997b).

In the Democratic Republic of the Congo, formerly Zaire, HIV prevalence has not shown a rise as dramatic as in neighbouring countries. Since 1986, infection rates in prenatal women have remained consistently between 6% and 7%, and it has been suggested that the prevalence of HIV is stable in large parts of the country (Gayle *et al.*, 1994; Piot and Laga, 1994). Most recent figures report nearly 30,000 AIDS cases for the country in 1996 (UNAIDS/WHO, 1997a).

In South Africa, an estimated number of 2.4 million people were HIV-infected by early 1997, an increase of more than a third since 1996. In Botswana, seroprevalence among the adult population doubled over the last 5 years; 43% of pregnant women in Francistown were seropositive (UNAIDS/WHO, 1997a).

NORTH AFRICA. The total number of HIV-infected individuals in Algeria, Chad, Egypt, Libya, Morocco, Sudan and Tunisia was estimated at 225,800 at the end of 1994, resulting in HIV prevalence rates of 0.1%, i.e. much lower than in the rest of the African continent (Table 1.3). The total number of AIDS cases in this region was reported to be 9037 in 1997. Two-thirds of these live in Chad (UNAIDS/WHO, 1997b). Initially, the infection mainly affected men who have sex with men, and to a lesser extent haemophiliacs and intravenous drug users, but, lately, heterosexual transmission of HIV is increasing in importance. This is illustrated by the shift in male to female ratio of infected individuals in Algeria, which changed from 4.3 in 1985 to 1.5 in 1991 (Benslimane and Sekhat, 1994).

WEST AFRICA. Some features distinguish the AIDS epidemic in West Africa from that in the other parts of sub-Saharan Africa. Here reports of AIDS cases were made early in the pandemic, but the epidemic spread of HIV infections in West Africa is relatively recent (Mboup and Gershy-Damet, 1994). Prevalence rates of HIV-1 differ considerably between different countries in the region, but are generally lower than in East, Central and South Africa, the exception being Côte d'Ivoire where 12% of pregnant women and 91% of prostitutes were found to be infected. Nigeria, the most populous country of Africa, is also situated in the region, and it is estimated that 2.2 million people are currently HIV-infected (UNAIDS/WHO, 1997a). A unique feature in this region is the frequent occurrence of dual infection with HIV-1 and HIV-2. The latter is endemic in West Africa but rarely found in the rest of the world, except for Angola and Mozambique. HIV-2 is the predominant HIV type both in the general population and in high-risk groups in the extreme west of the area, including Mauritania, Senegal, The Gambia, Cape Verde, Guinea and Sierra Leone, with the highest prevalence of 9.5% among the adult general population in Guinea-Bissau.

Latin America and the Caribbean

The HIV epidemic in Latin America and the Caribbean commenced in the late 1970s, as in North America. It is assumed that of the 12.9 million AIDS cases worldwide by the end of 1997, about 5% were in Latin America and the Caribbean, with over 1.3 million people living with HIV/AIDS. Projected figures for this region indicate the possibility of a levelling off and possibly a decline in the number of new HIV infections for the second half of the 1990s, which as a result of the long incubation period of the disease will still be accompanied by an upward trend in the number of AIDS cases.

At this stage, the patterns of spread of the infection are very heterogeneous and subject to rapid changes in various parts of the region (Mertens *et al.*, 1994; Piot and Laga, 1994; Zacarías *et al.*, 1994). For instance, the Caribbean region which has some of the highest incidence rates of AIDS in the world (as high as 100 new cases per 100,000 inhabitants in 1992 in the Bahamas) has since 1987 experienced a shift from sex between men as the first mode of transmission to a situation where most of new infections are caused by heterosexual contact (Zacarías *et al.*, 1994). The same has been observed in Central America after 1988, and the male to female ratio in some countries is 1 : 1. At present, homosexual or bisexual contacts are still contributing most to the incidence of HIV in other parts of the region, but this situation is expected to change in a few years.

For the whole region, newly infected men still greatly outnumber women, with overall ratios of 4.3 : 1 in Latin America, 2.2 : 1 in the Caribbean and 12 : 1 in the Andes region. The rising number of AIDS cases among women, and consequently among children under the age of 2, demonstrates that the epidemic is being firmly established among the general population. HIV rates in pregnant women have reached levels of 1% in Honduras and more than 3% in Porto Allegre, Brazil (UNAIDS/WHO, 1997a). However, the prevalence in the general population is considerably higher in the Caribbean. One of the first countries where this was documented is Haiti, where in the early 1990s, 10% of pregnant women and 40% of prostitutes were found to be seropositive. Brazil, with a cumulative total of 110,845 AIDS cases up to May 1997, has the second highest number of reported AIDS cases, after the USA.

Asia and the Pacific

This area covers a vast territory and is home to 55% of the world's population, China and India alone constituting 40%. Although the number of reported AIDS cases was still very low (82,932, or 4.7% of the world's total) in November 1997, WHO estimated the number of people living with HIV/AIDS for the entire region to be approximately 6.5 million (or 21% of the world's total) at the end of 1997. The discrepancy between number of AIDS cases reported and the UNAIDS/WHO estimates on the prevalence of people with HIV/AIDS for the region can be explained by it being in the early stage of the epidemic, as compared with other continents. The dynamics of the AIDS epidemic in Asia and the Pacific have some characteristics which distinguish it from the rest of the world (Kaldor *et al.*, 1994).

Whereas homosexual contact accounts for the majority of infections in

Australia and New Zealand, heterosexual transmission in which prostitution plays an important role is the predominant way individuals become infected in India and Southeast Asia. The situation is different in Myanmar, where over 65% of AIDS cases have been linked to intravenous drug use, and in Japan where a similar proportion was due to receipt of infected blood products. For the whole of the area, however, the importance of infection through heterosexual contact is increasing and is now already the most important mode of transmission (Piot and Laga, 1994; UNAIDS/WHO, 1997a).

OCEANIA. The vast majority of the 12,000 people living with HIV/AIDS on the continent of Oceania can be found in Australia and New Zealand, where 87% of reported AIDS cases are homosexual or bisexual men. HIV prevalence in the general population is still very low, with a prevalence rate among Australian blood donors of 0.9% (Crofts *et al.*, 1994).

The situation for the majority of the Pacific Islands is still poorly documented, but available data indicate that HIV is still not widespread. For the whole of Oceania excluding Australia and New Zealand, 494 AIDS cases were reported to WHO by November 1997, of which 62% were in Papua New Guinea (UNAIDS/WHO, 1997a).

Data from the Pacific Island countries showed homosexual contacts to be responsible for 38% of HIV infections by the end of 1993 and heterosexual contacts for 26%. The male to female ratio was 4 : 1 (Osuga and Chang, 1994). In contrast, more than half of the AIDS cases in Papua New Guinea are caused by heterosexual contact, the male to female ratio of HIV infection being 1 : 1, and injecting drug use is reported to be non-existent (Malau *et al.*, 1994).

INDIA. Recent figures report a total of cumulative AIDS cases of only 4980 to have occurred in India. With a population of over 16% of the world's total and expected to exceed 1 billion at the beginning of the 21st century, the future spread of HIV in India could strongly determine the course of the global AIDS pandemic (Jain *et al.*, 1994). It is estimated that between 3 and 5 million people were living with HIV in 1997, i.e. 11 years after the first serological evidence of infection was found in commercial sex workers in different areas of the country. Already in 1992, 41.2% of the prostitutes in Bombay were found to be seropositive. During the same period, the prevalence among intravenous drug users escalated in the north-eastern state of Manipur, bordering Myanmar, to 73% in 1996 (UNAIDS/WHO, 1997a). The rates in the general population still seem to be low; antenatal screening in Bombay in 1992 yielded a seroprevalence of below 1%, but in 1996, infection rates of around 2.4% were found in Mumbai (Bombay) and of around 4% in Pondicherry.

Rates of HIV infection are low in many Southeast Asian countries. In Indonesia, Malaysia, the Philippines and Singapore, infection rates remain well under 1%.

THAILAND (see also Chapter 6.1). Starting as late as 1988 as an infection restricted to homosexual and bisexual men, HIV quickly affected injecting drug users and, after that, commercial sex workers. Thailand has gone through all phases of the AIDS epidemic at very high speed, and HIV infection is now firmly rooted among the general population. By the end of 1994, Thailand had reported 22,135 AIDS cases, or 77.3% of all cases reported in Asia (Brown *et al.*, 1994). A high frequency of sexual contacts outside regular relationships, 10–20 times more frequent among men compared with women, could explain this rapid increase. The prevalences in the northern provinces of Chiang Mai, Chiang Rai and Phayao consistently have been the highest in the country, all with mean seroprevalence among antenatal clinic attenders above 6.0% and annual sero-incidence rates among male villagers as high as 8.5%. At present, the total number of infected individuals is estimated at 750,000, or 2.3% of the adult population.

There is increasing evidence of a fall in new infections, especially among sex workers and their clients (UNAIDS/WHO, 1997a). This results from intensive campaigns, increasing condom use among heterosexuals, boosting respect for women, discouraging men from visiting sex workers, and offering young women better educational and other prospects to discourage their entry into commercial sex. Prevalence rates among intravenous drug users have stabilized at around 40%.

CHINA. Only 150 AIDS cases had been reported by November 1997 for the whole of China, the most populous country in the world. HIV is now starting to spread in the country. The government estimated that at the end of 1996 up to 200,000 people were infected with HIV, a figure that probably doubled by the end of 1997.

At present, there are two epidemics occurring in China. The first is an HIV/AIDS epidemic among injecting drug users in the southern province of Yunnan which borders Myanmar, and which is spreading to neighbouring areas. The second, newer epidemic of STI is now surfacing among the heterosexual population, particularly along the south and the south-eastern seaborder (Xinhua *et al.*, 1994). In these more prosperous provinces, prostitution is re-emerging and the spread of STI could be followed by an HIV epidemic.

Genital herpes simplex virus infection

Genital herpes is one of the main causes of genital ulcer disease (GUD) in the world, including developing countries, and as such it is of particular importance in the transmission of HIV infection. Genital herpes was diagnosed in 49% of patients attending an STI clinic in Uganda with GUD, and 65% were HIV positive (Kamya *et al.*, 1995). Neonatal herpes infection has a considerable mortality, and transmission in most cases occurs during vaginal delivery. The sero-epidemiology of HSV infections, based on type-specific testing in 18 countries spread over the five continents showed that prevalence rates of HSV-2 in Asia are, in general, lower than those for sub-Saharan Africa (Nahmias *et al.*, 1990). In Taiwan, for instance, 13.5% of pregnant women had HSV-2 antibodies, but prevalence rates among adult general populations in Africa varied from 33.3% for Rwanda to 71.2% in Congo. Of two groups of low-risk women in Costa Rica and Haiti, 43.1 and 55.0%, respectively, had antibodies to HSV-2.

Human papillomavirus infection and cervical cancer (see also Chapter 11.3)

Poor feasibility of HPV detection tests and absence of a serological assay are responsible for paucity of data on the epidemiology of HPV infection in developing countries. The epidemiology of cervical cancer, the most common type of cancer in women in much of the developing world and the second most common cancer worldwide, is better documented. Patterns of high and low endemicity of cervical cancer show great similarity to those of most conventional STI, with most of sub-Saharan Africa, Asia and Latin America having a prevalence of over 20 cases per 100,000 women (Parkin *et al.*, 1993). Incidence rates vary considerably, from 5.6 per 100,000 in Pakistan to 96.5 in Brazil.

Hepatitis B virus infection

More than two billion people alive today have been infected with HBV, and it is estimated that approximately 350 million of them are chronic HBV carriers (WHO, 1996). Of the latter, about 95% live in developing countries, particularly in Africa and Asia (Norkrans, 1990). Important long-term complications of chronic HBV infection are development of cirrhosis and hepatocellular carcinoma which together kill approximately 1 million people each year. Hepatocellular carcinoma is associated with HBV infection in 80% of cases, and this explains the very high incidence of this cancer in areas of HBV endemicity (15–30 cases per 100,000 inhabitants per year).

Sexual contact is considered the main mode of transmission in low endemic industrialized countries, i.e. where HBV markers occur in less than 10% of the population. Thus, over 35% of HBV infections in the USA are attributable to sexual contact with an infected partner [Organisation Mondiale de la Santé (OMS), 1990]. However, in areas of intermediate or high endemicity, i.e. most of the developing world, a large proportion of the population is exposed to HBV much earlier in life, either through perinatal or non-sexual person to person contact, and sexual transmission therefore accounts for a smaller part of new infections. Nevertheless, the absolute number of sexually transmitted HBV infections even in these areas remains high (OMS, 1990). Perinatal, also referred to as vertical or mother to child, transmission occurs in 90% of pregnancies when the mother is HBV e-antigen positive, and as a rule results in chronic HBV carriage, but rarely in symptomatic hepatitis (Norkrans, 1990). This mode of transmission accounts for the majority of HBV infections and for 50% of the carriers in Southeast Asia. Although HBV prevalence seems to be stabilizing in certain parts of this area, such as Indonesia, Thailand and Malaysia, there is still an increasing trend in most countries of the Indian subcontinent (Tandon, 1996).

Non-sexual horizontal or person to person transmission, usually in early childhood, is also very important in Asia and is the predominant way in which people get infected in Africa. In these countries, horizontal transmission contributes considerably to HBV carriage prevalence up to the age of 10, but much less so after that age, in part because the risk of becoming a carrier reduces with infection at older age. It is estimated that of the approximately 470 million Africans, about 77% are exposed to HBV during their lifetime, and some 10% become chronic carriers (Kew, 1996).

Regional epidemiology of bacterial STI

Gonorrhoea

The WHO estimates that 62 million cases of gonorrhoea occurred worldwide among the adult population in 1995, with almost half of these in South and Southeast Asia, a quarter in sub-Saharan Africa and one-tenth in Latin America and the Caribbean (Table 1.2; WHO, 1995a).

Gonorrhoea is the number one cause of urethritis in the men in developing countries, occasionally resulting in urethral stricture. In women, it can result in salpingitis or PID, which occurs in 5–10% of untreated infections (Over and Piot, 1991). The importance of gonorrhoea for societies lies, apart from the healthy life days lost due to symptomatic disease, mainly in its effect on reproductive health, and infertility due to PID-induced tubal occlusion (Wasserheit, 1989). Infection with *N. gonorrhoeae* is the commonest cause of PID in most parts of the developing world, and 20–50% of PID cases in Africa are associated with gonococcal cervicitis (Wasserheit, 1989).

The overall prevalence of *N. gonorrhoeae* in African countries, where it is most likely the commonest STI, is higher than in Asia or Latin America. The median prevalence of gonococcal cervicitis among African women presenting at family planning, prenatal or gynaecologic clinics was 10%, compared with 1% in Asia. Reported prevalence rates in Latin America range between 2 and 18% (Wasserheit, 1989). However, in approximately 10% of men and 80% of women, infection with *N. gonorrhoeae* remains without symptoms. Thus, the number of infected individuals who would normally go unnoticed is substantial: studies on apparently asymptomatic antenatal and family planning clinic attenders in Durban, South Africa, found infection with *N. gonorrhoeae* in 4.1 and 10.0% of women respectively (Pham-Kanter *et al.*, 1996).

The high infectivity of *N. gonorrhoeae*, with a risk of infection following penile–vaginal intercourse of 30–40% for men and 50–80% for women (Over and Piot, 1991), combined with the existence of a large pool of asymptomatic infected individuals, complicates population-based control of gonorrhoea (WHO, 1995a).

Chlamydial infections

C. trachomatis was estimated to account for 89 million new cases of STI in 1995, the vast majority in the developing world (Table 1.2). Genital infection with *C. trachomatis* causes essentially the same clinical picture as does *N. gonorrhoeae* but, as infection rarely produces sufficient inflammation to result in clinical symptoms, many cases go unnoticed (Weinstock *et al.*, 1994).

The median prevalence of chlamydial infections of the cervix among African women presenting at family planning, antenatal or gynaecology clinics was 7%, with an upper level of over 20% in some areas. Mixed infections with *C. trachomatis* and *N. gonorrhoeae* are very common, as was seen for instance in South African studies where in 44–95% of cases with *C. trachomatis* infection, *N. gonorrhoeae* was present as well (Pham-Kanter *et al.*, 1996).

PID is at least as common, though clinically milder, a complication of *C. trachomatis* cervicitis, as of *N. gonorrhoeae*, and occurs in 5–10% of infections (Over and Piot, 1991). Some have suggested that due to the often subclinical progression of *C. trachomatis* infection and hence the longer treatment delay in cases of PID, the contribution of *C. trachomatis* to infertility might be higher than that of *N. gonorrhoeae.* A large multicentre study on bilateral tubal occlusion (WHO, 1995b) confirmed that women with serologically demonstrated past infection with *C. trachomatis, N. gonorrhoeae* or a combination of the two were much more likely to have bilateral tubal occlusion than those without such evidence. An interesting finding was that prevalence of anti-*C. trachomatis* immunoglobin G (IgG) was nearly as high in the group of infertile women without tubal occlusion but with other tubal abnormalities, suggesting that other mechanisms might play a role in the development of infertility as a result of *C. trachomatis* infection.

Several studies have documented an association between chlamydial PID and the risk of ectopic pregnancies, and one cohort study in women with acute salpingitis found that 7% of first pregnancies were ectopic in these women, as opposed to less than 1% in the control group (Weström *et al.*, 1981).

Transmission during delivery can result in ophthalmia neonatorum, of which it is a major cause in Africa, and in pneumonia in the newborn, but otitis media and gastroenteritis can also occur.

Syphilis

On a global scale, infections with *T. pallidum* remain a major health problem, especially in view of the facilitating role of ulcerative STI in HIV transmission. However, as a cause of genital ulceration, syphilis in most developing countries is secondary to infection with *H. ducreyi* (Goeman *et al.*, 1991). Several studies have reported coinfection with other pathogens such as *H. ducreyi* or HSV in up to 30% of GUD patients with positive serology for syphilis (Pham-Kanter *et al.*, 1996).

In spite of the fact that syphilis can be diagnosed easily and treated cheaply, and the risk of transmission through penile–vaginal intercourse is less than 30% (Over and Piot, 1991), it is estimated that in 1995, 12 million new cases of syphilis occurred worldwide among adults, nearly half being in South and Southeast Asia (Table 1.2; WHO, 1995a). Active syphilis has been found in 1–20% of pregnant women in some developing countries (Laga *et al.*, 1994). In studies among antenatal clinic attenders in South Africa, a median prevalence rate of positive syphilis serology of 7.6% has been reported (Pham-Kanter *et al.*, 1996).

Based on prevalence rates of syphilis in Africa, it has been estimated that 5–8% of all pregnancies of longer duration than 12 weeks will result in syphilis-induced spontaneous abortion, perinatal or infant death, or congenital syphilis in the newborn (Schulz *et al.*, 1986). In Mozambique, 32.5% of women with second trimester miscarriage were found to *be T. pallidum* haemagglutination assay (TPHA) positive, compared with 18.3% of women attending antenatal care (Lindstrand *et al.*, 1993).

It is encouraging that in Lusaka, Zambia, a programme of large-scale testing and treatment of syphilis infection during pregnancy, initiated after a strong association with abortion, stillbirth, low birth weight and congenital syphilis had been demonstrated, resulted in a significant decrease of these adverse pregnancy outcomes (Hira *et al.*, 1990).

Syphilis incidence rates are poorly documented in most developing countries. Prevalence rates in Asia are in general lower than in Africa; for instance, positive Venereal Disease Reference Laboratory (VDRL) tests in 0.7 and 3.3% of pregnant women in Indonesia and Malaysia respectively (De Schrijver and Meheus, 1990; Joesoef *et al.*, 1996). In Singapore, an incidence rate of 40 cases per 100,000 inhabitants was found for the year 1986 (Lee and Thirumoorthy, 1987).

Chancroid

The epidemiology of chancroid is poorly documented, mainly as a result of the absence of a reliable easy diagnostic test, and prevalence data are extremely rare. However, data on the proportion of genital ulcerations caused by *H. ducreyi* are available for a number of countries and, based on the ratios of chancroid to syphilis, WHO has estimated that approximately 7 million new cases of the disease occurred in 1995 (WHO, 1995a).

Chancroid is more prevalent in sub-Saharan Africa, where it is the most common identifiable cause of GUD. Between 20 and 70% of patients presenting in STI clinics in some African countries have a genital ulcer (Laga *et al.*, 1995) and, in a study in Swaziland, as many as 42% were found to be due to chancroid. In Durban, South Africa, this was found to be 14% in women and 22% in men (O'Farrell *et al.*, 1991a,b).

Few studies have been conducted on the prevalence of chancroid in general populations in Africa. In Mozambique, IgG antibodies against *H. ducreyi* were found in 20.4% of pregnant women, and 6% had an active GUD at the time of the survey (Vuylsteke *et al.*, 1993). In Ethiopia, chancroid is considerably less prevalent than in other East African countries, and antibodies indicating past infection were found in 10% of antenatal clinic attenders (Duncan *et al.*, 1994).

During the 1980s, the incidence of chancroid rose in seven out of 18 countries of Latin America according to a survey by the Pan-American Health Organization (PAHO) conducted between 1987 and 1991. There were marked regional differences, the rates varying from 0.1 per 100,000 for Cuba to 1229 for the Bahamas (Betts and Zacarias, 1994). This increasing trend most likely started a few years earlier, as can be assumed from data from El Salvador, where in one particular dermatology clinic the number of chancroid cases rose from 37 in 1981 to 144 in 1985. The vast majority of these (100% in 1981 and 95% in 1985) were men (Orellana-Díaz and Hernández-Pérez, 1988).

For Asia, the epidemiology of chancroid is largely unknown, except for Singapore where a clear decrease in incidence was seen following the country's economic development (Goh, 1987).

Regional epidemiology of protozoan STI

Trichomoniasis

Trichomoniasis is a rather benign condition and may be asymptomatic in up to 50% of infected women. Infections with *Trichomonas vaginalis* are extremely common in women in developing countries, with prevalence rates of 10–30% in most African studies of pregnant women, and a median prevalence of 20% in several studies of low-risk women (Wasserheit, 1989; Laga, 1994). Prevalence rates are generally lower in Asia and Latin America.

There were approximately 170 million new cases of *T. vaginalis* infection in 1995, and trichomoniasis has a higher prevalence and incidence than any other STI in both the developed and the developing world (WHO, 1995a).

Little attention has been given to this infection because of its mild symptomatology and absence of long-term sequelae. However, as is the case for other STI, the role of *T. vaginalis* infection as a facilitator of HIV transmission has been documented (Laga *et al.*, 1995) but needs further confirmation.

Interaction between HIV infection and other STI

(see also Chapter 11.4)

HIV transmission in STI-infected individuals

It is clear that when assessing the relationship between HIV transmission and the presence of other STI, sexual behaviour patterns which independently influence the epidemiology of both infections are important confounders that have to be considered. From a purely biological point of view, there are grounds for assuming that individuals who suffer from certain STI are more susceptible to HIV infection in the case of sexual contact with an infected person. This is obvious in the case of ulcerative STI, where the damaged mucosa or skin increases the probability of blood contact with infected genital fluids from the partner during sexual intercourse. The situation is more complex and less clear in non-ulcerative STI, but it has been postulated that here the increased susceptibility is facilitated by micro-ulcerations and friability, such as can be found in cervicitis and vaginitis, in combination with an increased presence of HIV-susceptible macrophages and lymphocytes in STI-infected genital mucosa and underlying tissues.

Furthermore, it has been suggested that HIV-infected individuals concurrently suffering from another STI are more infective to their partners, as a result of increased shedding of free virus particles and a higher presence of infected cells in their genital fluids. This has an important impact on female to male transmission, as HIV concentrations in female genital fluids are very low in women free from conventional STI. It has been observed that in areas highly endemic for STI, female to male transmission occurs more easily. For instance, in Thailand, the risk of infection of the male partner following a single sex contact was 5.6%, which was nearly 190 times higher than in steady couples in Europe (Laga *et al.*, 1994).

Longitudinal studies taking into account the confounding effect of sexual behaviour have demonstrated that STI may increase the risk of HIV transmission by a factor of 2–6.

Altered natural history of STI during immune depression

So called 'classical' STI commonly occur concurrently, but thus far no impact has been demonstrated of one STI on the progress or treatment outcome of another STI occurring in the same individual. In the case of HIV infection, however, the development of immune depression does seem to influence natural progression and response to antimicrobial therapy of some STI. For further details of these interactions, the reader is referred to the relevant sections of the chapters in Part II. There is little evidence of changes in natural history or treatment outcome of genital infections with *N. gonorrhoeae, C. trachomatis* or *T. vaginalis* in HIV-infected individuals, although it has been reported that severity of PID might be increased.

References

Belsey, M.A. (1976) The epidemiology of infertility: a review with particular reference to sub-Saharan Africa. *Bulletin of the World Health Organization* 54, 319–341.

Benslimane, A. and Sekhat, S. (1994) HIVs and AIDS in North Africa. In: Essex, M., Mboup, S., Kanki, P.J. and Kalengayi, M.R. (eds), *AIDS in Africa.* Raven Press, New York, pp. 603–611.

Bergström, S. (1990) Genital infections and reproductive health: infertility and morbidity of mother and child in developing countries. *Scandinavian Journal of Infectious Diseases* 69 (Suppl.), 99–105.

Betts, C. and Zacarias, F. (1994) Regional assessment of STD trends in Latin America and the Caribbean. *Sexually Transmitted Diseases* 21 (Suppl.), S108.

Brown, T., Sittitrai, W., Vanichseni, S. and Thisyakorn, U. (1994) The recent epidemiology of HIV and AIDS in Thailand. *AIDS* 8 (Suppl. 2), S131–S141.

Brunham, R.C. and Ronald, A.R. (1991) Epidemiology of sexually transmitted diseases in developing countries. In: Wasserheit, J.N., Aral, S.O. and Holmes, K.K. (eds), *Research Issues in Human Behaviour and Sexually Transmitted Diseases in the AIDS Era.* American Society for Microbiology, Washington, DC, pp. 61–80.

Brunham, R.C. and Embree, J.E. (1992) Sexually transmitted diseases: current and future dimensions of the problem in the third world. In: Germain, A., Holmes, K.K., Piot, P. and Wasserheit, J.N. (eds), *Reproductive Tract Infections.* Plenum Press, New York, pp. 35–58.

Bugingo, G., Ntilivamunda, A., Nzaramba, D., Van De Perre, P., Ndikuyeze, A., Munyantore, S., Mutwewingabo, A. and Bizimungu, C. (1988) Étude sur la séro-positivité liée à l'infection au virus d'immunodéficience humaine au Rwanda. *Revue Médicale Rwandaise* 20, 37–42.

Carpels, G., Fissette, K., Limbana, V., Vandeum, A., Vandenbulcke, W. and Portaels, F. (1995) Drug resistant tuberculosis in sub-Saharan Africa: an estimation of incidence and cost for the Year 2000. *Tubercle and Lung Disease* 76, 480–486.

Cates,W., Farley, T.M.M. and Rowe, P.J. (1985) Worldwide patterns of infertility: is Africa different? *Lancet* 2, 596–598.

Crofts, N., Ballard, J., Chetwynd, J., Dickson, N., Lindberg, W. and Watson, C. (1994) Involving the communities: AIDS in Australia and New Zealand. *AIDS* 8 (Suppl. 2), S45–S53.

D'Costa, L.J., Plummer, F.A., Bowmer, I., Fransen, L., Piot, P., Ronald, A.R. and Nsanze, H. (1985) Prostitutes are a major reservoir of sexually transmitted diseases in Nairobi, Kenya. *Sexually Transmitted Diseases* 12, 64–67.

De Cock, K.M., Soro, B., Kouliblay, I.M. and Lucas, S.B. (1992) Tuberculosis and HIV infection in sub-Saharan Africa. *Journal of the American Medical Association* 268, 1581–1587.

De Schrijver, A. and Meheus, A. (1990) Epidemiology of sexually transmitted diseases: the global picture. *Bulletin of the World Health Organization* 68, 639–654.

Duncan, M.E., Roggen, E., Tibaux, G., Pelzer, A., Mehari, L. and Piot, P. (1994) Seroepidemiological studies of *Haemophilus ducreyi* infection in Ethiopian women. *Sexually Transmitted Diseases* 21, 280–288.

Gayle, H.D., Heyward, W.L. and Nzila, N. (1994) HIVs and AIDS in Central Africa. In: Essex, M., Mboup, S., Kanki, P.J. and Kalengayi, M.R. (eds), *AIDS in Africa.* Raven Press, New York, pp. 651–667.

Goeman, J., Meheus, A. and Piot, P. (1991) Epidémiologie des maladies sexuellement transmissibles dans les pays en développement à l'ère du SIDA. *Annales de la Société Belge de Médecine Tropicale* 71, 81–113.

Goh, C.L. (1987) Chancroid – a review. *Annals of the Academy of Medicine* 16, 680–682.

Grosskurth, H., Mosha, F., Todd, J., Mwijarubi, E., Klokke, A., Senkoro, K., Mayaud, P., Changalucha, J., Nicoll, A., Kagina, G., Newell, J., Mugeye, K., Mabey, D. and Hayes, R. (1995) Impact of improved treatment of sexually transmitted diseases on HIV infection in rural Tanzania: randomised controlled trial. *Lancet* 346, 530–536.

Hira, S.K., Bhat, G.J., Chikamata, D.M., Nkowane, B., Tembo, G., Perine, P.L. and Meheus, A. (1990) Syphilis intervention in pregnancy: Zambian demonstration project. *Genitourinary Medicine* 66, 159–164.

Jain, K.M., John, T.J. and Keusch, G.T. (1994) Epidemiology of HIV and AIDS in India. *AIDS* 8 (Suppl. 2), S61–S75.

Joesoef, M.R., Knapp, J.S., Idajadi, A., Linnan, M., Barakbah, Y., Kamboji, A., O'Hanley, P. and Moran, J.J. (1994) Antimicrobial susceptibilities of *Neisseria gonorrhoeae* strains isolated in Surabaya, Indonesia. *Antimicrobial Agents and Chemotherapy* 38, 2530–2533.

Joesoef, M.R., Wiknjosastro, G., Norojono, W., Sumampouw, H., Linnan, M., Hansell, M.J., Hillis, S.E. and Lewis, J. (1996) Coinfection with chlamydia and gonorrhoea amongst pregnant women with bacterial vaginosis. *International Journal of STD and AIDS* 7, 61–64.

Kaldor, J.M., Sittitrai, W., John, T.J. and Kitamura, T. (1994) The emerging epidemic of HIV infection and AIDS in Asia and the Pacific. *AIDS* 8 (Suppl. 2), S1–S2.

Kamya, M.R., Nsubuga, P., Grant, R.M. and Hellman, N. (1995) The high prevalence of genital herpes among patients with genital ulcer disease in Uganda. *Sexually Transmitted Diseases* 6, 351–354.

Kew, M.C. (1996) Progress towards the comprehensive control of hepatitis B in Africa: a view from South Africa. *Gut* 38 (Suppl. 2), S31–S36.

Laga, M. (1994) Epidemiology and control of sexually transmitted diseases in developing countries. *Sexually Transmitted Diseases* 21 (Suppl. 2), S45–S50.

Laga, M., Diallo, M.O. and Buvé, A. (1994) Inter-relationship of sexually transmitted diseases and HIV: where are we now? *AIDS* 8 (Suppl. 1), S119–S124.

Laga, M., Nzila, N. and Goeman, J. (1995) The interrelationship of sexually transmitted diseases and HIV infection: implications for the control of both epidemics in Africa. *AIDS* 5 (Suppl. 1), S55–S63.

Lee, C.T. and Thirumoorthy, T. (1987) Epidemiology of syphilis in Singapore over three decades (1955–1986). *Annals of the Academy of Medicine, Singapore* 16, 622–626.

Lind, I. (1990) Epidemiology of antibiotic resistant *Neisseria gonorrhoeae* in industrialized and developing countries. *Scandinavian Journal of Infectious Diseases* 69 (Suppl.), 77–82.

Lindstrand, A., Bergström, S., Bugalho, A., Zanconato, G., Hegesson, A. and Hederstedt, B. (1993) Prevalence of syphilis infection in Mozambican women with second trimester miscarriage and women attending antenatal care in second trimester. *Genitourinary Medicine* 69, 431–433.

Malau, C., O'Leary, M., Jenkins, C. and Faraclas, N. (1994) HIV/AIDS prevention and control in Papua New Guinea. *AIDS* 8 (Suppl. 2), S117–S124.

Marlink, R. (1994) The biology and epidemiology of HIV-2. In: Essex, M., Mboup, S., Kanki, P.J. and Kalengayi, M.R. (eds), *AIDS in Africa*. Raven Press, New York, pp. 47–65.

Mboup, S. and Gershy-Damet, G.M. (1994) HIVs and AIDS in West Africa. In: Essex, M., Mboup, S., Kanki P.J. and Kalengayi, M.R. (eds), *AIDS in Africa*. Raven Press, New York, pp. 613–649.

Meheus, A. (1992) Women's health: importance of reproductive tract infection, pelvic inflammatory disease and cervical cancer. In: Germain, A., Holmes, K.K., Piot, P. and Wasserheit, J.N. (eds), *Reproductive Tract Infections*. Plenum Press, New York, pp. 61–92.

Meheus, A., Schulz, K.F. and Cates, W. (1990) Development of prevention and control programs for sexually transmitted diseases in developing countries. In: Holmes, K.K., Mårdh, P.A., Sparling, P.F., Wiesner, P.J., Cates, W.J., Lemon, S.M. and Stamm, W.E. (eds), *Sexually Transmitted Diseases*. McGraw-Hill, New York, pp. 1041–1046.

Mertens, T.E., Burton, A., Stoneburner, R., Sato, P., Beer, D.L., Carael, M. and Belsey, E. (1994) Global estimates and epidemiology of HIV infections and AIDS. *AIDS* 8, (Suppl. 1), S361–S372.

Moses, S., Manji, F., Bradley, J.E., Nagelkerke, N.J.D., Melisa, M.A. and Plummer, F. (1992) Impact of user fees on attendance at a referral centre for sexually transmitted diseases in Kenya. *Lancet* 340, 463–466.

Murray, C.J.L., Styblo, K. and Rocillon, A. (1990) Tuberculosis in developing countries: burden, intervention and cost. *Bulletin of the International Union of Tuberculosis and Lung Disease* 65, 6–24.

Nahmias, A.J., Lee, Francis K. and Beckman-Nahmias, S. (1990) Sero-epidemiological and sociological patterns of herpes simplex virus infection in the world. Scandinavian Journal of Infectious Diseases 69 (Suppl.), 19–36.

Narain, J.P., Raviglione, M.C. and Kochi, A. (1992) HIV associated tuberculosis in developing countries: epidemiology and strategies for prevention. WHO/TB/92.164, World Health Organization, Geneva.

Norkrans, G. (1990) Epidemiology of hepatitis B virus (HBV) infections with particular regard to current routes of transmission and development of cirrhosis and malignancy. *Scandinavian Journal of Infectious Diseases* 69 (Suppl.), 43–47.

O'Farrell, N., Hoosen, A.A., Coetzee, K.D. and van den Ende J. (1991a) Genital ulcer disease in women in Durban, South Africa. *Genitourinary Medicine* 67, 322–326.

O'Farrell, N., Hoosen, A.A., Coetzee, K.D. and van den Ende, J. (1991b) Genital ulcer disease in men in Durban, South Africa. *Genitourinary Medicine* 67, 327–330.

Orellana-Díaz, O. and Hernández-Pérez, E. (1988) Chancroid in El Salvador. *International Journal of Dermatology* 27, 243–245.

Organisation Mondiale de la Santé (1990) *Consultation sur l'Hépatite B en tant que Maladie Sexuellement Transmissible.* OMS, Geneva.

Osuga, K. and Chang, C. (1994) AIDS in the Pacific Islands. *AIDS* 8 (Suppl. 2), S111–S116.

Over, M. and Piot, P. (1991) Health sector priorities review: HIV infection and sexually transmitted diseases. In: Jamison, D.T. and Mosley, W.H. (eds), *Disease Control Priorities in Developing Countries.* Oxford University Press, New York, pp. 18–34.

Parkin, D.M., Pisani, P. and Ferlay, J. (1993) Estimates of the worldwide incidence of eighteen major cancers in 1985. *International Journal of Cancer* 54, 594–606.

Pham-Kanter, G.B.T., Steinberg, M.H. and Ballard, R.C. (1996) Sexually transmitted diseases in South Africa. *Genitourinary Medicine* 72, 160–171.

Piot, P. and Laga, M. (1994) Epidemiology of AIDS in the developing world. In: Broder, S., Merigan, T.C. and Bolognesi, D. (eds), *Textbook of AIDS Medicine.* Williams and Wilkins, Baltimore, Maryland, pp. 109–132.

Rahlenbeck, S.I., Yohannes, G., Molla, K., Reifen, R. and Assefa, A. (1997) Infection with HIV, syphilis and hepatitis B in Ethiopia: a survey of blood donors. *International Journal of STD and AIDS* 8, 261–264.

Schulz, K.F., Cates, W. and O'Mara, P.R. (1987) Pregnancy loss, infant death, and suffering: legacy of syphilis and gonorrhoea in Africa. *Genitourinary Medicine* 63, 320–325.

Serwadda, D., Mhalu, F., Karita, E. and Moses, S. (1994) HIV and AIDS in East Africa. In: Essex, M., Mboup, S., Kanki, P.J. and Kalengayi, M.R. (eds), *AIDS in Africa.* Raven Press, New York, pp. 669–689.

Sewankambo, N.K., Wawer, M.J., Gray, R.H., Serwadda, D., Li, C.J., Stallings, R.Y., Musgrave, S.D. and Kondelule, J. (1994) Demographic impact of HIV infection in rural Rakai District, Uganda: results of a population-based cohort study. *AIDS* 8, 1707–1713.

Tandon, B.N. (1996) Ninth triennial international symposium on viral hepatitis and liver diseases. Rome 21–25 April 1996. *Tropical Gastroenterology* 17, 77–83.

Tapsall, J.W. (1995) Surveillance of antibiotic resistance in *Neisseria gonorrhoeae* and implications for the therapy of gonorrhoea. *International Journal of STD and AIDS* 6, 233–236.

Trees, D.L. and Morse, S.A. (1995) Chancroid and *Haemophilus ducreyi*: an update. *Clinical Microbiology Reviews* 8, 357–375.

UNAIDS/WHO (1997a) Report on the global HIV/AIDS epidemic. www.unaids.org.

UNAIDS/WHO (1997b) Global AIDS surveillance, part 1. *Weekly Epidemiological Record* 72, 357–364.

UNAIDS/WHO (1997c) Global AIDS surveillance, part 2. *Weekly Epidemiological Record* 72, 365–372.

Van Dyck, E., Roussau, R., Duhamel, M., Behets, F., Laga, M., Nzila, M., Bygdeman, S., Van Heuverswijn, H. and Piot, P. (1992) Antimicrobial susceptibility of *Neisseria gonorrhoeae* in Zaire: high level plasmid mediated tetracycline resistance in Central Africa. *Genitourinary Medicine* 68, 111–116.

Van Dyck, E., Laga, M., Manoka, A.T., Behets, F. and Piot, P. (1995) Epidemic spread of plasmid-mediated tetracycline resistant *Neisseria gonorrhoeae* in Zaire. *International Journal of STD and AIDS* 6, 345–347.

Van Gorkom, J. and Kibuga, D.K. (1996) Cost-effectiveness and total costs of three alternative strategies for the prevention and management of severe skin reactions attributable to thiacetazone in the treatment of human immunodeficiency virus positive patients with tuberculosis in Kenya. *Tubercle and Lung Disease* 77, 30–36.

Vuylsteke, B., Bastos, R., Barreto, J., Crucitti, T., Folgosa, E., Mondlane, J., Dusauchoit, T., Piot, P. and Laga, M. (1993) High prevalence of sexually transmitted diseases in a rural area in Mozambique. *Genitourinary Medicine* 69, 427–430.

Wasserheit, J.N. (1989) The significance and scope of reproductive tract infections among third world women. *International Journal of Gynecology and Obstetrics* (Suppl. 3), 145–168.

Wasserheit, J.N. and Holmes, K.K. (1992) Reproductive tract infections: challenges for international health policy, programs and research. In: Germain, A., Holmes,K.K., Piot P. and Wasserheit, J.N. (eds), *Reproductive Tract Infections – Global Impact and Priorities for Women's Reproductive Health.* Plenum Press, New York, pp. 7–33.

Weinstock, H., Dean, D. and Bolan, G. (1994) *Chlamydia trachomatis* infections. *Infectious Disease Clinics of North America* 8, 797–819.

Weström, L., Bengtsson, L.P.H. and Mårdh, P.A. (1981) Incidence, trends and risk of ectopic pregnancy in a population of women. *British Medical Journal* 282, 15–18.

World Bank (1993) AIDS: a threat to development. In: *The World Bank. World Development Report 1993 – Investing in Health.* Oxford University Press, New York, pp. 99–107.

World Bank Policy Research Project (1997) *Confronting AIDS – Public Priorities in a Global Epidemic.* Oxford University Press, New York, p. 353.

World Health Organization (1993) AIDS. The current global situation of the HIV/AIDS pandemic. *Weekly Epidemiological Record* 68, 9–11.

World Health Organization (1995a) An overview of selected curable sexually transmittable diseases. WHO/GPA/STD/95.1.

World Health Organization Task Force on the prevention and management of infertility (1995b). Tubal infertility: serologic relationship to past chlamydial and gonococcal infection. *Sexually Transmitted Diseases* 22, 71–77.

World Health Organization (1996) *The World Health Report 1996: Fighting Disease, Fostering Development.* World Health Organization, Geneva.

Xinhua, S., Junhua, N. and Qili, G. (1994) AIDS and HIV infection in China. *AIDS* 8 (Suppl. 2), S55–S59.

Ye, S.Z. (1994) Survey on antibiotic sensitivity of *Neisseria gonorrhoeae* strains isolated in China, 1987–1992. *Sexually Transmitted Diseases* 21, 237–240.

Zacarías, F., González, R.S., Cuchi, P., Yanez, A., Peruga, A., Mazin, R., Betts, C. and Weissenbacher, M. (1994) HIV/AIDS and its interaction with tuberculosis in Latin America and the Caribbean. *Bulletin of the Pan American Health Organization* 28, 312–323.

CHAPTER 2
Anatomy of the genitalia and other organs

O.P. Arya
Department of Medical Microbiology and Genitourinary Medicine, University of Liverpool, Liverpool, UK

As some STI may cause multisystem disease, the clinicians may consult an appropriate text book for a working knowledge of the anatomy and physiology of the corresponding system(s). In this chapter, the relevant aspects of the anatomy of the genitalia, and of the extragenital sites serving as portals of entry of causative organisms of STI are described.

Male genitalia (Fig. 2.1)

Penis

The penis has three masses of erectile tissue – the two corpora cavernosa, one on either side of and dorsal to the third mass – the corpus spongiosum. The glans penis is the terminal enlargement of the corpus spongiosum. The fraenum is a fold of mucous membrane extending from the undersurface of the prepuce on to the glans, up to the edge of the urethral orifice.

Communicating with the preputial sac, on the superior surface of the corona of the glans penis and on either side of the fraenum, are the glands of Tyson. These glands secrete sebaceous material called smegma (Plate 1) which emanates a characteristic odour. These glands atrophy following circumcision.

Urethra

The urethra is divided into two main parts – anterior and posterior. The anterior urethra lies in the substance of corpus spongiosum. It is subdivided further into two parts: the distal pendulous or the penile urethra and the proximal fixed bulbous urethra, into which, respectively, open the ducts of Littre's glands and Cowper's glands. The external urethral orifice is the narrowest part of the urethra, and the urethral enlargement just behind it forms the fossa navicularis. Situated on the upper wall of the fossa navicularis is a large crypt called the lacuna magna. The paraurethral ducts (present in some) are small blind channels running parallel to the terminal urethra within

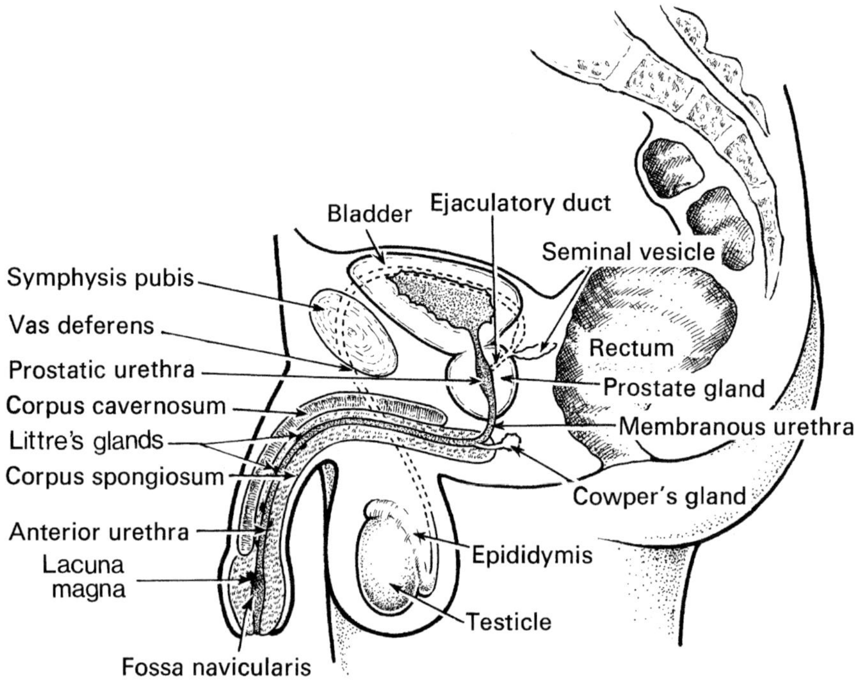

Fig. 2.1. Anatomy of the male genitourinary tract.

the glans penis which open within or close to the external urinary meatus.

The fossa navicularis is lined by stratified squamous epithelium, and the rest of the anterior urethra and the ducts of Littre's and Cowper's glands are lined by columnar epithelium.

The posterior urethra has also two further subdivisions: the membranous urethra and the prostatic urethra. The membranous urethra runs from the prostate to the bulb of the penis, is 1.25 cm long and is lined by transitional epithelium. Cowper's glands, located in the urogenital diaphragm, lie on either side of the membranous urethra. The prostatic urethra runs through the prostate gland, is 3 cm long and is lined by transitional epithelium.

Hypospadias is a congenital ventral defect in the terminal urethra. It increases the liability to infection and relapse in urethritis.

Prostate gland

The prostate gland, located between the bladder neck and the urogenital diaphragm, is a firm structure composed of glandular tissue within a fibromuscular stroma. It has the shape and size of a chestnut. About 4 cm from the anus, its posterior surface is in contact with the anterior rectal wall through which the gland may be palpated. It has three zones: a periurethral zone around the urethra, a central zone between the urethra and ejaculatory duct, and a peripheral zone palpable on rectal examination. (Some experts recognize a fourth zone, i.e. a narrow transitional zone located between the central and peripheral zones, and the site of benign hypertrophy in older men.) The glandular tissue is lined by columnar epithelium. The ducts of the prostatic acini, which are short in the central zone and rather tortuous in the peripheral zone, drain into the prostatic urethra. The peripheral zone is the one most susceptible to development of inflammation and carcinoma.

Seminal vesicles and ejaculatory ducts

The seminal vesicles are two convoluted pyramid-shaped pouches, each about 5 cm long and situated between the base of the bladder and rectum. Their mucous coat is lined by columnar epithelium. At its lower end, each vesicle narrows into a straight duct which joins with the corresponding vas deferens to form the common ejaculatory duct, which pierces the prostate and opens into the urethra at the verumontanum.

Vasa deferentia

The vasa deferentia ascend from the lower ends of the epididymes, run upwards in the posterior part of the spermatic cords, traverse the inguinal canal, enter the pelvic cavity and eventually reach the base of the prostate where they join the ducts of the seminal vesicles (see above). They are lined by columnar epithelium.

Testes and epididymes

The testes are oval structures suspended in the scrotum by the spermatic cords. The left testis hangs somewhat lower than the right. Their glandular component consists of many lobes containing convoluted seminiferous tubules which manufacture spermatozoa. These tubules unite to form a number of efferent ductules which join the upper pole or the head of the epididymis. The epididymis, which consists of the head (globus major), body and tail (globus minor), lies along the lateral part of the posterior border of the testis. A groove can usually be felt between the epididymis and the testis except superiorly. The epididymes are lined by columnar epithelium.

Female genitalia (Figs 2.2 and 2.3)

Vulva

The vulva includes the mons pubis, the clitoris, the labia majora and minora, the vestibule and Bartholin's glands. The mons pubis, covered with hair at puberty, is a rounded eminence of fatty tissue in front of the pubic symphysis. The clitoris, an analogue of the penis, is an erectile structure located between and behind the anterior ends of the labia minora. The labia majora are two

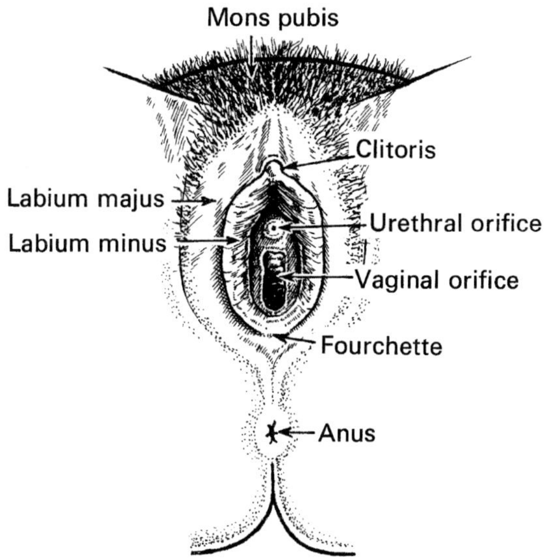

Fig. 2.2. The vulva.

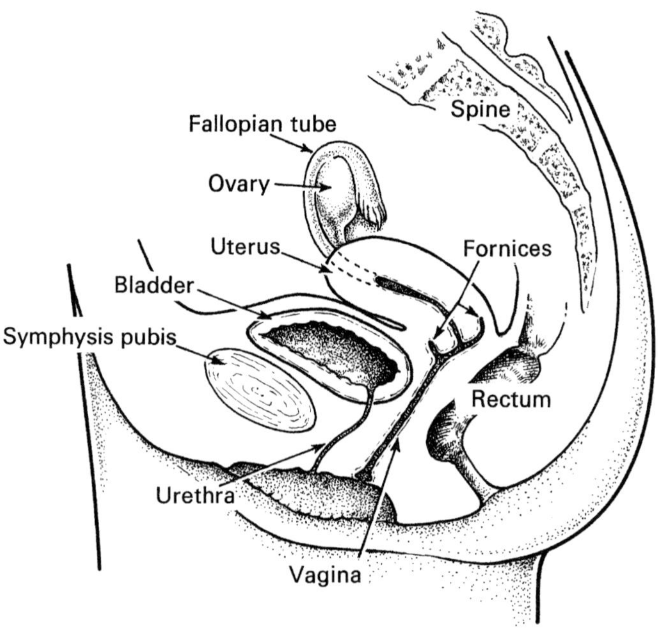

Fig. 2.3. Female pelvic organs.

prominent folds of adipose tissue extending from the mons pubis to the perineum. Their outer pigmented part is covered by pubic hair, while the inner smooth part contains many sebaceous follicles. The labia minora, situated between the labia majora, are two small mucocutaneous folds, extending from and ensheathing the clitoris and uniting posteriorly to form the fourchette. The vestibule is a cleft between the labia minora, and situated in it are the orifices of the urethra, vagina and Bartholin's ducts. Bartholin's glands, which are the homologues of Cowper's glands in the male, are small mucus glands, situated deep in the posterior part of the labia majora. Their ducts are about 2 cm long and open on the sides of the vestibule at the junction of the middle and posterior third of the labia minora. They are lined by columnar epithelium.

Urethra

The female urethra is about 4 cm long. Many small urethral glands open into the urethra. Skene's glands, which are the homologues of the prostate gland in the male, are paraurethral glands, situated near the lower end of the urethra, and their ducts open on either side of the external urethral orifice. The urethra near the bladder is lined by transitional epithelium, while the rest is lined by stratified squamous epithelium. The ducts of the urethral and Skene's glands are lined by columnar epithelium.

Vagina

The vaginal canal extends from the vestibule to the uterus. Its anterior and posterior walls are respectively 7.5 and 9 cm long. It is situated behind the bladder and in front of the rectum. Its upper end surrounds the vaginal part of the cervix, forming anterior, posterior and two lateral fornices. In the newborn infant, the vagina has many layers of squamous epithelium due to the presence of the mother's oestrogens. After a few weeks, with the decreasing levels of oestrogens, the squamous epithelium is replaced by immature thin columnar or cuboidal epithelium. The oestrogen level rises as puberty approaches and the vaginal mucous membrane in the adult is lined by stratified squamous epithelium which is by then several layers thick. The oestrogen levels fall after menopause and, consequently, the vaginal mucosa becomes thin and atrophic.

The pH of the vagina is determined by the glycogen content, the Döderlein bacilli, the oestrogen level and menstruation. The normal vaginal pH of the premenopausal non-pregnant vagina at other than menstrual times is ≤ 4.5. The acidity and the stratified squamous epithelium provide protection against pathogenic bacteria.

Uterus and fallopian tubes

The uterus lies in the pelvic cavity between the urinary bladder in front and the rectum behind. It has two parts, the body and the cervix, separated by the internal os. In the body of the uterus, the mucous membrane, often termed the endometrium, is covered on its free surface with columnar epithelium. The endocervix is also lined by columnar epithelium while the ectocervix, i.e. the vaginal surface of the cervix, is lined by stratified squamous epithelium.

In young girls, the ectocervix may appear red (ectopy) because of a single layer of ectopic columnar epithelium (continuous with that of endocervix) overlying the stromal capillary bed. Pregnancy and oral contraceptives may also be associated with a similar appearance, which may be mistakenly described as ‘erosion’ but in reality is an eversion of the endocervical columnar epithelium. The site of the squamocolumnar junction in older women is often higher up in the cervical canal.

On each side of the upper part of the uterus open the fallopian tubes. Each tube is about 10 cm long and terminates in a fimbriated end close to the ovary. The fallopian tubes are lined by columnar epithelium.

The ovaries, each about 3 cm long, 1.5 cm wide and 1 cm thick, are situated, one on each side of the uterus, lying in relation to the posterior layer of the broad ligament below the fallopian tubes.

Lymphatic drainage of genitalia

Males

The lymph vessels of the penis, the penile urethra, the scrotum and the perineal skin drain into the inguinal lymph glands. The lymphatics of the posterior urethra, the vas deferens and the seminal vesicles end in the external and the internal iliac glands, and those of the prostate terminate mainly in the internal iliac and the sacral lymph glands. The testes drain into the aortic group of lymph glands.

Females

The lymphatic drainage of the vulva, the lower part of the vagina and the perineal skin is into the inguinal lymph glands, and that of the upper part of the vagina and cervix into the external iliac, internal iliac and the sacral lymph glands. The lymphatics of the body of the uterus, the fallopian tubes and the ovary drain mainly into the aortic group of lymph glands.

Other organs which may be portals of entry of STI organisms

Anus, anal canal and rectum

The anus or anal orifice is the lower opening of the anal canal. It is surrounded by folds of skin which converge and continue into the lower part of the anal canal. The anal canal is 2–3 cm long. The upper part of the anal canal and the rectum is lined by columnar epithelium.

The lymph vessels from the anus and the lower part of the anal canal drain into the inguinal lymph glands. The lymphatics of the rest of the anal canal and the lower part of the rectum terminate in the internal iliac lymph glands, whereas those of the upper part of the rectum drain into the pararectal and the preaortic lymph glands.

Pharynx and mouth

The nasal part of the pharynx is lined by ciliated columnar epithelium, the oral and laryngeal parts by stratified squamous epithelium while the part in between these regions is lined by cuboidal epithelium.

The lymph vessels from the lower lip, the floor of the mouth and the tip of the tongue drain into the submental group of lymph glands. The lymphatic drainage of the rest of mouth, the tongue and the tonsils is into the submandibular and the deep cervical lymph glands.

Conjunctivae

The conjunctivae are the mucous membranes lining the eyelids which are then reflected on to the eyeball. The palpebral conjunctivae are lined by columnar epithelium and the ocular conjunctivae by stratified squamous epithelium.

The lymph vessels draining the eyelids and conjunctivae end in the parotid and submandibular group of glands.

Further reading

Williams, P. (ed.) (1995) *Gray's Anatomy*, 38th edn. Churchill Livingstone, Edinburgh.

CHAPTER 3
Immunity and the genital tract

C.A. Hart
Department of Medical Microbiology and Genitourinary Medicine, University of Liverpool, Liverpool, UK

The human body constantly is bombarded with disease-causing bacteria, yet infection is the exception rather than the rule. Unfortunately, the most pathogenic microorganisms have evolved strategies for avoiding immune defences. In general, immune defences may be divided into non-specific (or innate) and specific (or adaptive) arms (Box 3.1).

Non-specific immunity

This arm of the immune system acts as a barrier at skin and mucus surfaces to prevent ingress of microorganisms. Should this fail, then there are a number of non-specific tissue defences. The non-specific immune system is directed at all pathogens; new components are not synthesized in response to a pathogen nor is there memory of a particular pathogen.

Skin and mucosa

The skin of the genital tract is keratinized stratified squamous epithelium and there are very few if any microorganisms that can penetrate intact skin. Of course, ulcerative disease or any break in skin or mucosa will increase the risk of infection. Sebaceous secretions contain fatty acids, have a high NaCl content and are acidic and thus inhibit most pathogenic microorganisms except staphylococci. The skin of the genitalia has a rich normal flora consisting of resident *Staphylococcus epidermidis*, propionibacteria, peptococci and peptostreptococci. In addition, microorganisms such as *Escherichia coli*, *Candida albicans* and enterococci will colonize skin transiently from the faecal flora.

The fossa navicularis of the male urethra and most of the female urethra are lined by stratified squamous epithelium, and higher up is columnar or transitional epithelium. The distal 2–3 cm of the urethra has a normal flora, consisting of staphylococci and, in some cases, *E. coli*. The vagina and ectocervix are lined by stratified squamous epithelium which may be keratinized, depending upon age and hormonal status. The cervical os is lined by columnar epithelium. The type of epithelium determines susceptibility to

Box 3.1. Non-specific and specific immunity.

Non-specific

A. At body surface
1. Skin and mucous membranes: lack of receptors, impermeability.
2. Secretions
- mucus – trap, false receptor, blocking receptor.
- lysozyme – digests peptidoglycan.
- lactoferrin – starves bacteria of iron.
- zinc (in prostate) – inhibits a range of pathogens.
- polyamines (spermine) – bactericidal.
- pH – acidic environment inhibitory to some pathogens.

3. Inflammatory response: brings blood defence components (neutrophils, complement, antibody, etc.) to site of invasion.
4. Normal flora.

B. In tissue
1. Bactericidal activity of plasma: complement, properdin, C-reactive protein.
2. Phagocytes: principally neutrophils and monocytes.
3. Febrile response: increased temperature slows replication of pathogens and enhances immune activities.
4. Natural killer cells: non-specific killing of virus-infected cells.

Specific

A. Humoral (or antibody-mediated: IgG, IgM, IgA, IgE)
1. At body surfaces: secretory IgA – inhibits microbial attachment, does not fix complement or attract neutrophils.
2. In tissues: IgM, IgG, IgA, IgE (against nematodes) – activates complement cascade, attracts and activates neutrophils.

B. Cell-mediated: cytotoxic lymphocytes, antibody-dependent cytotoxicity, macrophages. Its role in defence against genital tract infection is unclear.

infection, for example *Chlamydia trachomatis* infects columnar but not squamous epithelia. This may be dependent both upon receptor expression by the cells and their state of maturation. Vaginal secretions contain lysozyme, lactoferrin and mucin. Lysozyme cleaves the bacterial peptidoglycan backbone rendering them more susceptible to osmotic lysis. Most bacteria have an absolute requirement for iron, and lactoferrin is a high-affinity iron-binding protein that starves the bacteria of iron. Unfortunately gonococci, for example, have iron-binding proteins of even higher affinity. The vagina also has a rich normal flora. There are 10^8–10^9 microorganisms per millilitre of secretions, and many are adherent to the mucosa. The normal flora has a role in preventing ingress of pathogens, but some components of normal flora such as group B streptococci are potential pathogens.

The inflammatory response is a most important part of the non-specific immune system. Although it is, in part, responsible for the signs and symptoms of infection, its role is to bring blood defence components to the site of microbial attack. Serum factors include antibody, complement, properdin and C-reactive protein (CRP). The complement cascade can be activated by antibody–antigen complexes (classical cascade) or by direct interaction with the bacterial cell wall, properdin or CRP (alternative cascade). Activated complement proteins act as neutrophil chemoattractants, and opsonins, anaophylotoxins and the final components of the cascade (C6–C9) form a membrane attack complex which can lyse bacteria. Interestingly, congenital deficiency of the final components can result in disseminated gonococcal disease.

It is arguable that the neutrophil is the most important component of both the specific and non-specific defences. Neutrophils are professional killing cells. The majority of their killing activity is by production of reactive oxidants such as superoxide anions, singlet oxygen, hydrogen peroxide and hypochlorite. These are concentrated around the bacterium in the phagocytic vacuole. At the same time, lysosomal granules fuse with the phagosome and release their enzymes to complete microbial killing.

In the tissues and blood

Most of the sexually transmitted pathogens are adapted to infecting the genital mucosa, with little systemic spread. This is clearly not the case for others such as HBV, HIV or *Treponema pallidum*. In addition to mechanisms described in the inflammatory response, the febrile response provides a non-specific defence. Pyrogens such as interleukin-1 (IL-1), which is released by neutrophils, act on the thermo-regulatory centre in the hypothalamus. The rise in body temperature serves to inhibit growth of microorganisms and increases the activity of the immune system.

Specific immunity

With this, once a particular pathogen has been encountered, specific defence components are synthesized to combat it. In addition, cells carry memory (immunoglobulin on B lymphocytes, T-cell receptor on T lymphocytes) of the pathogen's antigenic make-up and, each time it is encountered again, a more rapid and powerful response is produced. Three sorts of cells are involved in the specific immune response, namely antigen-presenting cells (APCs), thymus-derived lymphocytes (T cells) and bone marrow-derived lymphocytes (B cells). The APCs are dendritic cells, macrophages and B cells, of which the dendritic cells are the most important. Dendritic cells (which in skin and mucosa are called Langerhans cells) are bone marrow-derived and are mobile, but are most numerous where they can be in contact with T cells. APCs engulf antigenic molecules, process them into small fragments (often peptides) and present them on their cell surface in association with major histocompatibility complex (MHC) molecules to appropriate T cells. T cells are subdivided into two major types, $CD4^+$ and $CD8^+$ cells. $CD4^+$ cells recognize antigenic peptides in association with MHC class II molecules, whereas $CD8^+$ cells recognize those attached to MHC class I. The $CD4^+$ cells are T-helper cells and help B cells to produce antibody optimally. However, they also subserve cell-mediated immune functions by cytokine release and may also be cytotoxic killers. The $CD8^+$ cells are responsible for cytotoxic killing of virus-infected or tumour cells.

Humoral immunity

B cells produce antibody. They may be triggered directly by so-called T cell-independent antigens (e.g. polysaccharides such as the pneumococcal capsule), but this produces low-affinity IgM antibody which is not long lasting. The class switch to longer lasting and more specific IgG, IgA and IgE antibodies requires $CD4^+$ or T-helper cells. The $CD4^+$ responses can be T-helper-1 (T_H1) or T_H2. T_H1 responses involve IL-2, γ-interferon and lymphotoxin secretion, which lead to inflammatory responses. T_H2 responses involve IL-4, IL-5, IL-6 and IL-10 secretion and lead to antibody formation, including IgG and IgE. The major lymphoid systems involved in antibody production are the lymph nodes, spleen and the mucosal lymphoid tissue (Peyer's patches, tonsils, adenoids, and gut and bronchial-associated lymphoid tissue). In mucosal tissue, the antigen–antibody interaction is via secretory IgA and is non-inflammatory (i.e. T_H1 responses are damped down). Some genital tract pathogens, e.g. *Neisseria gonorrhoeae*, can evade IgA both by antigenic switching and by producing IgA protease.

Cell-mediated immunity

Cell-mediated immunity is a more destructive immunity; it kills both the pathogen and the cells it is infecting. Although it is clear that a T-cell response occurs after infection with most if not all STI, its role in protecting against re-infection is unclear.

CHAPTER 4
History taking, examination of patient, collection of specimens and common presenting symptoms

O.P. Arya
Department of Medical Microbiology and Genitourinary Medicine, University of Liverpool, Liverpool, UK

The attitude of the clinic staff must be friendly, welcoming and non-judgemental, as many patients who come to STI clinics are emotionally disturbed and embarrassed. The patient should be assured of confidentiality and interviewed with tact and care. The initial favourable impressions will facilitate good rapport and cooperation for accurate history and relevant physical, including genital, examination, which are all essential components for the appropriate management of STI.

History

A full history, aided by appropriate leading questions to fill gaps, should include the patient's own account of the symptoms and their duration, topical or systemic therapy (prescribed by an authorized person or self-administered), use of recreational drugs, drug allergies, past history of STI (including, if tested for HIV, date and result of test) or other important illness, last voided urine (especially in males) and all recent exposures including extra-marital, locality and source of infection whether known or unknown, gender of the partner(s), oral or rectal intercourse, and use of condom. In the case of the females, the additional information will include method of contraception, menstrual history, pregnancies and their outcome, and cervical cytology.

Examination of patient and collection of specimens

All patients should be given adequate explanation as to what the examination entails and the tests which will be carried out. The patients should be examined in privacy, preferably with a chaperone of appropriate gender, especially if the patient is female. The patients should be told of normal findings and informed of any abnormal signs.

Males

The patient is asked to strip to the ankle below and the chin above, and then examined in good light, standing up or lying down. One approach is to proceed as follows: inspect the skin on and around the genitals for any lesions; palpate the groin for lymph glands; inspect the pubic hair and lower abdomen for lice; examine the scrotum to ascertain the state of the testes, epididymes and vas; retract the prepuce (in those uncircumcized) and observe the condition of the reflex prepuce, the glans penis, the urethral meatus as well as the consistency, colour and amount of urethral discharge if present. If necessary, the urethra may be massaged gently a few times from the root of the penis to the urethral orifice.

The meatus may be cleaned with a dry sterile swab to ensure an uncontaminated sample. Material for smear and culture for *Neisseria gonorrhoeae* may be obtained with a cooled flamed platinum loop, a sterile disposable plastic loop or an appropriate sampling swab (Fig. 4.1). The sampling swabs chosen should be non-toxic or of low toxicity to the infecting organisms being investigated. For *Chlamydia trachomatis*, as cells rather than secretions are required, a swab such as cotton wool on a thin metal wire is used. The swab is inserted 2–4 cm into the urethra (each swab being inserted a little further for multiple specimens) and gently rotated several times before withdrawal. The swabs are then sent to the laboratory in appropriate transport media but for *N. gonorrhoeae* may be plated immediately in the clinic (see also Chapter 5). A wet preparation and culture for *Trichomonas vaginalis* may also be made. In the absence of urethral discharge, a thin swab,

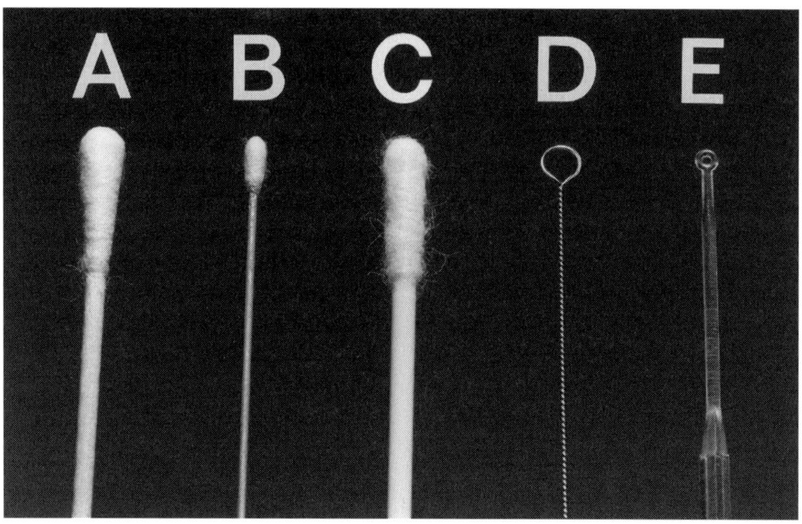

Fig. 4.1. Loops and swabs for urogenital specimens. A, Standard size cotton wool swab on a wooden stick; B, cotton wool on a thin metal wire; C, cotton wool on a rayon stick; D, nichrome wire loop; and E, disposable plastic loop.

such as cotton wool on a thin metal wire, may be moistened slightly with sterile water or saline to facilitate insertion, otherwise the passage of a standard cotton wool swab (Fig. 4.1) may be painful. The patient should be informed that the procedure may be painful as may also be the next urination.

The patient is then examined for any mucocutaneous lesions of the perianal region, mouth and throat and for enlargement of lymph glands (epitrochlear, axillary, cervical, posterior auricular and occipital), followed by examination of other systems as indicated.

The patient is then asked to urinate into two glasses, up to about 5 cm in the first and the remainder in the second glass. Any debris, threads or flakes are noted, followed by dip-stick testing to detect blood, protein, glucose, etc. The two-glass urine test roughly indicates the extent of urethritis. The haziness and/or flakes in only the first glass may indicate anterior urethritis (Chapter 7.5). Haziness in both glasses may be due to phosphates which dissolve with acetic acid; persistent haziness in the second glass may indicate infection of the posterior urethra and bladder.

Rectal examination, if indicated, may then be performed by inserting a lubricated gloved finger into the anal canal.

In homosexual males, a lubricated proctoscope, using an inert lubricant, is passed and rectal mucosa is examined. Material for smear and culture is then obtained for *N. gonorrhoeae* (and culture for *C. trachomatis* if indicated) from the rectal wall by rotating a swab several times from side to side. If proctoscopy is not possible, a cotton-tipped swab may be inserted 2.5 cm into the anal canal and rotated from side to side for several seconds for the material to be absorbed on to the swab. If there is too much faecal matter on the swab, it should be discarded and another specimen obtained.

Prostatic examination and massage

Prostatic examination is carried out to assess the state of the prostate with regard to its size, tenderness and consistency. Prostatic massage is carried out as a diagnostic procedure when chronic prostatitis is suspected. Prostatic massage is contraindicated in the presence of acute urethritis, urinary tract infection, acute epididymitis and acute prostatitis.

PROSTATIC EXAMINATION. The patient may be examined standing up with legs apart bending over the back of a low chair, or on the couch in the left lateral or a knee–elbow position. A well-lubricated gloved finger is inserted gently into the rectum. A normal prostate gland is smooth, non-tender, of rubbery consistency and about 4 cm in length and width. An acutely tender, enlarged, boggy prostate indicates an abscess and should not be massaged. In chronic prostatitis, the prostate may feel normal or may be slightly tender with nodular enlargement. The diseased seminal vesicles may be enlarged and palpable above the prostate, but normal seminal vesicles cannot be detected easily.

PROSTATIC MASSAGE. The patient should be informed of the procedure and assured that, although uncomfortable, it is not painful. The patient should not have ejaculated for 3 days, nor received antibacterial agents for at least 1 week and not urinated for at least 6 h before the collection of specimens. The prepuce, in those uncircumcized, is cleaned and retracted, and the glans penis is cleaned with sterile saline or water. The patient is then asked to void 5–10 ml (urine 1) and, after voiding a further 200 ml, a second 5–10 ml specimen (midstream urine) is collected (urine 2). (The foreskin should be retracted while voiding to obtain urine specimens.) The patient then adopts a knee–elbow position on the couch. A gloved finger is then inserted and the prostate massaged from above and lateral to the gland, six times on each side, by gentle and firm pressure of the finger directed downwards and inwards, followed by a few strokes in the middle from above downwards. The prostate fluid (expressed prostatic secretion, EPS) may be seen at the urethral meatus. The fluid should be allowed to drop on to the slides for microscopy of wet film and Gram staining, and on a culture plate, and then spread evenly with a loop for the isolation of *N. gonorrhoeae*, and/or the material may be obtained on swabs to be sent to the laboratory in appropriate transport media. If necessary, the prostatic secretion flow may be aided by milking the urethra. After obtaining specimens of the prostatic secretion, the glans penis is again cleaned as before, and a third specimen of urine, 5–10 ml (post-massage urine or urine 3), is collected.

Smears are made for examination for pus cells, Gram-negative diplococci and *T. vaginalis*, and cultures for *N. gonorrhoeae*, *T. vaginalis* and other organisms. The presence of more than 15 pus cells in a fresh wet preparation on a slide using a × 40 objective or clumps of pus cells in the EPS smear suggests prostatitis.

The above method called 'segmental culture technique' is designed to determine the site of infection. Thus, bacterial prostatitis may be diagnosed if prostatic secretion or urine 3 shows at least a tenfold increase in the bacterial count in comparison with the urine 1 and urine 2, or if bacteria are isolated from the EPS of patients whose urine 2 is sterile.

Females

The patient should be in a lithotomy position for examination of the female genitalia. If possible, an angle-poise lamp is directed appropriately. After inspecting the skin of the pubic, vulval, perianal areas and thighs, the inguinal glands are palpated and the pubic hair examined for lice and nits. The labia minora are then separated and any discharge from the introitus noted. The urethral meatus is wiped clean and inspected for redness and urethral discharge, which may become obvious only after massaging the urethra with the index finger in the vagina. Beads of pus may be seen at the paraurethral duct orifices if Skene's glands are infected. Gram-stained smear and culture may be made from this pus. Specimens for chlamydia if possible, and for smear and culture for gonorrhoea, should also be obtained from the urethra by insertion and gentle rotation of the appropriate swabs 1–2 cm into the terminal urethra. This procedure often is painful and should be performed with care after the patient has been so informed. Bartholin's glands are then palpated with the finger in the introitus and the thumb on the outer side. The normal glands are not palpable. If infected, the gland(s) may be tender and a bead of pus may be seen at the duct orifice(s) which may be inflamed. The ducts may need to be massaged on each side, and any discharge should be sampled for smear and culture. Even clear mucus may, occasionally, yield *N. gonorrhoeae* and/or *C. trachomatis* (see below for specimens for *C. trachomatis*).

A bivalve vaginal speculum moistened with warm water is then passed, directed towards the posterior vaginal fornix. The vaginal walls are inspected and the quality and quantity of any vaginal discharge noted. Specimens are obtained to ascertain the vaginal pH and for the amine test, wet film for the detection of *T. vaginalis*, yeasts and clue cells, Gram stain for yeasts, clue cells and other morphotypes and, if possible, culture for *Candida* spp. and *T. vaginalis*. Vaginal material for pH determination should be obtained with care so as to avoid contamination with cervical mucus which has a pH of about 7.0. A narrow range pH paper is touched with the vaginal swab or placed on the surface of the speculum after removal from the vagina. Alternatively, the pH indicator held in a forceps, may be applied to the vaginal wall near the lateral fornix. A cervical cytology smear may now be taken, if appropriate.

The external os of the cervix is then wiped clean with cotton wool held in a sponge-holding forceps. The condition of the cervix with regard to ectopy, congestion, etc., and the character of the cervical discharge are noted. Nabothian cysts or follicles, sometimes seen on the cervix, are a normal finding and are formed when the ducts of the glands in the cervix are blocked by the surface epithelial cells. Cervical specimens are then obtained by inserting cotton-tipped swabs about 1–2 cm into the endocervix and firmly rotating them for about 10 s to obtain adequate material. For *N. gonorrhoeae*, a smear is spread thinly on a microscopic slide for Gram staining and a swab for culture is sent to the laboratory in a suitable transport medium, or the material may be inoculated on to the culture plate in the clinic and then sent to the laboratory (see also Chapter 5). As chlamydiae are obligate intracellular organisms, the swabs are rubbed against the mucous membrane to obtain the infected cells for culture and antigen detection tests. The swab for culture is then placed in the *Chlamydia* transport medium and stored in the refrigerator at 4°C until sent to the laboratory the same or the next day. If inoculation is not possible within 24 h, the specimen should be frozen at –70°C. The swabs for antigen detection are placed in the appropriate transport medium and need not be refrigerated.

A bimanual pelvic examination is then carried out to ascertain the condition of the uterus and appendages. Movement of the cervix and examination of fornices are not normally painful. For women who have undergone hysterectomy, the specimens may be obtained from the urethra, vaginal fornices and the rectum. A thorough physical examination is then performed as in the case of men.

Rectal specimens are taken if indicated (with or without proctoscopy as described above for homosexual males). Because of cultural taboos, rectal examination may have to be restricted to proven gonorrhoea contacts.

A urine specimen should be tested for albumin and sugar.

Female children

The genital examination must be very gentle. A speculum should not be used, and the specimens may be obtained with a platinum or plastic loop or a cotton wool swab from the vagina, urethra and the rectum.

Both sexes

A blood specimen is taken for syphilis serology to indicate past or present infection and to serve as a baseline for future tests. After appropriate information/counselling, a hepatitis screen and HIV serology should be offered to all patients. Other investigations, including darkfield examination for *T. pallidum* (see Chapter 7.1), throat swab, urine culture, blood counts, blood chemistry, lumbar puncture, radiology, etc., are carried out as indicated.

Records

The patient's records should be legible and include the history, clinical findings, results of investigations, the treatment given and compliance, any side effects, the dates of follow-up appointments, partner notification, and outcome of treatment such as cured, referral to a higher medical centre/other specialists, or lost to follow-up.

Common presenting symptoms

Some men and women with STI have no symptoms. They attend STI clinic as contacts of patients known to have had an STI or to be checked for STI after they have exposed themselves to the risk of STI. They could be harbouring one or more STI agents and hence should be examined and tested as thoroughly as those with symptoms.

The common presenting symptoms and some of their possible causes are shown in Table 4.1. As expected, patients with extragenital symptoms may first attend other out-patient departments, e.g. those with skin rash may first be seen at the skin clinic. A high index of suspicion is, therefore, necessary. Conversely, not all patients with anogenital symptoms attending STI clinics have STI. All of these features and the differential diagnoses are described in Part II. The reader is also referred to Chapter 10 (Problem-oriented approach), and Chapter 11 (Special topics).

Further reading

Mears, E.M., Jr and Stamey, T.A. (1968) Bacteriological localization patterns in bacterial prostatitis and urethritis. *Investigative Urology* 5, 492–518.

Stamey, T.A. (1981) Prostatitis. *Journal of the Royal Society of Medicine* 74, 22–40.

Table 4.1. Common presenting symptoms of STI and their possible common causes.

Symptom	Cause(s)[a]
Dysuria and/or penile discharge	Gonorrhoea, chlamydial infection, *Ureaplasma* infection, non-specific urethritis, sub-preputial discharge associated with balanoposthitis
Anogenital ulceration	Chancroid, syphilis, herpes, lymphogranuloma venereum, Donovanosis, pyoderma, trauma
Vaginal discharge	Bacterial vaginosis, trichomoniasis, gonococcal and/or chlamydial infection, candidiasis, foreign body, chemical irritation, physiological, atrophic vaginitis, neoplasm
Itching on or around genitalia	Candidiasis, trichomoniasis, pediculosis, scabies
Anogenital lumps or warts	HPV infection, molluscum contagiosum, syphilis, prominent coronal papillae, sebaceous cysts
Scrotal pain or swelling	Gonococcal and/or chlamydial epididymo-orchitis, epididymal cysts, hernia, hydrocele, mumps, torsion of testes, testicular cancer, filariasis
Lower abdominal pain in women	Gonococcal and/or chlamydial infection associated with PID, cystitis (usually associated with dysuria and frequency), appendicitis, ectopic pregnancy, ovarian cyst
Generalized skin rash	Syphilis, HIV infection, other dermatoses
Spots, redness of glans penis/prepuce	*Candida* balanitis/balanoposthitis, poor genital hygiene, other genital dermatoses
Inguinal swelling	Chancroid, pyoderma, syphilis, lymphogranuloma venereum, gonorrhoea in men, genital herpes, hernia
Other anorectal symptoms (painful defaecation, anal discharge, etc.)	Gonococcal and chlamydial infections, herpes, Donovanosis, HPV infection, *Shigella*, *Salmonella* and *Campylobacter* infections, amoebiasis
Neonatal conjunctivitis	Chlamydial, gonococcal and other bacterial infections

[a]The list is not comprehensive.

CHAPTER 5
Laboratory aspects

C.A. Hart
Department of Medical Microbiology and Genitourinary Medicine, University of Liverpool, Liverpool, UK

Laboratory investigations are no substitute for careful history-taking and clinical examination by an experienced physician. However, since several different microorganisms can cause the same clinical presentation, for a definitive diagnosis of STI, laboratory help is necessary. In order to obtain maximum benefit from laboratory tests, the clinician needs to ensure that the specimens are taken properly and that they are transported to the laboratory as rapidly as possible and with sufficient relevant information. In order to interpret the results, the clinician also needs to have an understanding of what is normal and what is abnormal.

What is normal?

It is estimated that the adult human body contains approximately 10^{14} cells, but only 10% (10^{13} cells) are human. The remaining 90% make up the normal flora that colonizes skin and mucosal surfaces (Table 5.1). The normal flora is not distributed uniformly over body surfaces, for example the colon and vagina are heavily colonized whereas the hands, stomach and oesophagus have scanty, normal flora. The normal flora is not immutable but changes as individuals are exposed to different exogenous bacteria, given anti-microbials or even become ill. The type of colonizing microorganisms vary according to the site sampled. In general, anaerobes greatly outnumber aerobes at most mucosal surfaces. Indeed, it is generally accepted that the anaerobic flora provide colonization resistance. This is the ability of our normal flora to prevent colonization and thus infection by more pathogenic microorganisms. The use of antibiotics with an anti-anaerobic spectrum (e.g. ampicillin, augmentin, clindamycin, cefoxitin) can greatly disturb colonization resistance.

The vagina has a rich and diverse normal flora. Strict anaerobes such as anaerobic streptococci, *Prevotella* and *Porphyromonas* spp. (previously named *Bacteroides*), *Fusobacteria*, *Clostridia* and *Eubacterium* spp. can be found in large numbers, together with facultative anaerobes such as *Staphylococcus epidermidis*, *Lactobacillus* spp., enterococci, *Actinomyces* spp., *Escherichia coli* and other coliforms that have gained access from the large bowel. In addition,

Table 5.1. Normal flora.

	Colonization density	Predominant microorganisms
Skin		
Hands	100–200 cm^{-2}	Staphylococci and transients by touching
Forehead	$1–1.5 \times 10^4$ cm^{-2}	Staphylococci, anaerobic streptococci, corynebacteria
Axilla	10^5 cm^{-2}	Staphylococci, anaerobic streptococci, propionibacteria
Groin/ perineum	$10^6–10^7$ cm^{-2}	Staphylococci, anaerobic streptococci, faecal flora
Mucosa		
Conjunctivae	$10^2–10^3$ cm^{-2}	*S. epidermidis*, corynebacteria
Oral cavity	$10^6–10^{10}$ ml^{-1}	α-Haemolytic streptococci, *Actinomyces* spp., *Eubacterium* spp., *Lactobacillus* spp., *Neisseria* spp., *Veillonella* spp., *Porphyromonas* spp., *Prevotella* spp., *Fusobacterium* spp., *Mycoplasma* spp., *Candida* spp.
Pharynx	$10^7–10^9$ cm^{-2}	Streptococci, pneumococci, *Neisseria* spp., *Haemophilus* spp., *Moraxella* spp., *Candida* spp.
Oesophagus/ stomach	$10^1–10^2$ ml^{-1}	Transients, ?*Helicobacter pylori*
Small intestine	$10^2–10^4$ ml^{-1}	Transients, lactobacilli, bifidobacteria
Large intestine	$10^{10}–10^{12}$ ml^{-1}	Anaerobes (*Bacteroides*, *Prevotella*, *Eubacterium*, *Clostridium* spp.) predominate, *E. coli*
Urethra	Only distal 2 cm	*Lactobacillus* spp., staphylococci, α-streptococci, corynebacteria, *E. coli*
Vagina	$10^8–10^9$ ml^{-1}	Staphylococci, lactobacilli, streptococci, *Haemophilus* spp., peptococci, *Porphyromonas* spp., *Prevotella* spp., *E. coli*

Normally sterile areas are sinuses, middle ear, bronchial tree below vocal chords, proximal urethra, bladder, ureters, prostate, epididymis, uterine cavity, fallopian tubes, peritoneum, gall bladder, liver, blood, cerebrospinal fluid, muscle, joints and bone.

potential pathogens such as group B streptococci, *Gardnerella vaginalis*, *Haemophilus influenzae*, *Mobiluncus* spp., *Ureaplasma urealyticum*, *Mycoplasma hominis* and even *Chlamydia trachomatis* can be isolated from women with no signs of infection. *Candida albicans* can also be part of the normal flora. Viruses such as herpes simplex type 2 (HSV-2 or HHV-2) cytomegalovirus (CMV or HHV-5; see Table 6.3.1) and even HIV are excreted into the vagina in the absence of disease, but whether these are normal flora is a matter for debate.

Taking and transporting samples (see also Chapter 4)

To obtain the best sample, the area must be clearly visible and this will need, in the case of females, speculum examination. This will ensure that the maximum amount of infective material is obtained with the least contamination by normal flora. For many genital pathogens, both the purulent exudate and the underlying cells need to be sampled, thus it is important to rub the swab on the area rather than just dipping it in the pus. The material used in some swabs can interfere with, for example, antigen detection or polymerase chain reaction (PCR) amplification, and often manufacturers supply the correct swabs for their test. For detection of gonococci by culture, the ideal is to plate out at the bedside. However, this is not always possible, and a variety of transport systems (e.g. Gonoline) or media have been produced in order to improve the survival of these fragile bacteria. For cultures of *Chlamydia*, mycoplasma and viruses, transport media (usually tissue culture media or phosphate-buffered saline) containing appropriate antibiotics are used. The antibiotics are used to suppress the growth of contaminating bacteria during transport. Samples for culture, immunofluorescent antigen test (IFAT) or PCR should be stored and, ideally, transported at 4–8°C. Samples for culture should not be frozen at -20°C but will survive if frozen at -70°C or below. Finally, it is most important that the request form contains as much information as possible, including suspected diagnosis, since many of the laboratory tests are pathogen-specific.

Diagnostic methods

The aim of the diagnostic laboratory is to perform highly sensitive and specific tests as rapidly as possible in order to provide the physician with information to manage the patient correctly. Often, and especially in developing countries, there has to be a balance between this aim and the availability of resources (Table 5.2). In some settings, diagnostic facilities will have simple staining and microscopy only, whereas others at the tertiary level will have facilities for culture, antigen detection or even genome detection.

In general, the tests available can be subdivided into non-specific and specific (Box 5.1).

Non-specific tests

These tests confirm the clinical suspicion that an infection is present, but do not detect the pathogen. For STI, the most frequently used tests are peripheral blood white cell counts and differentials, measurement of acute phase response [most often erythrocyte sedimentation rate (ESR) or C-reactive protein (CRP)], white cell counts in genital tract secretions and the leukocyte esterase dip-stick (LED) test. In general, the peripheral blood white cell count will be raised with a neutrophilia, often with a left shift in bacterial infection and with lymphocytosis in viral infection. Exceptions include neutropenia in

Table 5.2. Appropriate provision of laboratory services[a].

Level	Technology
Village	Nil
Peripheral health centre	Microscopy: Gram-stain, wet-mounts, Ziehl–Neelsen
District hospital	Microscopy Simple ELISA (e.g. HIV, hepatitis B)
Regional hospital	Microscopy: as above plus immunofluorescence ELISA: antigen detection and serology Culture: bacterial, fungal Antimicrobial susceptibility Serology
National laboratory	As in the regional hospital *plus* Genome detection Viral culture Viral and bacterial typing

[a]Ideally, appropriate quality control schemes of media production, the various methods of pathogen detection and susceptibility testing should also be implemented.

severe bacterial infection (e.g. gonococcal or meningococcal septicaemia) and lymphopenia in AIDS. Indeed, lymphocyte and $CD4^+$ counts are often used as surrogate markers of disease progression in AIDS. A very high neutrophil count can indicate a collection of pus, for example pelvic abscess. Of the measurements of acute phase proteins, estimation of CRP (normal <1 mg l^{-1}) is that used most often. CRP is raised in bacterial infections or tissue damage but not in viral infections.

The LED is a dip-stick test that can be used on urine samples to detect inflammation. It detects the esterases that are present in neutrophils, thus a positive result indicates the presence of an inflammatory response. It is positive in urinary tract infection and urethritis, and may also be positive with calculi, or renal tuberculosis.

Specific tests

With these, the aim is to determine the nature of the infecting microorganism. The tests available vary greatly in sensitivity, specificity and rapidity.

Direct visualization

Microscopy is used to detect microorganisms in either unstained or stained material. These are 'catch-all' techniques aimed at detecting any pathogen that is present. There must be between 10^4 and 10^5 microorganisms ml^{-1} in a sample for them to be detected by light microscopy, and 10^6 ml^{-1} by electron microscopy. Electron microscopy with its higher resolving power is used to detect viruses. Examples include detection of HHV-1 and -2, varicella-zoster virus (HHV-3) and molluscum contagiosum virus in lesions or HHV-5 in urine. It is also used as a confirmatory test following viral culture. It requires

Box 5.1. Laboratory diagnostic tests.

A. Non-specific (is infection present?)

Blood:	White cell count and differential
	Acute phase response (ESR, plasma viscosity, C-reactive protein, cytokines, orosomucoid, α_1-antitrypsin)
CSF:	Cell count, protein, glucose, lactate estimations
Urine:	Cell count, protein, nitrite, leukocyte esterase
Vagina:	Cell count, amine test, clue cells

B. Specific (what is the pathogen?)

1. Rapid (20 min–4 h)

Direct visualization

Light microscopy (stained brightfield, dark ground or phase-contrast)
Electron microscopy
Fluorescent microscopy (auramine phenol)

Antigen detection

Enzyme-linked immunosorbent assay	(ELISA)
Latex particle agglutination	(LPA)
Radioimmunoassay	(RIA)
Countercurrent immunoelectrophoresis	(CIE)
Immunofluorescent antibody test	(IFAT)

Genome detection

DNA hybridization	
Polymerase chain reaction	(PCR)
Ligase chain reaction	(LCR)
Branched DNA detection	(BDNA)

2. Culture (slower, minimum of 12–18 h)
Viral culture (not all cultivable, needs cell culture)
Bacterial culture (most pathogenic bacteria cultivable in 24–48 h)
Fungal culture (can take up to 1 week depending on fungus)
Antimicrobial susceptibility (takes a further 18–24 h)

3. Antibody detection
Usually provides retrospective evidence of infection rather than acute diagnosis, except for a few infections (e.g. hepatitis or syphilis).

expensive equipment and trained staff, and this is only available in a few centres in tropical countries. In contrast, light microscopy is available in most parts of the developing world. Ideally the microscope should have ×10, ×40 and ×100 (oil-immersion) objective lenses and a good light source. It is a powerful tool when used correctly and properly maintained. Material for microscopy can be prepared as simple wet mounts to detect *Trichomomas vaginalis* (motile protozoa 10–12 μm × 7–10 μm), *Candida albicans* (non-motile spheres or budding spheres ~5 μm) before or after culture and *Treponema pallidum* by dark ground microscopy (spiral bacteria 0.15 × 6–15 μm with flexuous motility). A variety of simple staining methods are available (Box 5.2). Gram stain will allow visualization of polymorphs and lymphocytes, and bacteria can be differentiated by shape (cocci, bacilli), arrangement (chains, streptococci; clusters, staphylococci; pairs, diplococci) and cell wall (Gram-positive, blue–purple or Gram-negative, pink–red); the human cells will always be Gram-negative. However, because of the rich normal flora, pathogens can only be detected by some distinctive feature. For the specific diagnosis of *N. gonorrhoeae*, Gram-negative diplococci must be seen within pus cells (neutrophils). Although extracellular, Gram-negative diplococci could be gonococci, they could also be commensal *Neisseria*.

Giemsa stain binds to nucleic acid and has been used to detect bacteria and bacterial inclusions within infected cells. Its sensitivity in detecting chlamydial inclusions is low (~50%). Acid-fast stains [Ziehl–Neelsen (Z-N), auramine phenol] are used for the detection of mycobacteria and *Cryptosporidium parvum*. In general, auramine phenol, which is fluorescent, provides better sensitivity than Z-N.

Antigen detection

Antigen detection tests depend upon the availability of good quality antibody against the particular pathogen sought. The tests are pathogen-specific, they will only detect one particular pathogen, and a set of tests is required to cover all possible pathogens. Nowadays, most of these tests are commercially available. This improves quality control and ease of use but, inevitably, means increased cost. The enzyme-linked immunosorbent assay (ELISA) format is used most frequently. It has the advantage of being less labour intensive and able to examine large numbers of samples but the disadvantage of being more difficult to adapt for small numbers of samples and of not actually visualizing the pathogen. The usual format is antigen capture. The wells of microtitre

Box 5.2. Staining techniques.

Preparation of smears
Swabs should be spread gently on a clean glass slide or suspensions of bacteria from plates similarly spread using a sterile loop. The slides should be air-dried (not by heating) and then fixed by passing through the bunsen flame four or five times.

Gram stain
The slide is flooded or immersed in crystal violet (1% v/v) for 30–60 s. It is then washed in tap water. Then it is flooded with Lugol's iodine (1% v/v) for 30–60 s which cross-links the crystal violet to the Gram-positive bacterial cell wall. The slide is again washed in tap water and decolorized for less than 10 s in acetone (100%) or 95% ethanol. Longer periods can over-decolorize the Gram-positive bacteria rendering them Gram-negative. Finally, the slide is counterstained with safranin (0.5–1.0% v/v) for 30 s. The slide is then allowed to dry and examined using the oil-immersion (×100) objective lens.

Methylene blue
The slide is flooded with methylene blue (1%) for 1 min, allowed to dry and examined as for the Gram stain. This will detect pus cells and bacteria, but all will be stained blue.

plates are coated with antibody to the particular pathogen. Samples are then added and, if the pathogen is present, it will be trapped by the antibody. The wells are washed thoroughly to remove material that has stuck non-specifically to the plastic. Then a second antibody against the pathogen to which an enzyme has been chemically attached is added. If antigen (the pathogen) has been captured, then the second antibody–enzyme conjugate will also bind. The wells are again washed thoroughly and the enzyme's substrate added. This is usually a compound that changes colour when hydrolysed by the enzyme, thus the wells and therefore the samples containing the pathogen can be detected. Antigen-capture ELISAs are available for detection of HIV (p24), HBV (HBSAg, HBeAg), CMV, HHV-1 and -2, *C. trachomatis*, *N. gonorrhoeae* and *T. vaginalis*. Each has varying degrees of sensitivity and specificity but are usually above 80–85%. Of the other immunoassays, radioimmunoassay (RIA) is little used since it requires radioactivity and expensive equipment. Latex particle agglutination (LPA) uses latex particles coated with antibody to a pathogen. If the pathogen or its antigens are present, the antibody binds to them and this cross-links the latex particles causing the milky suspension to clump. It is generally less sensitive and specific than ELISA.

IFAT has the advantage that the infectious agent is visualized but has the disadvantage of being labour intensive and requiring expensive equipment (ultra-violet microscope) which can be difficult to maintain. IFAT is used to detect *C. trachomatis*, and CMV, and to confirm and type HHV-1 and -2 following tissue culture.

Genome detection

This is a developing area for pathogen detection and provides the most sensitive test. In general, the DNA hybridization tests have been disappointing, often proving less sensitive than culture. Of the genome amplification tests, PCR is that most often used. Theoretically, it can detect as little as one copy of a genome in a sample. In practice, the sensitivity is lower because of inefficient extraction of nucleic acid. PCR amplifies double-stranded DNA targets, thus for detection of RNA viruses [e.g. HIV, hepatitis C virus (HCV)] their genomic RNA must be converted to cDNA using reverse transcriptase (RT). The target sequences are generally less than 500 base pairs (bp) and they are usually chosen from a part of the genome that shows little sequence variability. Targeting is done by using synthetic oligonucleotides (usually 20 bases) that bind to the sense and antisense strands of the DNA (Fig. 5.1). The target sequence is copied using a DNA polymerase enzyme which is heat stable so that it is not denatured by the high temperatures used in PCR. The enzyme most often used is *Taq* polymerase (from the heat-tolerant bacterium *Thermus aquaticus*). The reagents (sample DNA, oligonucleotide primer, individual nucleotides, *Taq* and buffer) are placed in a tube. This is first heated (to ~95°C) to separate the two strands of target DNA, and then allowed to cool to 55°C to allow the primers (which are in excess) to bind to the target. The temperature is then raised to 70°C to allow the *Taq* polymerase to add bases to the primer complementary to the target DNA sequence. At each repeated

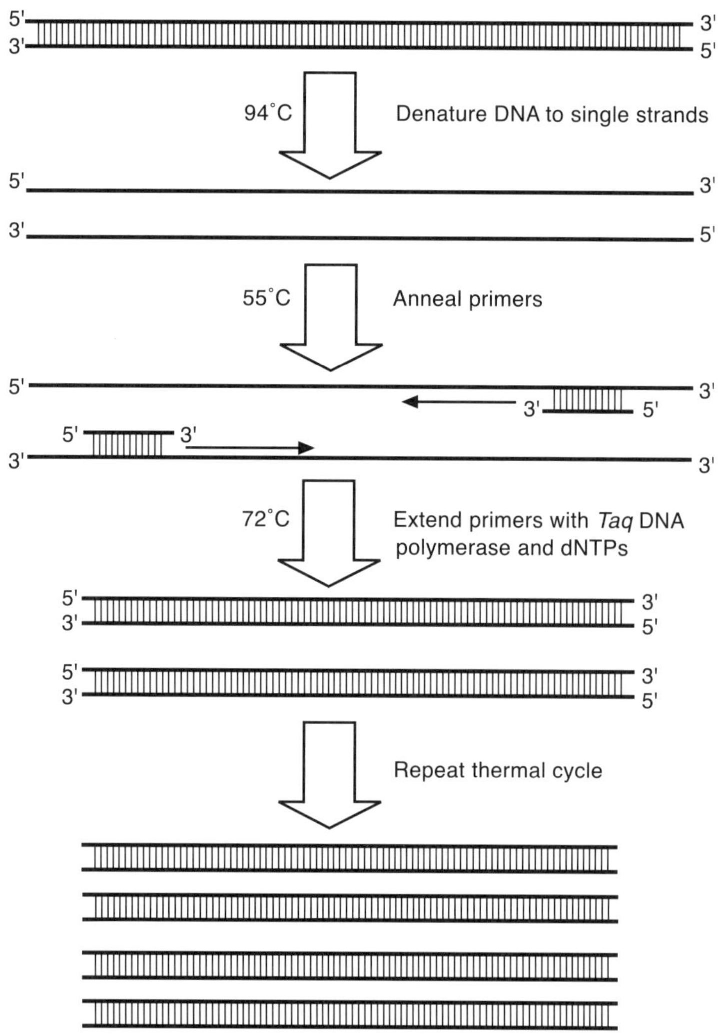

Fig. 5.1. The polymerase chain reaction.

cycle, the amount of target DNA is doubled. At the end of 35–40 cycles, there will be sufficient target DNA (amplicon) to be detected by gel electrophoresis or modified ELISA technology. The technology is very sensitive, e.g. in detecting *C. trachomatis* it is 10–20% more sensitive than culture or immunoassay. Great care must be taken to prevent cross-contamination between samples since only tiny amounts of contamination can result in false-positives. For this reason, it is advisable to have sample and reagent preparation areas in different rooms from each other and from the thermal cyclers. PCRs are commercially available for detection of HIV, HBV, HCV, HPV, HHV-1 and -2, CMV, *C. trachomatis*, *N. gonorrhoeae* and *T. pallidum*.

They are quite expensive. PCR technology can also be adapted to give estimates of amounts of virus in the blood. For example, measurement of HIV load is used to predict disease progression and monitor response to therapy in AIDS. Estimation of HCV load is used to determine who and when to treat with interferon.

A number of other genome and signal amplification methods including ligase chain reaction (LCR), Qβ , branched DNA, nucleic acid sequence-based amplification (NASBA) and transcription-mediated amplification (TMA) have been devised. Of these, LCR has proved highly sensitive and specific for detecting *C. trachomatis*, equal to or better than PCR.

Culture

In general, culture techniques are 'catch-all' rather than pathogen specific. However, they become pathogen-specific when selective media are used. They are slower techniques in that they require time for the pathogen to grow. For medicolegal purposes, it is often necessary, where possible, to culture the pathogen and store it frozen at –70°C or below.

VIRUSES. Viruses vary in their ease and speed of culture. Some are not cultivable (e.g. HCV, molluscum contagiosum), others with difficulty [e.g. HBV, HIV, Kaposi's sarcoma-associated (HHV-8)] and some with ease (e.g. HHV-1, HHV-2, CMV). HHV-1 and -2 can be cultured within 24 h, whereas CMV can take 5–7 days. It is expensive to run a viral culture diagnostic service, as a variety of different cell lines must be maintained. In addition, especially in tropical countries, contamination of tissue culture suites by airborne moulds and fungi is difficult to control. Some but not all viruses produce a characteristic cytopathic effect on cultured cells. Nevertheless, it is still necessary to confirm the identity of the isolated virus. This is usually done by electron microscopy and/or immunoassay.

BACTERIA. Bacterial culture is often more readily available and certainly is less expensive. Most of the sexually transmitted pathogens can be grown in 24–48 h. The exceptions include *C. trachomatis* (3–4 days), *M. hominis* and *U. urealyticum* (2–3 days). *C. trachomatis* is an obligate intracellular pathogen and will only grow in tissue culture. Protein synthesis in the cells (e.g. McCoy cells) is inhibited by cycloheximide (so that they do not outgrow the *C. trachomatis*) and the sample is centrifuged on to the cells. Over the next 48–72 h, the bacterium grows to produce large inclusions which can be detected by simple stains (e.g. Giemsa, periodic acid–Schiff; PAS) or IFAT. This method is at least as sensitive as antigen detection methods but less sensitive than PCR. It is of course 100% specific.

N. gonorrhoeae is a fastidious and fragile bacterium which has to be isolated against a background of robust normal flora. For this, the culture media must be both enriched (to support growth) and selective (to kill normal flora), and cultures must be done in CO_2 (4–6%) in humidified air at 35–36°C. A variety of different media have been used. Most often they contain peptone starch agar base buffered with phosphate (36 g l^{-1}), haemoglobin (1%) or horse blood, a growth supplement, e.g. Iso-vitalex (1%) or yeast extract and horse or pig serum (10%). However, serum blood agar (chocolatized by heating in a boiler until it turns brown) is the most readily available medium. The medium is made selective by adding antibiotics to kill the normal flora. Most often, vancomycin (which kills Gram-positive bacteria), colistin (which kills Gram-negatives other than *Neisseria* spp.), trimethoprim (which inhibits swarming *Proteus* and other bacteria) and either nystatin or amphotericin B (which inhibit fungi) are incorporated. The concentrations vary between media but, for example, modified Thayer–Martin contains vancomycin (3 mg l^{-1}), colistin (7.5 mg l^{-1}), trimethoprim (5 mg l^{-1}) and nystatin (12.5 mg l^{-1}). Following incubation, suspect colonies must be identified as gonococci. Gonococci are Gram-negative oxidase-positive diplococci that hydrolyse glucose but not maltose, lactose, sucrose or fructose to produce acid. Further confirmation can be obtained by immunoassays (IFAT or LPA). Antimicrobial susceptibility testing is usually done by controlled disc diffusion, but rapid detection of penicillinase-producing *N. gonorrhoeae* can be done by using the chromogenic cephalosporin, nitrocefin.

The diagnosis of chancroid depends upon culture of *Haemophilus ducreyi*. Large numbers of bacteria (10^7–10^8 ml^{-1}) are present in pus from ulcers and buboes. Isolation requires selective enriched media and incubation at 33–35°C in humified 10% CO_2 in air. To optimize isolation, the use of two separate isolation media is advised. Selection is obtained by incorporating vancomycin (3 μg ml^{-1}) into enriched media such as chocolate agar containing Iso-vitalex (1%) or GC agar plus haemoglobin and fetal calf serum. *H. ducreyi* forms solid colonies that can be pushed across the agar plates.

Mycoplasma hominis and *U. urealyticum* can be grown in beef-heart infusion broth (PPLO, pleuropneumonia-like organism broth) incorporating yeast extract (10% v/v) and horse serum (20% v/v). Separate broths are prepared containing arginine, glucose and urea together with phenol red (0.002%, a pH indicator). *M. hominis* metabolizes arginine to produce ammonia which increases the pH and causes a colour change in the broth. *U. urealyticum* has a powerful urease enzyme which converts urea to ammonia, again increasing the pH. Culture takes up to 1 week.

FUNGI. *Candida albicans* and other *Candida* spp. will grow on blood agar, but the selective medium most readily available is Sabouraud's which will detect smaller numbers of yeasts.

PROTOZOA. *T. vaginalis* can be detected by direct wet-mount preparations. Greater sensitivity is achieved by culture overnight at 37°C in Kupferberg medium or modified Diamond medium, followed by microscopic examination.

Serology

With these tests, a specific antibody (IgM, IgG or IgA) response to the pathogen is sought. Following initial infection, it can take 7–14 days for sufficient specific antibody to be produced for detection, and paired acute and convalescent sera are required. Therefore, serology is less useful for acute diagnosis since it provides evidence that an infection has happened. There are exceptions, for example an IgM response to hepatitis A virus (HAV) can be detected as soon as the patient becomes jaundiced and, in patients with primary syphilis, serological tests can be positive at presentation. Serology provides epidemiological information and, for some pathogens, detection of antibody usually means that the patient continues to be infected and is probably infective. Examples include detection of antibodies to any of the herpesviruses, HIV and HCV. A variety of formats are available.

Probably the least sensitive and most labour intensive is the complement fixation test. The most versatile is ELISA in which antigen coats the wells of microtitre plates. The patient's serum is then added and if they have antibody to the pathogen, it will bind to the well specifically. After extensive washings (to remove non-specifically binding antibody), enzyme-conjugated anti-human immunoglobulin is added, followed by substrate. A change in colour and intensity reflects the presence and amount of antibody in the patient's serum. The ELISA can be made class-specific (to detect specific IgG, IgA or IgM antibodies) either by using class-specific antibody–enzyme conjugates or initially coating the wells with the various class-specific anti-human antisera.

The serological tests for syphilis are subdivided into non-treponemal (or non-specific) and treponemal (or specific) tests. The former detect antibody against antigens released from host tissue by syphilis and the latter detect antibody against antigens from *T. pallidum*. The two most frequently used non-treponemal tests are VDRL (Venereal Disease Reference Laboratory) and RPR (rapid plasma reagin) tests. Both employ cardiolipin, lecithin and cholesterol as antigens which are mixed with patient's serum on a solid matrix (microscope slide or card). The mixture must then be rotated for 10 min before reading. The VDRL is read using a microscope looking for flocculant clumps. The RPR has charcoal added to the antigen mixture, and a positive test is seen as clumps of charcoal which have been trapped by the antigen–antibody complex. The test can be made quantitative by using dilutions of the patient's serum. These tests are sensitive (they detect most true-positives) but not very specific (they detect a number of false-positives). They are thus used for initial screening of sera and positives confirmed using the *Treponema*-specific tests. The non-treponemal tests are also useful for monitoring response to therapy (see also Chapter 7.1). Occasionally (<2% of cases), and especially in secondary syphilis, truly positive sera give a weak positive or rough appearance due to a prozone phenomenon. This occurs with flocculation and clumping tests (e.g. VDRL and RPR) and is due to an excess of antibody. Dilution of the serum will reveal a positive reaction. Thus, all sera showing the slightest reactivity should be diluted and re-tested.

The *Treponema*-specific tests include the *T. pallidum* haemagglutination assay (TPHA), the fluorescent treponemal antibody absorption (FTA-ABS) test and antibody-capture ELISA. Each utilizes *T. pallidum* as antigen. In the TPHA, fixed red cells are coated with antigen. These are added to serial dilutions of patient's serum. If antibody is present, then the red cells agglutinate and form a layer over the bottom of the microtitre wells. If there is no antibody (or it has been diluted out), the red cells form a button in the well. A disadvantage of TPHA is that it does not differentiate IgG and IgM antibodies. This is possible with FTA-ABS and ELISA. The FTA-ABS is an indirect immunofluorescent test. The patient's serum is first mixed with a suspension of Reiter treponemes (to absorb antibody to non-*T. pallidum* treponemes). Then it is placed on a microscope slide on which is fixed *T. pallidum*. The slide is then washed and either anti-human IgG or IgM–fluorescein conjugate is added. On viewing the slide using a UV microscope, fluorescent spirochaetes indicate a positive result. The ELISAs are recently available tests and are usually in the IgG or IgM antibody-capture or competitive formats. They appear sensitive and specific and are much easier to perform than the FTA-ABS.

Chlamydial antibody can be detected using microimmunofluorescence (MIF) tests. These employ antigens (elementary bodies) grown in egg yolk or tissue culture sacs, and antibody is detected by using anti-human isotype-specific fluorescein conjugates. It is a laborious and time-consuming test but can detect antibody against the various *C. trachomatis* serogroups including LGV.

Tables 5.3 and 5.4 outline the laboratory tests available for diagnosis of bacterial, viral, fungal and protozoal STI.

Table 5.3. Diagnosis of bacterial STI.

Bacterium	Culture	Non-cultural
Bacterial vaginosis	? Benefit	Amine test, clue cells and various morphotypes on stain of smear[a]
Calymmatobacterium granulomatis	In tissue culture[b]	Biopsy or scrape of lesion stained by Giemsa[a]
Chlamydia trachomatis	On McCoy cells (~72 h)	Giemsa stain, antigen detection (ELISA, IFAT), PCR[a], serology not of much use except possibly for LGV
Gardnerella vaginalis	On fastidious anaerobic agar[a]	See bacterial vaginosis above
Haemophilus ducreyi	On chocolate agar[a]	PCR[b]
Mobiluncus spp.	On fastidious anaerobic agar[a] (6–7 days)	Gram stain, see bacterial vaginosis above
Neisseria gonorrhoeae	On enriched selective media[a] (e.g. Thayer–Martin)	
Mycoplasma hominis	PPLO medium[a]	PCR[b]
Treponema pallidum	Not available	Dark ground microscopy[a] PCR[b], Serology[a] (RPR, VDRL, TPHA, FTA IgG or IgM antibodies, ELISA)
Ureaplasma urealyticum	PPLO medium[a]	PCR[b]

[a]Most sensitive and specific test available.
[b]Indicates research technique not commercially available.

Table 5.4. Diagnosis of viral, fungal and protozoal STI.

	Culture	Non-cultural
RNA viruses		
HAV	—	IgM anti-HAV[b]
HIV	$CD4^+$ T lymphocytes[c]	Serology (ELISA)[a], antigen detection (p24), PCR[b] or RT-PCR[b] (also possible to measure viral load)
HCV	—	Serology (ELISA)[a], RT-PCR[b] (also possible to genotype and measure viral load)
DNA viruses		
HHV-1 and -2	Tissue culture[b] (Vero) HHV-1 and -2 differentiated by IFAT	Giemsa, Tzank or Papanicolau stains (poor sensitivity), IFAT, PCR[b], electron microscopy
HHV-5 (CMV)	Tissue culture (MRC-5)	Serology (ELISA)[a], IFAT[b], PCR[b], RT-PCR (for viral mRNA), viral load
HHV-8	Tissue culture[c]	Serology[a], PCR[b]
Molluscum contagiosum	—	Electron microscopy[b] (if needed)
HPV	—	PCR[b], *in situ* hybridization, Papanicolau stain
Fungi		
Candida spp.	Sabouraud's agar[b]	Gram-stain
Protozoa		
Trichomonas vaginalis	In liquid media (Feinberg Whittington or Kupferberg)	Wet-mount or phase-contrast microscopy, PCR[c], antigen detection (ELISA)

[a]Does not provide evidence in acute infection.
[b]Most sensitive and specific method.
[c]Research only.

PART II
Infections and Microorganisms

CHAPTER 6
Viral infections

CHAPTER 6.1
HIV infection and AIDS

P. Phanuphak[1] and D.M. Serwadda[2]
[1]Department of Medicine, Chulalongkorn University, Bangkok, Thailand; [2]Institute of Public Health, Makerere University Medical School, Kampala, Uganda

Human immunodeficiency virus (HIV) infection and acquired immune deficiency syndrome (AIDS) follow the path of other infectious diseases by being more prevalent in the tropics than in other parts of world. The reasons include low income, low education, poor hygiene and lack of resources. These factors can partially explain the rapidly spreading epidemic of HIV and AIDS in sub-Saharan Africa and South and Southeast Asia. The socioeconomic impact of HIV/AIDS, in turn, further compromises the resource and development of countries in the tropics.

Clinical manifestations of HIV infection in the tropics may differ from those in other parts of the world due to the differences in endemic or environmental pathogens, genetic susceptibility and nutritional and immunological status. *Penicillium marneffei*, for example, is the unique AIDS-defining systemic fungal infection in northern Thailand. As a result, the natural history of HIV infection in the tropics is likely to be different from in the non-tropics. Patients may also have shorter survival due to lack of adequate care. In addition, unique HIV-1 subtypes present in the tropics may explain differences in infectivity and clinical course.

This chapter first covers some basic aspects, followed by clinical and management experiences largely in Thailand, and then the picture in sub-Saharan Africa.

Epidemiology (see also Chapter 1)

As compared with the HIV epidemic in the developed world where HIV infection is predominantly a disease of homosexual and bisexual men and intravenous drug users (IVDUs), the infection in the tropics occurs mainly among heterosexuals. Although IVDUs are also a risk group in many countries in the tropics such as Thailand, India and Myanmar, the heterosexuals form the largest risk group, especially if they have high-risk sexual behaviour. Heterosexuals account for 80–90% of the entire HIV-infected population in India and Thailand.

The HIV epidemic in Thailand clearly illustrates how the infection can rapidly escalate when there is inadequate control. It began in 1984 in foreign and Thai homo/bisexuals. The second wave of the epidemic started in 1988 among the IVDUs (Table 6.1.1). This was followed by the third wave of the epidemic in 1989 among female sex workers, and clients of sex workers, in 1990 as the fourth wave. Finally, the fifth wave occurred in 1991 among housewives and newborns. Lessons to be learnt from the Thai epidemic are that all potential risk groups should be considered as targets for simultaneous prevention campaigns irrespective of how low the prevalence is in that group at that moment. Promiscuous heterosexual behaviour poses the greatest threat of large epidemics simply because heterosexuals are potentially the largest group in the population.

Pathogenesis

Although some still feel that HIV may be a mere passenger in AIDS, most now accept that HIV is the primary infectious agent leading to AIDS. The virus is abundant in the blood, semen and the vaginal secretions which makes the exchange of, or the contamination with, blood and genital fluid the most important routes of HIV infection. After entry, HIV can infect several cell types, but most importantly the $CD4^+$ T-helper cells. It may remain dormant in the infected cells for a variable period of time or may replicate constantly in the body, particularly within cells in the lymph nodes. The immune system, on the other hand, is also stimulated constantly by the invader and produces the humoral and cell-mediated immune responses to the virus. The final outcome, which is also the general outcome of such a battle, is a progressive

Table 6.1.1. Five waves of HIV epidemic in Thailand and the estimated numbers with HIV infection in individual risk groups.[a]

Wave	Starting year	Population group	Size of the population	Estimated number of HIV infection in 1997
1	1984	Male homo/bisexuals	100,000	10,000 (10%)
2	1988	IVDU	100,000	40,000 (40%)
3	1989	Female sex workers	200,000	56,000 (28%)
4	1990	Clients of female sex workers	4,000,000	320,000 (8%)
5	1991	Non-married women, housewives and newborns	18,000,000	324,000 (1.8%)

[a]Adapted from the sentinel surveillance data, Ministry of Public Health in Thailand. A total of 750,000 HIV-infected individuals were estimated to be present throughout Thailand by the end of 1997, whereas the cumulative estimate was 1 million.

deterioration of the cell-mediated immune system leading to secondary infection with a variety of opportunistic pathogens and to the development of neoplastic growths, the hallmarks of AIDS. Therefore, it is essential to dissect the pathogenesis of HIV infection into viral factors, host factors and their interactions.

The viral factors

HIV is a member of the retrovirus family in subfamily lentivirinae. It contains two copies of a single-stranded RNA genome which encodes three polycistronic structural genes (*gag*, *pol* and *env*) and a number of regulatory genes. The *gag* precursor protein, p55, is cleaved by viral protease to p24 (inner core protein or capsid antigen), p17 (outer core protein or matrix antigen) and p15, which is cleaved further into two nucleic acid-binding proteins (p9 and p7). The *pol* precursor protein gives rise to reverse transcriptase (RT, p51), the protease and the integrase (p31) proteins. The *env* precursor glycoprotein, gp160, gives rise to gp120 (surface glycoprotein) and gp41 (transmembrane glycoprotein) which, in combination, form the 'spikes' projecting out from the lipid bilayer or the viral envelope (Fig. 6.1.1).

Among the various regulatory proteins of HIV are Tat (transactivator of transcription), Rev (regulator of expression of virion proteins) and Nef (negative factor, whose function is unclear). The accessory proteins Vif, Vpr, Vpu, Vpx and Vpt are involved in the production of infectious virus, such as in the process of assembly and budding.

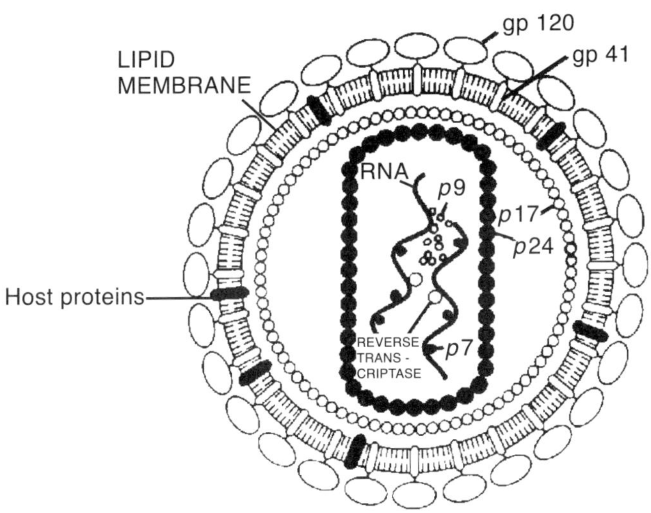

Fig. 6.1.1. HIV-1: schematic structure (adapted from Shaw *et al.*, 1988).

HIV life cycle

The CD4 antigen on the host cell surface serves as the primary receptor for HIV. It binds via the CD4-binding site on gp120. This results in displacement of gp120 and proteolytic cleavage of the third variable loop (V3) which allows interaction between a fusion domain on gp41 and a fusion receptor on the cell surface. Following membrane fusion, viral RNA enters into the cell and is reverse-transcribed into DNA by reverse transcriptase. The transcribed viral DNA provirus is transported into the nucleus and integrated into chromosomal DNA (see Fig. 6.1.2). The proviral DNA may remain latent in the cell for a variable period of time before starting to produce viral genomic RNA and viral mRNA. The viral mRNA is used to synthesize viral polypeptides. The viral genomic RNA is packaged into the viral capsid and buds through the cell membrane while incorporating the viral envelope glycoprotein present on the cell membrane.

During the initial phase of HIV infection, approximately 10^9 virions are produced per day, of which 10^6 are mutant variants.

Cell tropism

Besides $CD4^+$ T lymphocytes, HIV can also infect B lymphocytes, monocytes, macrophages, megakaryocytes, natural killer cells, eosinophils, Langerhans cells of skin, fibroblasts, laryngeal and bowel epithelial cells, dendritic cells, microglia, astrocytes, and brain capillary and thymic endothelial cells. Many of these cells do not have surface CD4. HIV entry into $CD4^-$ cells may be mediated through the fusion between the fusion domain at the amino terminus of gp41 and the fusion receptor on the cell surface, such as galactosyl ceramide on brain and bowel cells. In addition, HIV entry may also be mediated through the Fc and complement receptors when antibody to HIV is present, i.e. opsonization as is the case for monocytes and macrophages.

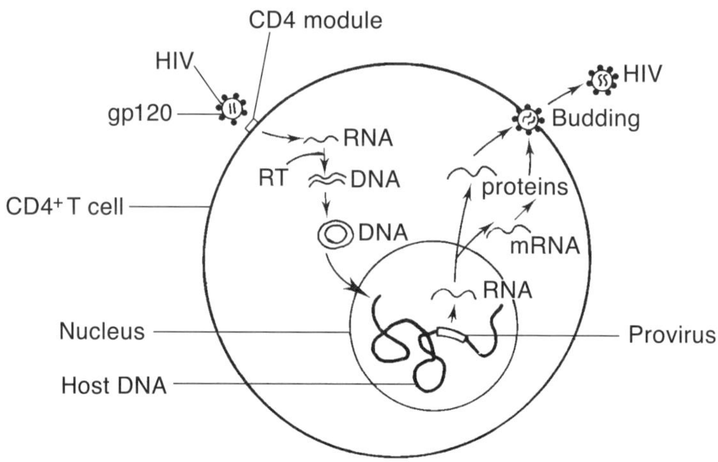

Fig. 6.1.2. HIV life cycle.

HIV variants

There are two main variants of HIV designated HIV-1 and HIV-2. HIV-1 is the predominant variant in most parts of the world. HIV-2 is endemic mainly in West Africa. The latter is 55% genetically different from HIV-1 and is more closely related to simian immunodeficiency virus (SIV) than to HIV-1. HIV-2 is believed to be less transmissible and less pathogenic than HIV-1 and may have a protective role against superinfection with HIV-1.

Within HIV-1 and HIV-2, biological and serological heterogeneity exist but the HIV-1 subtypes or clades are better studied. HIV-1 has been classified into two major groups: group M which is more common and contains at least eight genetic subtypes (clades) (Table 6.1.2), and group O which contains several heterogeneous viruses. Recent genetic analyses of HIV-1 subtypes have indicated that some HIV-1 strains of a particular subtype may in fact be mosaic or recombinant forms of two or more different subtypes as a result of genetic recombination in individuals coinfected with two or more HIV subtypes.

Intrasubtype variation does occur, termed 'isolates'. The genetic differences within subtypes will usually not exceed 15% whereas inter-subtype variation will lie beyond the 25% range. A variant of the B subtype has been identified from Thai IVDUs, initially termed Thai genotype B (B_B). The tetrapeptide motif at the tip of the V3 loop on gp120 from most B_B isolates is GPGQ whereas that of the classical B subtype from the western hemisphere is GPGR.

The peptide sequence which initially was used to serotype the B subtype in Thai IVDUs (B_B) could not identify most of the HIV in Thai homo/bisexual men who theoretically should also be infected with the B subtype. However, when the peptide sequence of the classical B subtype (B_{MN}) was used, 52% of homo/bisexual men could be identified as having B_{MN} infection. This suggested that there were at least two B subtypes in Thai patients, B_B in IVDUs and B (or B_{MN}) in homo/bisexuals. In Thailand, the E subtype is predominant among heterosexuals.

The reasons for HIV-1 subtype segregation in certain risk groups are not clearly understood. It may just be a chronological event, namely, successive

Table 6.1.2. Geographic distribution of HIV-1 subtypes.

Subtype (Clade)	Predominant geographic distribution
A	Central and West Africa
B	North America, South America, Europe, Australasia
C	South and Central Africa, India
D	Central and West Africa
E	Thailand, Central Africa
F	South America, Central Africa, Europe
G	Central Africa, Taiwan, Russia
H	Central Africa
O	West Africa, France

infection with subtype B_{MN} at the beginning of the epidemic in Thailand, followed by B_B and then lastly E. This is supported by the findings that more Thai IVDUs currently are being infected with the E subtype than 4–5 years ago. The other reason may be the relative ease of infection with different subtypes at a particular route of entry. For example, it was noted that subtype E was much more efficient than subtype B_{MN} in infecting Langerhans cells of the vaginal mucosa and of the foreskin of the penis. This was supported by the finding that sexual partners of subtype E-infected individuals were more likely to be infected concordantly than partners of B-infected subjects. However, this unique subtype-specific infectivity still remains controversial.

The clinical significance of heterogeneity of HIV-1 subtypes also remains speculative. Patients infected with different HIV-1 subtypes may have different clinical courses. This could be due either to differences in lifestyles or to biological difference in the viruses. Evidence is forthcoming from ongoing large cohort studies in Africa and Asia where more than one HIV-1 subtype is spreading. In addition, genetic diversity of HIV within the population makes the design of an effective, broad-coverage HIV vaccine more difficult.

Host factors (the immune response to HIV infection)

Humoral immune response

Like any antigen, HIV induces a spectrum of antibodies following infection. The antibodies are directed against the various components of the virion as evident in Western blot assay. These antibodies form the basis for serodiagnosis. IgG antibodies are the main class present in the patients, but IgM, IgA and IgE antibodies have also been described.

What functional role these antibodies play is incompletely understood. They may be neutralizing, cytotoxic (ADCC = antibody-dependent cell-mediated cytotoxicity) or enhancing antibodies. Although enhancing antibody can be demonstrated *in vitro*, its *in vivo* role is unclear. Some of the antibody responses to HIV may contribute to the allergic or autoimmune processes found in some patients.

Cell-mediated immune response

Like B cells, T cells also respond to HIV infection. Both $CD4^+$ and $CD8^+$ T cells are involved. $CD4^+$ T cells can either be T_H1 cells or T_H2 cells. T_H1 cells produce interleukin 2 (IL-2) and γ-interferon (γ-IFN), which results in cellular immunity against the virus, partly through the activation of the $CD8^+$ cytotoxic T lymphocytes (CTL) and partly through the $CD4^+$ CTL. T_H2 cells produce IL-4, IL-6 and IL-10 which enhance antibody production, which may be responsible for the hypergammaglobulinaemia found in HIV infection. Although there are usually brisk and strong $CD4^+$ T-cell responses during early HIV infection, $CD4^+$ cell depletion is a common event in the late stage of HIV infection.

$CD4^+$ cell depletion may be a result of direct cell killing by cytopathic virus through altered cell membrane integrity during virus budding, through the intracellular accumulation of toxic unintegrated proviral DNA or as a result of syncytium formation between infected and uninfected cells. $CD4^+$ cell depletion may also be caused by antibody and CTL directed against virus envelope protein (gp120) expressed on the infected cells or on the uninfected cells via the binding of soluble gp120 on to the surface CD4. In addition, $CD4^+$ T cells may be depleted or rendered anergic by the exhaustive stimulation of a restricted set of V_β families of T-cell receptors by the HIV superantigen or by persistent stimulation of CD4 by the gp120–antibody complexes. Finally, apoptosis or programmed cell death of HIV-infected $CD4^+$ T cells may also contribute to the overall $CD4^+$ cell depletion in HIV infection. The clinical outcome of $CD4^+$ cell depletion is the onset of various opportunistic infections and neoplasms characteristic of HIV disease.

$CD8^+$ T cells are also activated initially by HIV. The numbers of $CD8^+$ cells are greatly increased during early HIV infection and then decreased at later stages, probably through mechanisms similar to $CD4^+$ cell depletion such as apoptosis and superantigen stimulation. Functionally, $CD8^+$ T cells are the main and the most effective CTL against HIV. Constantly exposed but uninfected individuals or patients who are long-term survivors are found to have strong CTL responses. In addition, $CD8^+$ T cells can secrete an antiviral factor which can suppress viral replication non-specifically.

The final outcome of viral and immune pathogenesis

The clinical outcome of the HIV infection depends upon the viral properties and protective immune responses. The virulence and the infecting dose play a vital role. Virulence is related to subtypes and biological characteristics of HIV, such as cell tropism, rate of replication, cytopathicity or syncytium-inducing properties, and the patterns of antiviral resistance. In addition, viral expression also depends upon expression of various cytokines which is in turn affected by various cofactors such as coinfections or the use of illicit drugs. It has been demonstrated that even in clinical 'latency', the virus multiplies rapidly in the lymph nodes. During this early phase of HIV infection, very few virions are found in the peripheral blood. This discrepancy in the viral load between peripheral blood and lymphoid tissues is a result of an intact immune system early in the infection. Many of the virions are trapped by the follicular dendritic cells which present the virus to T and B cells within the lymph nodes. The humoral and cell-mediated immune responses thus stimulated, such as neutralizing antibodies and CTL, will keep the virus load in check. Subsequently, as a result of dysfunction of the dendritic cells, including decreased ability to present the antigens to the immune system and of HIV-related depletion of $CD4^+$ and $CD8^+$ cells, virus will pass into the blood, signalling the onset of HIV disease.

Clinical manifestations (see also Appendix 6.B and Chapter 10.4)

Acute HIV seroconversion syndrome

This mononucleosis-like syndrome occurs in 60% of individuals with a documented time of HIV infection. It develops within 3–6 weeks after infection and lasts 1–2 weeks before resolving spontaneously. The symptoms and signs include fever, headache, sore throat, oral ulcers, diarrhoea, generalized maculopapular erythematous skin rash, lymphadenopathy, myalgia and meningoencephalitis. The clinical illness is usually accompanied by a transient but marked decline in $CD4^+$ cell count. Resolution of the acute illness will be followed by positive anti-HIV serology. Such acute HIV seroconversion syndrome is rarely detected in Thai patients. The reasons are unclear and could include the lack of awareness by the patient and the physicians.

Asymptomatic infection

More asymptomatic HIV infections are diagnosed in Thailand than symptomatic infections. This is probably true in many other countries where HIV infection is relatively recent and surveillance is the main activity. In Thailand, most of the asymptomatic HIV cases are detected through pre-employment screening, pre-operative screening, screening at drug addiction treatment centres, at antenatal care clinics, during blood donation and during mass screening in various risk groups. Most of such screenings are performed without proper counselling and without the patient's consent. The procedures also lead to lack of confidentiality and discrimination against seropositive individuals. This has prompted the establishment of the anonymous voluntary counselling and testing centres throughout Thailand as an alternative to mandatory testing.

Although asymptomatic, many HIV-infected Thai subjects were found to have $CD4^+$ cell count of less than 200 μl^{-1}. These are the more advanced asymptomatic patients and they usually will not have generalized lymphadenopathy which is found in the earlier stage of the disease. The fact that some asymptomatic patients may be so immunosuppressed underlines the value of educational campaigns for voluntary counselling and testing, preferably in an anonymous setting, for those with risk behaviours so that HIV infection can be detected early. In addition, efforts should be made to persuade the asymptomatic HIV-infected individuals to come for regular clinical and immunological (i.e. $CD4^+$ cell count) follow-up, so that earlier prophylactic and therapeutic interventions can be instituted.

Early symptomatic HIV infection

In Thailand, many symptoms and signs can be regarded as reliable clues to HIV infection. These include herpes zoster, oral candidiasis, oral hairy leukoplakia, prolonged fever, chronic diarrhoea, progressive weight loss and pruritic papular eruptions (PPEs). PPE is the descriptive term for a form of generalized pruritic eruption commonly found in patients with HIV infection in tropical countries. In addition to the above well-defined pre-AIDS clinical manifestations, some clinical manifestations are also recognized to be more frequent or more severe in HIV-infected individuals. These include psoriasis, psoriatic arthritis, seborrhoeic dermatitis, muscle wasting in the absence of significant weight loss, HSV-I and -2 infections, chickenpox, warts, mucocutaneous fungal and bacterial infections, skin hyperpigmentation and premature grey hair. (See Chapter 11.5 for details of mucocutaneous manifestations.)

AIDS

Box 6.1.1 lists the revised CDC 1993 AIDS-defining illnesses which are intended for surveillance. Of the list, *Mycobacterium tuberculosis* is the most common AIDS-definining opportunistic infection in Thailand, followed by *Pneumocystis carinii* pneumonia (PCP) and cryptococcal meningitis. There are geographic differences in the prevalence of various opportunistic infections, even within Thailand. PCP is consistently infrequent, while disseminated penicilliosis is consistently more prevalent in northern Thailand.

Box 6.1.1. CDC 1993 revised AIDS-defining illnesses.

Infections
Candidiasis of bronchi, trachea, lungs or oesophagus
Coccidioidomycosis, disseminated or extrapulmonary
Cryptococcosis, extrapulmonary
Cryptosporidiosis, chronic intestinal (>1 month duration)
Cytomegalovirus infection including retinitis (excluding liver, spleen or nodes)
Herpes simplex bronchitis, pneumonitis, oesophagitis or chronic ulcers (>1 month)
Histoplasmosis, disseminated or extrapulmonary
Isosporiasis, chronic intestinal (> 1 month)
Mycobacterium avium complex or other mycobacterium, disseminated or extrapulmonary
Mycobacterium tuberculosis, any site
Pneumocystis carinii pneumonia
Pneumonia, recurrent
Salmonella septicaemia, recurrent
Toxoplasmosis of brain

Malignancies
Cervical cancer, invasive
Kaposi's sarcoma
Lymphoma (Burkitt's, immunoblastic or primary brain)

Others
Encephalopathy, HIV-related
Progressive multifocal leukoencephalopathy
Wasting syndrome due to HIV
<200 $CD4^+$ T cells μl^{-1}

Compared with the Western world, some AIDS-defining illnesses are found more frequently in Thai patients, such as tuberculosis, cryptococcal meningitis, disseminated penicilliosis and recurrent *Salmonella* septicaemia, as shown in Table 6.1.3. Conversely, Kaposi's sarcoma, *Mycobacterium avium* complex infection and coccidioidomycosis are found significantly less frequently in Thai patients. Some other conditions, such as recurrent pneumonia, cervical cancer, lymphoma and progressive multifocal leuko-encephalopathy are either uncommon or not recorded accurately. The basis for such cross-cultural and cross-geographical differences in the incidence of AIDS-defining illnesses is multifactorial. This may be due to differences in endemicity of the pathogens in the environment. Secondly, they may be due to differences in the proportion of the various risk behaviours among AIDS patients, for example Kaposi's sarcoma is common in homosexuals and recurrent pneumonia is common in IVDUs. However, even among HIV-infected Thai homo/bisexuals, Kaposi's sarcoma is quite rare. This may be due to differences in exposure to the cofactors among the two culturally different groups of homo/bisexuals. Thirdly, the differences may be explained by the accessibility to the various diagnostic procedures such as endoscopy, magnetic resonance imaging and electron microscopy.

Three conditions which frequently are encountered in Thai patients are described briefly. For the other conditions see Appendix 6.B.

Tuberculosis

Mycobacterium tuberculosis is the most common mycobacterial infection encountered in HIV-infected patients in developing countries. However, the prevalence of other mycobacterial infections in many developing countries has not yet been investigated systematically. Of the 101 cases of tuberculosis collected from 200 AIDS patients at Chulalongkorn Hospital, 53 (50.5%)

Table 6.1.3. Comparison of AIDS-defining illnesses in developing countries such as Thailand in relation to the Western world.

Higher incidence in Thailand	Equal incidence in Thailand	Lower incidence in Thailand
Tuberculosis	PCP	Kaposi's sarcoma
Cryptococcal meningitis	*Candida* oesophagitis	*Mycobacterium avium*
Penicilliosis	Toxoplasmosis	Coccidioidomycosis
Salmonella septicaemia	HIV encephalopathy	Progressive multifocal leukoencephalopathy(?)
	CMV	
	Cryptosporidiosis	
	HIV wasting syndrome	
	Histoplasmosis	
	Disseminated herpes simplex	
	Isosporiasis	
	Recurrent pneumonia (?)	
	Cervical cancer (?)	
	Lymphoma (?)	

cases had pulmonary tuberculosis, 15 had tuberculosis of lymph nodes and 12 had disseminated tuberculosis. The remainder had tuberculosis of various other organs (percardium, six; pleura, five; meninges and peritoneum, two each; oesophagus, ileum and joints, one each; undetermined, three).

Cervical lymph nodes are the most common site of tuberculous lymphadenitis. It is characteristically unilateral, and one to three glands may be involved which may coalesce. Compared with the reactive lymphoid hyperplasia as seen in early HIV infection, tuberculous lymph glands are several times larger and show signs of inflammation. At a later stage, fluctuation develops when numerous acid-fast bacilli can be demonstrated on needle aspiration. Patients may have constitutional symptoms such as afternoon fever, night sweats and weight loss. Compared with other AIDS-defining opportunistic infections, patients with pulmonary tuberculosis as their first AIDS-defining illness will generally have a higher $CD4^+$ cell count, i.e. over 200 cells μl^{-1}. In addition, in spite of relative T-cell deficiency, the tuberculin test frequently will be strongly positive which aids the diagnosis of active tuberculosis.

The diagnosis of disseminated tuberculosis can be difficult. Patients are generally severely immunosuppressed and cachectic with protracted high fevers. Hepatomegaly is one of the most frequent findings with or without splenomegaly. The liver is firm and non-tender. Mild to moderate elevation of serum transaminases may be seen, but marked elevation of alkaline phosphatase frequently is found. Liver ultrasound is generally unrevealing and diagnosis is usually made by liver biopsy. Blood culture for *M. tuberculosis* is usually positive. In addition, tuberculosis of the skin, gastrointestinal tract and central nervous system may be part of the overall picture of disseminated tuberculosis.

The treatment and prophylaxis of tuberculosis are detailed below (see also Appendix 6.B).

NOSOCOMIAL SPREAD. There is a great concern in developing countries over nosocomial spread of *M. tuberculosis*, especially the multidrug-resistant bacteria. In Thailand, many cases of pulmonary and extrapulmonary tuberculosis (such as tuberculous lymphadenitis or tuberculous pharyngitis) have been documented among doctors, nurses and others directly involved with AIDS patient care. The most efficient and cost-effective methods for prevention of such nosocomial transmission in hospitals and households have yet to be determined.

Cryptococcal meningitis

The most common cause of meningitis in AIDS patients is *Cryptococcus neoformans*. It occurs in 20% of AIDS patients across Thailand. The incidence increases progressively with decreasing $CD4^+$ cell counts. Patients usually present with headache, nausea, vomiting, fever, blurred vision, mental changes and radicular pain referred to the legs and buttocks. Diagnosis is usually made by the examination of cerebrospinal fluid (CSF) with positive India ink stain and positive culture for *C. neoformans*. The CSF usually shows very little inflammation as reflected by little change in CSF protein, sugar and cells. CSF and serum cryptococcal antigen levels are seldom used to confirm the diagnosis. However, a negative cryptococcal antigenaemia in an individual with fever and headache will save the patient from lumbar puncture.

The treatment of cryptococcal meningitis is detailed below (see also Appendix 6.B).

Penicilliosis

Systemic infection with *P. marneffei* is considered as an AIDS-defining illness in Thailand. The organism is endemic in northern Thailand, southern China, Vietnam and Hong Kong. Bamboo rats are one of the natural reservoirs but its route of transmission to man is as yet uncertain. In Thailand, penicilliosis is found mainly in AIDS patients from the north. The infection is characterized by fever (92%), anaemia (77%), weight loss (76%) and skin lesions (71%). The skin lesions are usually papules with central umbilication or molluscum contagiosum-like lesions (Fig. 6.1.3). Presumptive diagnosis is made by microscopic examination of Wright-stained samples of bone marrow aspirate or touch smears of skin or lymph node biopsies showing intracellular and extracellular basophilic spherical, oval and elliptical yeast cells with clear central septation (Plate 2). The treatment of penicilliosis is described below.

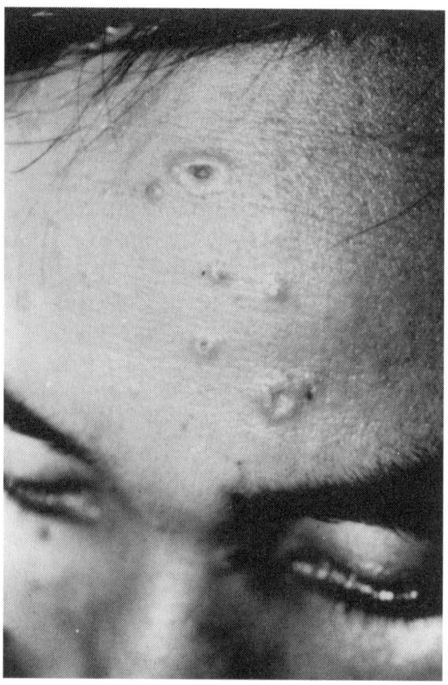

Fig. 6.1.3. Penicilliosis: molluscum contagiosum-like skin lesions of *P. marneffei* infection.

Natural course of HIV infection

In spite of differences in socioeconomic status, nutritional status and the endemic pathogens, HIV patients in Thailand do not seem to progress faster than patients in the Western world. The annual progression rate from asymptomatic to symptomatic HIV infection or AIDS in a small cohort in Bangkok was found to be 6.8% . In addition, $CD4^+$ cell counts declined at a rate of 20% per year. There is still controversy as to whether heterosexually acquired infections will progress faster than those acquired homosexually or via intravenous drug use.

Management of HIV/AIDS patients

(see Chapter 10.4 for management at PHC level)

The management includes diagnosis, treatment, prevention and community care aspects. Clearly, the best management of AIDS patients requires a multidisciplinary approach including specialists in sexually transmitted and other infectious diseases, chest diseases, dermatology, gastroenterology, ophthalmology, neurology, etc.

Diagnosis of HIV infection

A positive anti-HIV test makes the diagnosis of HIV infection. Enzyme-linked immunosorbent assay (ELISA) is the most frequently used assay for anti-HIV serology in Thailand. Gel particle agglutination (GPA) is used as a supplementary or confirmatory test. Samples with discordant results are re-tested by Western blot, which is much more expensive. Many rapid test kits and saliva test kits are also available in small clinics and in emergency rooms. However, these simple test kits are prohibited for direct sale to the public due to the concern over inadequate pre- and post-test counselling.

Baseline assessment and other considerations

A comprehensive baseline assessment of a patient with HIV infection will include a detailed history, clinical examination, STI screen including syphilis serology, hepatitis B screen, cervical cytology in women (see Chapter 4), full blood count, CD4 cell count, blood chemistry, HIV load, *Toxoplasma* antibody test, tuberculin skin test and chest X-ray. Other considerations include counselling, education, partner notification, nutrition, vaccination against hepatitis B and influenza, anti-HIV therapy and follow-up (all mostly determined by the patient's condition, circumstances and resources available).

Laboratory prognostic markers

The $CD4^+$ cell count is the most frequently used marker for immunological evaluation of HIV patients as well as for prognosis and assessment of therapeutic response. It can be determined using a fluorescent microscope which is available in every provincial hospital in Thailand, although not every provincial hospital provides such a service. Automated flow cytometry is available in all University hospitals and in all of the 16 regional hospitals throughout Thailand. The absolute $CD4^+$ cell counts are used to guide initiation of primary PCP prophylaxis and the initiation, change or addition of antiretrovirals.

Although levels of p24 antigen, β_2-microglobulin and neopterin can be of prognostic value, they are used infrequently in clinical practice. On the other hand, viral load measurements have been started in some research laboratories in Thailand and may prove practical for clinical use if the cost can be decreased.

Diagnosis, treatment and prophylaxis of opportunistic infections (see also Appendix 6.B)

Thailand can be categorized as a developing country with moderate resources. With such a definition, all opportunistic infections in HIV patients will be diagnosed and treated accordingly. Diagnosis may be hampered by the reluctance of some physicians to perform invasive diagnostic procedures such as biopsy. Consequently, the diagnosis is usually, and often correctly, made on a presumptive and therapeutic basis.

Fortunately, medications to treat the more common opportunistic infections are not too expensive. These include cotrimoxazole, ketoconazole, isoniazid, rifampicin, ethambutol, pyrazinamide, amphotericin B and aciclovir. Many drugs are also available as generic drugs. In Thailand, these medications are provided free of charge to all patients if they cannot self-support. However, some patients, even though covered by personal or employer's medical insurance, are afraid to claim reimbursement because of the stigma of HIV infection.

Itraconazole, fluconazole, ganciclovir, foscarnet and liposomal formulations of, for example, amphotericin and daunorubicin, some requiring prolonged administration, are expensive. As a result, even patients with moderate incomes cannot afford these drugs. The Thai government has set aside a central fund to purchase expensive drugs. How long this limited fund will last, when demand is increasing, is unclear. Concern over cost also prompts cost-saving therapeutic trials such as the use of itraconazole instead of fluconazole for the treatment and secondary prophylaxis of systemic fungal infections or the use of intravitreal injections of small amounts of ganciclovir and foscarnet compared with intravenous infusion.

Treatment and prophylaxis of tuberculosis

Fortunately, almost all Thai patients with tuberculosis respond satisfactorily to the standard antituberculous treatment regimen. The regimen used most frequently is a four-drug combination (isoniazid, rifampicin, ethambutol and pyrazinamide) for the first 2 months, followed by 7 months with isonizaid and rifampicin. Life-long isoniazid is usually not given in Thailand as 'secondary prophylaxis'. In spite of clinical response, the *in vitro* susceptibility of the 288 isolates tested at the Central Chest Hospital in Bangkok in 1993 revealed 11.5, 10.8, 1.7 and 8.5% resistance to isoniazid, rifampicin, ethambutol and pyrazinamide, respectively. Combined isoniazid and rifampicin resistance was found in 1.7%, and three-drug resistance was 1%. Isoniazid and rifampicin hepatotoxicity is generally uncommon in Thai patients and rarely requires dose reduction.

In developing countries, it is not known whether primary tuberculosis prophylaxis is effective, which drugs are effective, nor to whom prophylaxis should be given. There are similar uncertainties over secondary prophylaxis.

Treatment and prophylaxis of cryptococcal meningitis

The optimum treatment for cryptococcal meningitis is unclear. Amphotericin B is less expensive and somewhat more effective than fluconazole, especially for very ill patients, but its administration requires prolonged hospitalization. Therefore, in countries where there is a shortage of hospital beds, fluconazole is used as an alternative, either initially or after a short induction course of Amphotericin B. Itraconazole is less expensive than fluconazole and currently is being tested for both primary treatment and secondary prophylaxis of cryptococcal meningitis.

Treatment of penicilliosis

The infection responds well to amphotericin B or itraconazole but relapse is common.

Antiretrovirals (see also Appendix 6.A)

Currently, the nucleoside analogues [zidovudine (ZDV), didanosine (ddI), zalcitabine (ddC), stavudine (d4T) and lamivudine (3TC)] and the protease inhibitors (saquinavir, ritonavir and indinavir) have all been licensed in Thailand. They are expensive and are specifically excluded from almost all medical insurance policies. As a result, the Thai government has allocated a budget to provide antiretrovirals free of charge to 'low income' patients. In fact, almost all patients turn to this source of supply. It is interesting to note that with the availability of generic antiretrovirals, the price of an antiretroviral has decreased by several fold when a large volume government purchase is made by bidding.

Guidelines for the use of government-supplied antiretrovirals in Thailand are changing continually, along with global trends. The 1997 guidelines have shifted towards earlier treatment (i.e. $CD4^+$ cell count 500 cells μl^{-1}) and with double nucleoside therapy. Protease inhibitors are recommended only for those who can self-support. The same is also true for the use of viral load assay in guiding the therapy. When more antiretrovirals are available and when the price is lower, better treatment regimens can be designed for developing countries, at least for those with moderate resources such as

Thailand, Brazil and South Africa. In addition, strengthening of the infrastructure for clinical trials is also needed in order to make more effective drugs accessible to the patients free of charge.

Alternative treatment approaches

Alternate treatment approaches include unconventional treatment methods such as herbal medicine, and home and community care.

Herbal medicine

Because of its unresponsiveness to conventional care, HIV/AIDS has generated many myths in terms of treatment and care in Thailand. Many unconfirmed claims for various traditional, herbal and spiritual treatments are being made. Each claim is magnified by the mass media and attracts thousands of patients to that traditional or spiritual healer. Some patients do get better in terms of appetite, weight gain or diarrhoea. Such success stories draw many patients away from conventional treatments.

Home and community care

Non-institutionalized care has become an increasing need in many countries such as Thailand, India and Africa where AIDS patients outnumber the available hospital beds. More than half of the male medical beds in several hospitals in Thailand are occupied by AIDS patients. This necessitates rapid turnover of hospital bed occupancy. Many patients are discharged sooner and transferred to day-care centres for continued, but less intensive care. Patients' relatives and community volunteers have to be trained in basic HIV medicine in order to provide care to patients at home. The western style of organized home care is not possible in developing countries because of the shortage of professional home care providers. For those who cannot be cared for at home, community-organized care facilities are an alternative. Such a community care service requires much support and understanding from the community; otherwise rejection can occur (see also Appendix 6.D).

HIV prevention

Education (see also Chapter 12.1)

AIDS education is considered the most cost-effective means of HIV prevention. Education should be targeted to both the risk groups and the general public. The latter is a much larger group but the approach is somewhat easier. Special efforts should be given to ethnic minorities who may have language or cultural barriers. An example in Thailand are the hill tribe people. Similarly, attention should also be given to socially disadvantaged groups such as street children, homeless people, slum dwellers and factory workers.

However, knowledge does not always produce changes in risk behaviour.

Most Thais know about AIDS and its prevention but many still practise risk behaviour. Therefore, the modern effective approach to AIDS education is the type of knowledge and information dissemination that will attract an individual's concern for and commitment to behavioural change. Methods to develop rational thinking and judgement should be taught, as well as the techniques of self-empowerment in order to stand against risk behaviours. Less risky or safer alternatives should also be provided. Thailand does not implement needle and syringe exchange programmes but it provides instructions and cleansing solutions to IVDUs. The 100% condom use programme is another success story in Thailand where condoms are used in almost every commercial sex act in many provinces. This was made possible through the collaboration of all parties involved, such as public health officers, law enforcement officers, owners of the sex establishments, commercial sex workers and their clients. This has resulted in a dramatic decline in the incidence of sexually transmitted diseases and may also explain the slowing down of the HIV epidemic in some risk groups in Thailand from 1994.

Vaccination (see also Chapter 12.2)

Vaccination represents another facet of HIV prevention. Certainly, it cannot, ethically, be used alone without the intended change in risk behaviour. Enthusiasm for the HIV vaccine was very high initially. It generated such high expectation that the WHO Global Programme on AIDS in 1992 selected Thailand, Uganda, Brazil and Rwanda as sites for international HIV vaccine efficacy trials. This not well-planned announcement attracted considerable criticism of using volunteers from developing countries as human guinea pigs for vaccines made in the developed world. Enthusiasm for the prophylactic HIV vaccine has declined since 1994 when a small number of US vaccinees were found to be unprotected and when the proposal for the efficacy trials in US volunteers was turned down.

Nevertheless, phase I and II HIV vaccine trials in developing countries are essential. They help to establish the infrastructure of the host institutes, feasibility and public acceptance. Evaluation can also be made on the safety and immunogenicity of the vaccine in ethnically different populations, especially when the local HIV subtypes are incorporated into the vaccine. In fact, the first HIV vaccine trial in Thailand was started in June 1994 with very good acceptance from the public. It confirmed that an HIV vaccine trial could be carried out successfully in Thailand. When efficacy trials are ready, the ethical issue will be even more important, especially for developing countries. Volunteers have to be well informed about the risk, and major efforts in behaviour modification have to be implemented even though larger sample size or longer duration of study is necesssary. One cannot risk the life of the volunteers, even if they are from developing countries, for the sake of scientific merit. Of equal importance is the fair share of the benefits resulting from the study between investigators from the north and the south.

The use of vaccines in patients with HIV infection is described in Appendix 6.C.

African Perspective

Epidemiology (see also Chapter 1)

AIDS was first reported in Africa in 1985, but it is possible that patients with AIDS were seen as early as 1982. Since then, the syndrome has been reported from every African country. Africa is experiencing a serious HIV epidemic. According to the WHO estimates (at the end of 1997), of the 30.6 million HIV-positive individuals in the world, about 20 million (66%) belonged to sub-Saharan Africa.

At the time of writing, Africa could be divided into countries with HIV seroprevalences of <5%, 5–10% and >10% (Table 6.1.4). It is clear that Central and East Africa have some of the highest HIV seroprevalence rates in Africa and contribute to over 60% of AIDS patients reported to WHO. However, HIV seroprevalence rates change over time in any given locality. This may be due to the rapid spread of the epidemic and/or effective control measures. HIV seroprevalence is gradually rising in southern Africa.

Recently there have been reports that HIV seroprevalence is decreasing in some parts of Africa, notably Uganda where sentinel surveillance among pregnant women and three longitudinal studies in various parts of the country show a decrease in HIV prevalence. The reasons for the HIV decline are, however, not very clear. One reason might be the high mortality among HIV-positive individuals in their cohorts. In addition, there are numerous reports indicating a significant change in sexual behaviour following extensive health education messages over the last 10 years. It is possible, therefore, that the decline in HIV seroprevalence is multifactorial. However, any conclusive statement on the trends of HIV prevalence and incidence in Africa requires more time for further evaluation.

Table 6.1.4. HIV prevalence in Africa.

Low prevalence (< 5%)	Medium prevalence (5–10%)	High prevalence (>10%)
Algeria	Botswana	Burundi
Benin	Cameroon	Cape Verde
Burkina Faso	Côte d'Ivoire	Central African Republic
Chad	Gabon	Congo
Egypt	Ghana	Gambia
Ethiopia	Niger	Guinea Bissau
Guinea	Senegal	Kenya
Liberia	South Africa	Malawi
Mali	Swaziland	Rwanda
Morocco	Zaire	Tanzania
Mozambique	Zimbabwe	Uganda
Nigeria		Zambia
Sudan		
Tunisia		

HIV infection in Africa is caused by HIV-1 and HIV-2. However, HIV-1 is a significantly more predominant cause of HIV infection throughout Africa. Heterogeneity of HIV-1 subtypes has been reported throughout Africa. HIV-1 sequence analysis studies have revealed the presence of HIV-1 subtypes A, B and D throughout Africa and subtype O in West Africa. HIV-2 is mainly found in West Africa, and has been reported in some areas of Angola and Mozambique. Recently, there have been reports that even in countries in West Africa, e.g. Senegal, where HIV-2 was the predominant strain, HIV-1 is spreading very rapidly and may soon become the dominant strain. Thus, in these areas, dual infection with HIV-1 and HIV-2 is not uncommon.

Transmission

The three major modes of transmission are: heterosexual, accounting for 85–90%; mother to child, 10–15%; and blood transfusion 0–5%. Homosexual contact and intravenous drug abuse are uncommon in Africa. There is no evidence to incriminate social contact or insects in the transmission of the virus. There has been great interest in the factors that might increase susceptibility (or infectivity) of an individual to (or with) HIV infection during sexual intercourse. Potential factors include: STI, particularly those resulting in genital ulcers; traumatic ulceration of the genitalia during sex; sexual practices; stage of infection; oral contraceptives; circumcision; and non-sexually transmitted or systemic infectious diseases. Genital ulceration has proved to be the strongest possible cofactor.

Currently, a number of longitudinal studies are investigating the temporal relationship between STI and HIV infection. Recently, Grosskurth and colleagues (1995) working in the Mwanza region of Tanzania have shown in a longitudinal study a 40% reduction in HIV infection as a result of improved treatment of sexually transmitted diseases. In Uganda, the Rakai Project is undertaking a study to assess the effect of mass treatment of STI on the prevalence of STI and incidence of HIV in the rural villages of the Rakai district. This study will be useful to validate the Mwanza study and hopefully give us a more detailed understanding of the interaction between STI and HIV.

Women and HIV infection

The male to female sex ratio of AIDS in Africa is 1:1. The mean age of male AIDS cases is 32 years, while for females it is 27 years. In a number of HIV seroprevalence studies in Africa, females show a much higher seroprevalence at a younger age compared with males. In the Rakai district in Uganda, females aged 15–20 years had seroprevalence rates six times higher than males in the same age group.

The reasons for such high prevalence rates among young females are not clear. Several explanations have been put forward. These can be divided into socioeconomic and biological factors. Socioeconomic factors include: (i) women in Africa have significantly less financial resources and as a result they engage in risky sexual relationships for financial reasons, i.e. prostitution; (ii) women tend to have less formal education and thus are usually less well informed about ways to prevent HIV infection; (iii) African culture allows polygamy and inheritance of widows; in this situation all the women involved in this marriage are at particular risk of HIV infection; and (iv) many studies in Africa have shown that migrant workers, i.e. long-distance truck drivers or miners, usually men, bring back HIV infection to their partners.

Possible biological factors include: (i) females tend to have a higher proportion of asymptomatic STI that may render them more susceptible to HIV infection; and (ii) females in Africa tend to engage in sex at a relatively young age compared with males; it is, therefore, possible that the immature female genital tract is easily traumatized during sex and this can lead to increased risk of HIV transmission.

It is also important to note that unlike males who can use a condom, females in Africa have no effective, acceptable and self-controlled protection from HIV infection. Since males play a dominant role in sex, females are at a disadvantage in negotiating for safer sex.

Clinical presentation in adults

The clinical spectrum of HIV infection in Africa is wide. It is determined by the opportunistic organisms prevalent in that environment. In addition, the timing of the clinical manifestations of these opportunistic infections is a function of the immune system. There are, however, interesting differences in the major opportunistic infections seen in different parts of Africa. It is also important to observe that the predominant clinical presentation of HIV infection or AIDS in any locality or country can change as HIV prevalence changes over time. For example, in Uganda, in the early course of the HIV epidemic, the skin, the oropharynx and the gastrointestinal tract were the sites predominantly affected at presentation. More recently, however, increasing numbers of patients have presented with respiratory or neurological disease. This may be due either to an increase in clinical awareness over time or to an increase in prevalence of a particular clinical presentation as more individuals get infected and live longer.

A high morbidity and mortality has been observed among HIV-positive individuals who do not fulfil the clinical WHO case definition of AIDS. A large number of HIV-positive individuals in Africa present and die of common bacterial infections well before they are identified clinically as AIDS patients. AIDS patients in Africa often present with multiple organ involvement, the gastrointestinal tract and the respiratory tract being the commonest combination.

Mucocutaneous manifestations

Mucocutaneous lesions are usually an early indicator of HIV infection (in up to 60% of those infected) and AIDS in Africa. They can be divided into lesions associated with HIV infection and lesions indicative of AIDS. The common lesions associated with HIV infection include a pruritic maculopapular rash with or without hyperpigmentation found especially in exposed parts, superficial mycoses, bacterial infections (pyoderma), folliculitis, parasitic and arthropod infestations (e.g. scabies), seborrhoeic dermatitis, molluscum contagiosum and HSV-2, and drug reactions especially to antituberculous drugs and sulphonamides. Lesions associated with AIDS include Kaposi's sarcoma, oral candidiasis, hairy leukoplakia, and herpes zoster.

Gastrointestinal manifestations

Gastrointestinal tract manifestations are a significant feature of HIV infection in Africa. The gastrointestinal tract is involved in up to 60% of AIDS patients at presentation. In Uganda, as elsewhere in Africa, gastrointestinal tract involvement-presenting symptoms include severe weight loss, chronic persistent liquid diarrhoea, anorexia, nausea and vomiting. The epidemic of people dying with severe weight loss in the early 1980s led the people of Uganda to refer to such a clinical presentation as 'slim disease'.

The aetiology of diarrhoea has been found to be a variety of intestinal pathogens. These include *Isospora belli*, *Cryptosporidium parvum*, microsporidia, CMV and *Strongyloides stercoralis*, identified in the stool and/or endoscopic biopsy. HIV infection of the gastrointestinal tract (HIV enteropathy) may be the cause in cases of diarrhoea where no pathogen can be isolated. *Shigella* and *Salmonella* species are also associated with HIV infection. Conspicuously absent infections in the gastrointestinal tract of AIDS patients include amoebiasis and schistosomiasis. Likewise, infection with *Mycobacterium avium* complex, unlike in Europe or North America, is extremely rare.

Autopsy studies have shown extensive *M. tuberculosis* in patients with clinical features of 'slim disease'. The commonest intestinal malignancy seen in AIDS patients in Africa is Kaposi's sarcoma. The gastrointestinal tract is the most commonly affected organ, often without any visible skin lesions. Gastrointestinal tract lymphomas and colon cancer are rarely seen in African AIDS patients.

Respiratory manifestations

The most significant respiratory infection in Africa is tuberculosis, seen in up to 60% of patients with HIV infection. Africa currently is experiencing an epidemic of tuberculosis as a result of the HIV epidemic. This relationship has significantly influenced the clinical presentation of HIV infection and AIDS in Africa. Often pulmonary disease is associated with disseminated tuberculosis.

Pneumococcal pneumonia appears to be more prevalent in HIV-infected individuals without any AIDS-defining illness. Sometimes it can be severe enough to cause death. Other infections that have been described include nocardiosis, cryptococcosis, candidiasis and PCP. PCP shows an interesting distribution in Africa. It is very rare in many parts of East and Central Africa. However, it appears to account for up to 10% of respiratory infections in parts of Zimbabwe and South Africa. In West Africa, PCP does occur, but it is rare except in Abidjan where it is seen in up to 10% of AIDS patients.

Nocardiosis is seen in up to 15% of patients with respiratory disease, and can be confused with tuberculosis. Multiple infection with two or even three organisms does occur and this makes management, especially in the African setting, rather difficult.

Kaposi's sarcoma is the commonest malignancy seen in the respiratory system. Lymphomas and bronchial carcinomas have not been reported to any significant extent.

Neurological manifestations

Involvement of the nervous system in HIV-infected individuals is being increasingly recognized in Africa. Clinical manifestations may result from HIV infection of the brain, spinal cord or peripheral nerves. The patient may present with dementia, or involvement of one or more intracranial nerves, especially the 3rd, 6th, 7th and 9th. Myelopathy presenting as paraplegia is commonly seen, and the clinical picture of Guillain–Barré syndrome has been reported.

Opportunistic infection of the CNS is usually serious and often fatal. Commonly encountered infections include cryptococcal meningitis and bacterial meningitis. Cryptococcal meningitis is seen more commonly in East and Central Africa compared with West Africa. Toxoplasmosis is seen on autopsy. Antemortem diagnosis of this infection is difficult in most parts of Africa due to lack of diagnostic facilities. A few serological studies in East and West Africa do indicate toxoplasmosis prevalence rates of 40–80% in the general population. West Africa has a higher prevalence.

Other reported infections include progressive multifocal leuko-encephalopathy (PML), CMV, herpes simplex and syphilis. Tuberculous meningitis does occur in AIDS patients but not as frequently as would be expected. In one large postmortem series in Abidjan, tuberculous meningitis accounted for only 10% of all CNS infections.

Kaposi's sarcoma has very rarely been found to involve the CNS in Africa. CNS lymphomas have been reported in West Africa. Postmortem reports from East Africa indicate that they are very rarely encountered.

Lymphorecticular system

Lymphadenopathy is one of the early sign of HIV infection in Africa. Usually cervical lymphadenopathy is noted first. Common biopsy findings include tuberculosis, Kaposi's sarcoma, cryptococcosis and toxoplasmosis. Up to 30% of the lymph nodes show non-specific inflammation. There is evidence now to suggest active immunological activity in lymph nodes against HIV infection.

Lymphomas are not common in HIV infection in Africa compared with homosexuals in North America. It is not clear why this is the case. One reason may be that Africans do not live long enough in an immunosuppressed state to develop lymphomas.

Cardiovascular manifestations

Pericardial effusion is a common clinical finding in AIDS patients. This is often due to tuberculosis. Kaposi's sarcoma has also been found on postmortem to be a cause of pericardial effusion. Echocardiographic features of myocardial dysfunction are often seen. Myocarditis probably due to HIV and opportunistic viral infections, such as herpes, has been reported. Endocarditis is not commonly seen in HIV-infected individuals, even with pre-existing valvular damage from rheumatic fever.

Many HIV-infected patients in Africa present with anaemia and fever. This often results in palpitations and tachycardia.

Management

Over the last 10 years there has been a significant increase in the understanding of clinical presentation, laboratory diagnosis and care of HIV infection. This has led to improved clinical management of HIV infection. In Africa, treatment is entirely targeted at opportunistic infections. There is no significant use of antiretroviral agents because they are not affordable. Two major aspects of clinical care have been introduced to manage HIV-infected patients in the African environment, namely: (i) HIV counselling and (ii) home-based care. (See also Chapter 10.4 for management at the primary health care level.)

Counselling

Counselling as a component of clinical management of any disease was not widely practised in Africa before the HIV epidemic. However, following the HIV epidemic, counselling has become a very significant component of management. HIV counselling/information/discussion services are now used extensively in many parts of Africa. Countries such as Uganda have been able to establish organizations like The AIDS Support Organization (TASO) and AIDS Information Centre (AIC) covering a large part of the country. In these centres individuals are able to obtain HIV testing and counselling. In addition, care and follow-up of AIDS cases is possible.

Home-based care

Home-based care, whereby the HIV-infected patients are managed at home through mobile clinics, increasingly is becoming a significant mode of provision of health services to AIDS patients in Africa. Organizations like TASO have demonstrated effectively that this approach benefits the patient and the relatives who help in the management. The need for this approach arises from the following facts: (i) the hospitals or health centres are few and thus are always overcrowded; (ii) as HIV infection is a chronic disease with frequent recurrences of febrile illness, many patients cannot afford the frequent visits to the health centre; and (iii) the involvement of the relatives in management at home is thought to be more cost effective since much less time is spent in hospitals. This approach, however, is not cheap for the health providers, and the sustainability of such a programme is not clear.

Role of traditional healers

The traditional healers have played a particularly strong role in the management of AIDS patients in Africa. They are widely available to patients, particularly in rural areas. The traditional healers throughout various parts of Africa have made claims that they can cure AIDS. Since modern Western medicine has not yet produced a cure, many AIDS patients flock to these traditional healers for help. The healers appear to listen, and give their patient more time than the hospital doctors to discuss their problems. In Uganda, a study to evaluate the treatment-seeking behaviour of individuals with STI showed that the majority of patients first visit a traditional healer; it is only when symptoms do not subside that they visit a health centre. This was true even for individuals who had easy access to modern health care.

Traditional healers usually provide patients with a cocktail of herbs, some of which the patients, apparently, find helpful. A systematic evaluation of the benefits of these herbs is urgently needed in Africa. It is important to note that traditional healers are not necessarily cheap to consult and may charge relatively high fees for their services.

Further reading

Clezy, K., Sirisanthana, T., Sirisanthana, V., Brew, B. and Cooper, D.A. (1994) Late manifestations of HIV in Asia and the Pacific. *AIDS* 8 (Suppl. 2), S35–S43.

Dore, G.J., Kaldor, J.M., Ungchusak, K. and Mertens, T.E. (1996) Epidemiology of HIV and AIDS in the Asia–Pacific region. *Medical Journal of Australia* 165, 494–498.

Essex, M., M'Boup, S., Kanki, P.J. and Kalengayi, M.R. (eds) (1994) *AIDS in Africa.* Raven Press, New York.

Folks, T.M. and Hart, C.E. (1997) The life cycle of human immunodeficiency virus type 1. In: De Vitta, V.T., Jr, Hellman, S. and Rosenberg, S.A. (eds), *AIDS: Etiology, Diagnosis, Treatment and Prevention,* 4th edn. Lippincott-Raven, Philadelphia, pp. 29–43.

Grosskurth, H., Mosha, F., Todd, H., Mwijarubi, E., Klokke, A., Kenkoro, K., Mayaud, P., Changalucha, J., Nicoll, A., Kagina, G., Newell, J., Mugeye, K., Mabey, D. and Hayes, R. (1995) Impact of improved treatment of sexually transmitted diseases on HIV in rural Tanzania: randomized controlled trial. *Lancet* 346, 530–536.

Hirsch, M.S., D'Aquila, R.T. and Kaplan, J.C. (1997) Antiretroviral therapy. In: De Vitta, V.T., Jr, Hellman, S. and Rosenberg, S.A. (eds), *AIDS: Etiology, Diagnosis, Treatment and Prevention,* 4th edn. Lippincott-Raven, Philadelphia, pp. 495–508.

Ho, D.D., Neumann, A.U., Perelson, A.S., Chen, W., Leonard, J.M. and Markowitz, M. (1995) Rapid turnover of plasma virions and $CD4^+$ lymphocytes in HIV-1 infection. *Nature* 373, 123–126.

Hogg, R.S., Strathdee, S.A., Craib, K.J.P., O'Shaughnessy, M.V., Montaner, J.S.G. and Schechter, M.T. (1994) Lower socioeconomic status and shorter survival following HIV infection. *Lancet* 344, 1120–1124.

Kunanusont, C., Foy, H.M., Kreiss, J.K., Rerks-Ngarm, S., Phanuphak, P., Raktham, S., Pau, C.P. and Young, N.L. (1995) HIV-1 subtypes and male-to-female transmission in Thailand. *Lancet* 345, 1078–1083.

Lucas, S.B., Hounnou, A., Peacock, C., Beaumel, A., Djomond, G., N'Gbichi, J.M., Yeboue, K., Hondé, M., Diomande, M., Giordano, C., Dorrly, R., Brattegaard, K., Kestens, L., Smithwick, R., Kadio, A., Ezani, N., Yapi, A. and DeCock, K.M. (1993) The mortality and pathology of HIV infection in a West African city. *AIDS* 7, 1569–1579.

Mulder, D., Nunn, A., Kamali, A. and Kengeya-Kayondo, J. (1995) Decreasing HIV-1 prevalence in young adults in rural Uganda cohort. *British Medical Journal* 311, 833–836.

Williams, O. (1991) *AIDS: an African Perspective.* CRC Press, New York.

Piot, P., Kapita, B., Ngugi, E., Mann, J., Colebunders, R. and Wabitsch, R. (eds) (1992)

AIDS in Africa. A Manual for Physicians. WHO, Geneva.
Rojanapithayakorn, W. and Hanenberg, R. (1996) The 100% condom program in Thailand. *AIDS* 10, 1–7.
Ruxrungtham, K., Muller, O., Sirivichayakul, S., Ubolyam, S., Teeratakulpisarn, S., Hanvanich, M. and Phanuphak, P. (1996) AIDS at a university hospital in Bangkok, Thailand. *AIDS* 10, 1047–1049.
Sewankambo, N., Wawer, M., Gray, R., Serwadda, D., Li, C., Musgrave, S. and Konde-Lule, J. (1994) Demographic impact of HIV infection in rural Rakai, Uganda: results of a population based cohort study. *AIDS* 8, 1707–1713.
Shaw, G.M., Wong-Staal, F. and Gallo, R.C. (1988) Etiology of AIDS: virology, molecular biology and evolution of human immunodeficiency viruses. In: Devita, V.T. Jr, Hellman, S. and Rosenberg, S.A. (eds), *AIDS: Etiology, Diagnosis, Treatment and Prevention*, 2nd edn. J.B. Lippincott, Philadelphia, pp. 11–31.
Sudre, P., Ten Dam, G. and Kochi, A. (1992) Tuberculosis : a global overview of the situation today. *Bulletin of the World Health Organization* 70, 149–159.
Supparatpinyo, K., Khamwan, C., Baosoung, V., Nelson, K.E. and Sirisanthana, T. (1994) Disseminated *Penicillium marneffei* infection in southeast Asia. *Lancet* 344, 110–113.
Ubolyam, S., Ruxrungtham, K., Sirivichayakul, S., Okuda, K. and Phanuphak, P. (1994) Evidence of three HIV-1 subtypes in subgroups of individuals in Thailand. *Lancet* 344, 485–486.

CHAPTER 6.2
HIV infection in pregnancy and children

J.B.S. Coulter[1] and J. Kayita[2]
[1]Liverpool School of Tropical Medicine, Liverpool, UK and [2]Department of Paediatrics and Child Health, Makerere University Medical School, Kampala, Uganda

WHO estimates that by the year 2000 there will be 30–40 million HIV-infected adults in the world, the majority in developing countries, half of whom will be women. In sub-Saharan Africa alone, 10 million children will have been infected and another 10 million children under the age of 10 years will have lost their mothers to AIDS, leaving them unprotected and inadequately cared and provided for. The infant and under five mortality rates are expected to increase significantly from the already unacceptably high levels.

Epidemiology

It is estimated that about 10,000 people are infected with HIV daily, 90% of them in developing countries. Annual incidence rates are up to 3% in some urban areas in sub-Saharan Africa. Many of the HIV infected are teenage girls and women in the active reproductive period. Several factors have fuelled the epidemic in Africa. These include prevalence of STI, increasing urbanization and migration, wars and social conflict, and the inadequate health infrastructure. The low status of women is one of several factors that make women and girls particularly susceptible to HIV infection in this region.

In sub-Saharan Africa, HIV prevalence is not distributed uniformly. In Uganda, where HIV is widespread, the average seroprevalence is about 10% in the rural areas and 25% in some urban centres. Females aged 15–19 years are up to 5–6 times more likely to be HIV-infected than their male counterparts. These trends of a disproportionate number of infections among young women and the increasing rural seroprevalence is of great concern. However, recent studies from Uganda suggest that there is a levelling off and even a reduction in seroprevalence rates in some areas, attributed, in part, to the very extensive public education campaigns and political will.

In sub-Saharan Africa, the seroprevalence rates among women attending antenatal clinics range from 5 to 35%, the highest figures being from large urban centres such as Blantyre, Kampala, Lusaka, Kinshasa and Abidjan.

Modes of transmission

In developing countries, perinatal transmission is the major mode of infection of infants and children. However, the contribution of infection from blood and blood products is not insignificant (up to 10% in some estimates). The role of unsterilized syringes and needles, and cultural practices such as ritual circumcision (of boys and girls) and scarification is unclear. Sexual child abuse may be a risk factor for young girls, particularly those left unprotected by the death of their parents.

Vertical transmission

Risk factors for vertical transmission are outlined in Box 6.2.1. Timing of HIV transmission is important regarding interventions to prevent transmission during pregnancy. Evidence for *in utero* transmission is based on the detection of HIV in aborted fetal tissues. However, transmission in early pregnancy is probably uncommon. Based on results of PCR, viral culture and HIV antibody measurements, it is estimated that about two-thirds of transmission occurs during the day of delivery and most of the remaining in the previous 2 months or so. Peripartum transmission is supported by the finding of higher transmission rates in the first- than the second-born twin, decreased transmission in infants delivered by Caesarean section reported in some studies, and the association of transmission with chorioamnionitis and STI.

Box 6.2.1. Risk factors for vertical transmission.

High viral load
- maternal symptomatic disease
- low $CD4^+$ cell counts
- p24 antigenaemia
- seroconversion during pregnancy

First-born twin

Prematurity
Chorioamnionitis
Sexual intercourse during pregnancy
STI
Vaginal delivery
Breastfeeding

Under investigation
Viral characteristics
- replication rate
- syncytium formation

Neutralizing maternal antibodies (deficiency)

Vitamin A deficiency

Genetic factors

These findings support the concept that infants are at risk of infection by HIV-infected blood and secretions in the genital tract during delivery and possibly also late pregnancy. Treatment of mothers with antiretroviral drugs in late pregnancy as well of their infants in the neonatal period decreases the transmission rates in infants. This supports the concept that the perinatal period is the most important time for vertical transmission.

Estimation of vertical transmission rates requires prospective controlled studies which are expensive and notoriously difficult to undertake because of the need to determine the presence or absence of HIV infection in infants who drop out or die. Published estimates from well-conducted studies for Africa are 25–32%, Europe 15–20% and the USA 20–30%. Mothers with a high viral load during pregnancy as manifest by symptomatic disease, low $CD4^+$ cell counts, p24 antigenaemia and seroconversion during pregnancy have an increased chance of infecting their infant. Mothers infected by HIV-2 have a lower vertical transmission rate.

Breastfeeding

Mothers who contract HIV infection while breast feeding may infect their infants in about 30% of cases. The additional risk of infection through breast milk if the mother has been infected before pregnancy, and presumably has some protective antibodies, is not clear (estimated to be 15%). Prospective studies comparing artificial and breast milk feeding are in progress. These may also help to ascertain the risk at different periods of breast feeding, i.e. postnatal or later. Present advice is that where no safe milk substitute is available (as in developing countries), mothers should breast feed, the rationale being that the chances of a bottle-fed infant dying from infection and malnutrition are considered to be much higher than those of dying from HIV infection contracted through breast milk. However, if the mother knows that she is HIV-infected, she should be counselled and given a choice between feeding methods.

HIV–pregnancy interaction

Pregnancy does not enhance HIV disease in asymptomatic infection. HIV-infected women are at risk of abortion, premature delivery and maternal death. Infected neonates may have a slightly lower birth weight than non-infected neonates born to HIV-seropositive mothers, but do not have an increased risk of congenital malformations. They may be prone to other transplacental and intrapartum infections, e.g. CMV, toxoplasmosis or HBV.

Clinical manifestations in children

It has been observed that high viral loads in the first months of life may speed up the progression of disease. Infected infants usually mainfest some clinical or immunological disorder within the first 12 months of life. A natural history study in Uganda showed that by 18 months of age, 90% of infected infants were symptomatic. Major signs associated with HIV infection are chronic diarrhoea, recurrent and persistent respiratory infections, skin disorders, generalized lymphadenopathy, hepatosplenomegaly, parotid enlargement, developmental delay and failure to thrive. Infants who present with severe forms of malnutrition are more likely to have marasmus than kwashiorkor.

Autopsy studies in African infants dying under 1 year of age have shown that *Pneumocystis carinii* pneumonia (PCP) may be detected in up to a third of cases. Coinfection with *Mycobacterium tuberculosis* is common but is difficult to confirm as tuberculin tests are often negative and facilities for culture are limited. However, judging from the number of children who do not respond to therapy, it may also be overdiagnosed. Malaria would appear to have the same incidence and expression in HIV-infected and non-infected children. There is an increased risk of acquiring measles before the age of immunization. Kaposi's sarcoma, though rare among HIV-infected children in industrialized countries, is relatively common in sub-Saharan Africa, and has overtaken Burkitt's lymphoma as the commonest malignancy of childhood in Uganda.

Diagnosis

Diagnosis in developing countries is based on the persistence of HIV antibodies after 15 months of age. Early diagnosis can be made by viral culture, antigen detection (by acid dissociation or heat treatment of p24 antigen–antibody complexes), polymerase chain reaction (PCR) and detection of HIV IgA-specific antibodies. After 1–2 months of age, PCR and culture have a high sensitivity (>90%). PCR is the standard method for early diagnosis. Most infants have HIV IgA antibodies by 6 months of age, and this can be a useful test in developing countries where resources are limited. For early diagnosis using the above techniques, at least two positive results should be obtained from separate blood samples.

Prognosis

Infant mortality is significantly higher among children born to HIV-infected mothers than those born to HIV-seronegative mothers regardless of the children's infection status. In a Ugandan prospective study, 53% of HIV-infected infants developed AIDS by 18 months of age and another 37% were symptomatic.

Management

Management at delivery

If not undertaken during the antenatal period, mothers should be screened in the perinatal period for tuberculosis, STI and other treatable diseases associated with HIV infection. If elective Caesarean section is contemplated, the problems of infection and other post-operative complications, particularly in mothers with advanced disease, should be considered. Where possible, artificial rupture of membranes, the use of scalp electrodes and fetal scalp tests, and episiotomy should be avoided.

At delivery, the infant should be washed with an antiseptic solution, e.g. chlorhexidine. Mouth-to-mouth resuscitation should not be undertaken. Care should be taken with handling of the placenta and body fluids. Decisions regarding breast feeding are discussed in the section on vertical transmission. Vitamin A supplements to the infant may reduce morbidity from HIV-related infections. Breast-feeding mothers should be given a vitamin A supplement postpartum.

Mothers should be counselled and support for the family provided. Follow-up should be emphasized, particularly regarding prophylaxis and management of PCP and other infections.

Management of infant

Early diagnosis is essential for the optimal management of HIV-infected infants, even in developing countries where interventions are limited. HIV/AIDS in children is a chronic disease, and a multidisciplinary, family-oriented approach is required as a child is usually one of several infected family members.

An infant born to an HIV-infected mother should be offered the best available child care, with emphasis on immunization, growth monitoring and neurodevelopmental assessment. Nutrition should be optimized, with emphasis on breast feeding, appropriately timed weaning and regular vitamin A supplementation to both prevent and treat malnutrition.

Chemoprophylaxis

PCP prophylaxis with cotrimoxazole is an essential part of management, particularly in early infancy. However, in developing countries, since few women know their infection status prenatally, prophylaxis is likely to be instituted too late to prevent PCP.

Antiretroviral therapy

Antiretroviral therapy, by decreasing the viral load, may enhance survival. In the USA, antiretroviral drugs, zidovudine (AZT) and didanosine (ddI) currently are licensed for use in children under 12 months of age, and protease inhibitors for those aged ≥2 years. However, antiretroviral therapy is not widely available nor is it affordable for the majority of patients in developing countries. The few who can afford it are unlikely to enjoy the desirable close laboratory support required to monitor progress and to detect the profound side effects on the bone marrow.

Routine immunization

In industrialized countries, bacille Calmette–Guérin (BCG) is omitted and killed polio vaccine is given to suspected HIV-infected infants. In developing countries, the usual extended programme of immunization (EPI) schedule is given (including neonatal BCG). Although, rarely, complications from BCG in HIV-infected infants have been recorded, it is generally considered safe to give in the neonatal period before the infant's immune system becomes depressed.

Haemophilus influenzae b and pneumococcal vaccines should be given as early as is feasible. Conjugate vaccines, when available for young HIV-infected infants, may help to reduce bacterial infections in the first few years of life.

Psychosocial support and counselling to families and children

This service is at best limited in sub-Saharan Africa, but children (infected and affected) need support to cope with the reality of chronic ill health, bereavement, discrimination and stigma, and separation from their siblings in the event of a parent's death. Parents need to be encouraged to plan for their children's future including nurturing a relationship between children and targeted guardians. Affected children are susceptible to all forms of exploitation and child abuse, and communities need to make a concentrated effort to protect and support these children.

Prevention of perinatal infection

Unless routine screening of women during pregnancy is practised, many asymptomatic mothers only discover their HIV infection when their infected infant develops symptoms. Detection of HIV infection in women provides the opportunity to investigate and treat STI and other infections such as tuberculosis, advise about contraception and offer termination. Infants born to HIV-infected women can be offered appropriate PCP prophylaxis and can be observed for development of symptoms of HIV-related disease.

Zidovudine given to HIV-infected mothers after 34 weeks' gestation, then parenterally during delivery, and for 6 weeks to their infants reduced the estimated vertical transmission rate by two-thirds. Further studies are examining the benefit of shorter regimens, e.g. administration during delivery only, and using a combination of retroviral drugs. Long-term effects on the fetus are unknown (see also Appendix 6.A).

The proportion of perinatal infections that can be reduced by elective Caesarean section is not yet established. It is estimated that 16 Caesarean sections may be necessary to prevent one infected infant. The difficulties and dangers of Caesarean section in developing countries, particularly in women with HIV infection, need to be emphasized.

Vitamin A levels are reduced in adults with well-advanced HIV disease.

Reduced vitamin A levels in the mother are associated with increased mother to child transmission and increased mortality in the infant. Trials of vitamin A and other micronutrients supplementation of women prenatally, and infants postnatally, are in progress in the hope of reducing HIV transmission. High doses of vitamin A given to women in early pregnancy may be teratogenic.

Use of vaginal disinfectants such as chlorhexidine during labour may reduce group B streptococcal perinatal infection. Studies so far have not shown benefit in decreasing HIV transmission.

There are ongoing studies of active immunization of pregnant women and newborns with HIV antigens, e.g. gp120, and of giving infusions of HIV hyperimmune serum or monoclonal antibodies against epitopes of HIV to the mother during delivery and to the newborn infant.

The future

Efforts to prevent paediatric HIV infections must focus on preventing infections among women, particularly young women who currently comprise the majority of new infections in developing countries. Comprehensive programmes of sex and reproductive health education targeting young people in and out of school, integration of STI treatment services in existing maternal and child health (MCH) services as well as making HIV screening services available to more women should contribute to the reduction of HIV infection among women and children. Women and girls should be empowered to take charge of their sexual and reproductive lives and participate more effectively with men in the development of culturally relevant strategies for protecting themselves and their families. Mothers should have greater access to health services where they can enjoy optimal management of labour and delivery. Community programmes to support child-headed households and households overwhelmed by the high dependency rate are badly needed in sub-Saharan Africa.

Screening of women at antenatal clinics for HIV and STI should be widely available. Thus HIV-infected infants can be identified before they present with AIDS-indicator diseases and be given PCP prophylaxis, and provided with growth and health monitoring. Uninfected children born to HIV-infected mothers will also benefit from improved health care and protection.

Further reading

Coulter, J.B.S. (1998) HIV in African children. *Journal of Medical Microbiology* (in press).

Scarlatti, G. (1996) Paediatric HIV infection. *Lancet* ii, 863–868.

UNICEF (1994) *Equity and Vulnerability: a Situation Analysis of Women, Adolescents and Children in Uganda.* UNICEF, Uganda.

US Bureau of Census (1995) *HIV/AIDS in Africa.* Research paper No. 20, Washington, DC.

CHAPTER 6.3
Herpes simplex virus infection

O.P. Arya and C.A. Hart

Department of Medical Microbiology and Genitourinary Medicine, University of Liverpool, Liverpool, UK

The herpesviruses are a family of viruses that, following primary infection, become established in latent or persistent form. Once infected, an individual is infected for life. The virus may re-emerge to produce recurrences from time to time. They may establish latency in neurones (neurotropic) or persist in white cells (lymphotropic or leukotropic). With the discovery of three new herpesviruses, their official nomenclature has been revised (Table 6.3.1).

Anogenital herpes

Anogenital herpes is a chronic, mainly sexually transmitted disease, characterized by recurrent episodes of anogenital ulceration and long periods of latency. Most cases are due to herpes simplex virus type 2 (HSV-2 or HHV-2), whereas type 1 is usually associated with orofacial and ocular lesions but can cause genital herpes. Its recurrent nature, although mostly a nuisance, may, however, cause significant psychosexual morbidity.

Table 6.3.1. The human herpesviruses (HHV).

Nomenclature			
New	Old	Diseases	Tropism
HHV-1	Herpes simplex virus-1	Orofacial herpes, genital herpes	Neurotropic
HHV-2	Herpes simplex virus-2	Genital herpes, orofacial herpes	Neurotropic
HHV-3	Varicella zoster virus	Chickenpox, shingles	Neurotropic
HHV-4	Epstein–Barr virus	Glandular fever	Lymphotropic
HHV-5	Cytomegalovirus	Asymptomatic, glandular fever	Leukotropic
HHV-6	B-cell lymphotropic virus	Exanthem subitum	Lymphotropic
HHV-7	RK virus	Exanthem subitum	Lymphotropic
HHV-8	Kaposi's sarcoma-associated herpesvirus	Kaposi's sarcoma	Lymphotropic

Epidemiology

Genital herpes is now the commonest type of genital ulceration in some of the Western countries where asymptomatic infection has also been reported to be significant. National prevalence rates of genital herpes (including subclinical carriage) are unknown in the tropics. However, genital ulceration is a common presentation in STI clinics in Africa and Asia, and genital herpes may be the cause in about 5–15% of these cases (see also Chapter 1). In common with other ulcerative diseases, it may facilitate transmission of HIV infection.

The virus

Herpesviruses are DNA viruses and all have an icosahedral nucleocapsid approximately 100 nm in diameter, surrounded by a loose lipid envelope (Fig. 6.3.1). The major antigens recognized by the immune system are the glycoproteins on the viral envelope. There are antigenic and biological differences, with a serological overlap, between HHV-1 and HHV-2. Thus, although orofacial HHV-1 infection does not protect against subsequent genital HHV-2 infection, it may lessen the severity of first attack.

Mode of transmission

Anogenital HSV infection is mainly sexually transmitted by direct physical contact including sexual intercourse, anal intercourse and orogenital or oroanal contact with an infected partner. The chances of transmission are much greater if the infected partner has herpetic lesions at the time than on occasions of subclinical viral shedding.

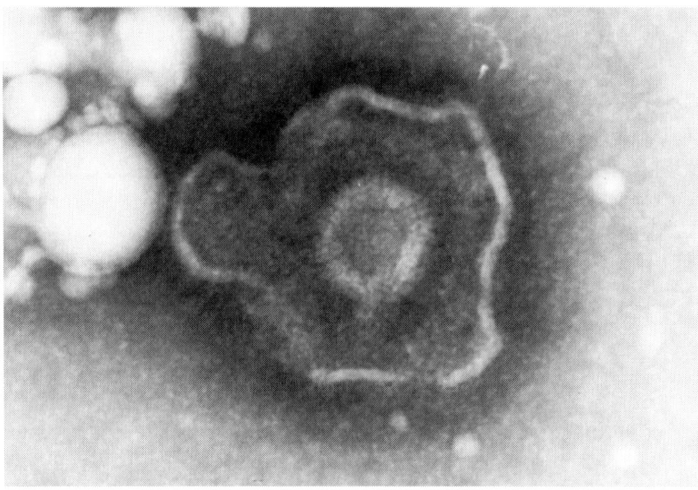

Fig. 6.3.1. Herpes simplex virus: negative stain electron micrograph.

Pathogenesis

The virus enters the body through a mucous surface or an abrasion of skin. While replicating locally, it spreads to the local sensory nerve endings and then migrates along the sensory nerves to the appropriate ganglia, e.g. to the sacral and trigeminal ganglia, respectively from genital and oral lesions. In the ganglia, the virus remains latent but may reactivate asymptomatically or symptomatically to cause recurrent disease.

Clinical features

Primary disease and first clinical attack

Primary infection may be asymptomatic. However, the first clinical attack in those who have no previously acquired antibody to HSV infection (primary symptomatic disease) is usually more severe than in those who show serological evidence of previous HSV infection.

After an incubation period of 2–10 days (or longer and difficult to determine), the patient develops erythema, red papules evolving into vesicles at the site of viral entry. The accompanying local symptoms include irritation, burning and pricking pain. Many also experience systemic symptoms including fever, headache, malaise and muscular pains. The thin-walled vesicles soon rupture, resulting in pleomorphic, shallow, mostly non-indurated, tender ulcers, followed by crusting of the skin lesions.

In men, the common sites are the glans penis, prepuce and the penile shaft (Plates 3–6). In women, who are generally more severely affected than men, the vulva, perianal region, vagina and cervix are the sites most frequently affected (Plates 7 and 8). Macroscopic lesions are seen infrequently on the cervix, but virus may be isolated from a cervical sample. In addition to the symptoms described above, severe vulvovaginitis and, rarely, necrotizing cervicitis may occur. The patient may complain of vaginal discharge, external dysuria (due to urine coming into contact with vulval ulcers), dyspareunia and lower abdominal pain. The pain due to ulceration is often very severe, and genital examination has to be carried out with extreme care. Symptoms are sometimes aggravated by concomitant candidiasis or trichomoniasis.

In both sexes, the inguinal glands may become enlarged and painful. Involvement of the urethra, more common in women, may result in internal dysuria, frequency, minimal clear mucoid urethral discharge and acute retention of urine – the last possibly due to trigonitis and reflex spasm of the vesical sphincter.

Extragenital lesions

Perianal and anal lesions, frequently encountered in women and homosexual men, are usually very painful. These may also be associated with proctitis with or without ulceration and/or rectal pain. Other symptoms include tenesmus, rectal discharge and blood in stools. Other extragenital sites, notably thighs, buttocks, groin and fingers, are mostly affected as a result of autoinoculation of the virus. Herpetic whitlows can be very painful. Lesions in the mouth (Plate 9) and throat are often associated with orogenital contact.

In immunocompetent persons and in the absence of secondary infection, most genital and extragenital lesions heal within 2–4 weeks.

Recurrent disease

About 50% of patients experience recurrent episodes which are generally milder than the primary attacks and of shorter duration. The symptoms are more severe in women but, in both men and women, the severity, duration and frequency may vary within the same patient.

Genital HHV-2 infection recurs more frequently than genital HHV-1 infection (exogenous re-infection among these patients appears to be rare). These recurrences may be triggered by emotional stress, trauma, fever, menstruation or some other unknown factor. There may or may not be prodromal symptoms, which include itching, tingling, burning, tenderness at the site of subsequent eruption, or radiating pain in the groin, buttock or leg. Occasionally the attacks may not progress beyond prodromal symptoms or local erythema. Some of these patients become anxious/depressed and frustrated. As time goes on, these relapses may become less frequent or even cease. A proportion, however, may continue to experience frequent recurrences for many years, whereas some may periodically shed the virus in the absence of clinically detectable lesions.

Complications

Local complications include secondary bacterial infection, sacral radiculitis and meningomyelitis. The secondary bacterial infection may result in scarring, which may progress to phimosis in men and labial adhesions in women. Sacral radiculitis and meningomyelitis, usually associated with anorectal herpes, may result in difficulty in micturition, constipation, inability to achieve penile erection, paraesthesiae around the thighs and buttocks, and diminution of skin sensations over the sacral region. In most cases, the symptoms and signs resolve within a few weeks.

The systemic complications include meningitis, encephalitis and disseminated HSV infection. Meningitis is seen more commonly in women and is usually associated with primary genital HHV-2 infection. The symptoms include headache, fever, vomiting and photophobia. The CSF is clear but on microscopy shows a lymphocytosis. The condition is usually benign and recovery is complete within a week. Encephalitis, which may occur in disseminated neonatal infection, is usually associated with non-genital HSV-1 infection in adults and older children.

Immunocompromised patients, such as those with AIDS, may experience more severe, prolonged, frequent and extensive attacks, including disseminated infection.

Some patients may develop erythema multiforme which is an allergic response to a number of drugs and infections including those due to HHV-1 and -2.

An association between the HHV-2 infection and carcinoma of the cervix remains unproven but it may be a cofactor promoting carcinogenesis by human papillomavirus.

Differential diagnosis

The differential diagnosis is from other causes of anogenital ulceration and is covered in the section on primary syphilis (Chapter 7.1). Syphilis must be considered in every case. Mixed infections may also occur. Hence, darkfield examination and repeated serological tests for syphilis should be carried out.

Diagnosis

Laboratory diagnosis of HSV will be largely beyond the means of most peripheral medical units in the tropics. In practice, therefore, the diagnosis has often to be made by exclusion and on clinical grounds. However, clinical differentiation from chancroid is often impossible.

The diagnostic methods include: (i) examination of the slides prepared from the scrapings of the lesions to demonstrate herpesvirus particles by electron microscopy; (ii) detection of the infected cells by fluorescent or peroxidase-labelled antibody staining which, with the use of HHV-1- and HHV-2-specific monoclonal antibodies, can also type the virus; (iii) viral isolation in tissue culture for which the swabs (after obtaining a specimen of vesicle fluid or by swabbing the base of the lesion or the scabbed lesion, or in the case of asymptomatic female, from the endo- and ectocervix and sweep of the labia) should be sent to the laboratory in viral transport medium; and (iv) demonstration of a fourfold rise in the serum antibody titre of the convalescent sample taken 2–3 weeks after the acute sample to support the diagnosis of a primary infection, especially if HHV-1- and HHV-2-specific antigens are used. The methods for detecting HSV are more sensitive in the early stages of the lesions.

Tests must also be done to exclude other STI. However, the first episode lesions in a female patient may be so painful and tender as to necessitate postponing some tests for other STI for a few days.

Antiviral drug susceptibility testing is carried out only in specialized centres. This surveillance is necessary in view of the development of resistance to aciclovir.

Management

Specific treatment

There is no curative treatment. The currently available drugs, i.e. aciclovir, famciclovir (prodrug of penciclovir) and valaciclovir (prodrug of aciclovir), active against herpesvirus, do not eradicate the virus from the ganglia. They reduce the duration of viral shedding, formation of new lesions and healing time, and have beneficial effect on pain and other symptoms if administered early in acute primary genital herpes, and at the onset of the prodrome in recurrent disease. Their benefit in recurrent genital herpes, when attacks are generally mild, is only marginal. They are all very expensive and their use in pregnancy and lactation is not established. Aciclovir has been in use for almost 10 years and, aciclovir-resistant mutants, which may be of clinical significance, especially in immunocompromised persons, have been described. Their indiscriminate use, therefore, should be avoided.

In view of the above limitations (especially the cost and failure to eradicate the virus from the ganglia), antiviral drugs are best reserved for patients with impaired immune responses, those with a severe initial episode of genital herpes with systemic and other symptoms, and those with severe frequent recurrences (more than six to eight per year).

Patients with severe local disease or disseminated infection requiring intravenous therapy will need to be hospitalized. The dose of aciclovir is 5 mg kg^{-1} intravenously 8-hourly (for patients with normal renal function) by slow infusion. For others, the oral regimens are aciclovir, 200 mg five times daily for 5 days (may be extended to 10 days for a severe first attack), *or*, famciclovir, 250 mg three times daily for 5 days, *or*, valaciclovir, 500 mg twice daily for 5–10 days. If treatment is considered necessary for a recurrent attack, the recommended oral regimens are: aciclovir as above for 5 days, *or*, famciclovir 125 mg twice daily for 5 days, *or*, valaciclovir as above for 5 days.

Suppressive therapy

The dose of aciclovir for suppressive therapy (prevention of repeated recurrences) is 200 mg orally four times daily, or 400 mg orally twice daily, and then possibly reduced to 200 mg two or three times daily for 6 months when it may be interrupted and the situation reviewed before resumption of therapy. valaciclovir, 500 mg orally once daily, has also been found to be effective. It should be noted that suppressive therapy may not eliminate viral shedding and may promote resistance.

Symptomatic treatment

In most tropical areas where antiviral treatment is unaffordable, the treatment of genital herpes remains largely symptomatic. Apart from the first attacks, especially in women, the genital infection in the majority of immunocompetent adults is usually mild, requiring simple measures such as maintenance of good local hygiene and frequent applications of salt solutions (a heaped teaspoonful of salt to a pint of warm water). Analgesics may be prescribed for pain. Some patients experience relief with ice (applied in a freezer bag). In the case of acute retention of urine, notably in females, urethral catheterization may spread the infection upwards and hence should be avoided. The patient should be encouraged to urinate in a warm bath, otherwise suprapubic catheterization may be considered. If there is a secondary infection, sulphadimidine, 1 g by mouth four times daily, or cotrimoxazole, two tablets twice a day for 5–7 days will usually suffice. One should be aware of the potential toxicity of these drugs. Concurrent candidiasis may aggravate symptoms and should be treated appropriately (see Chapter 8.1).

Other measures

Sexual intercourse or genital contact should be forbidden until the lesions heal. The role of subclinical viral shedding in transmission (including in patients on suppressive therapy) should also be discussed with the patient and partner. The patient should be advised to wash his/her hands after touching the lesions and not to share towels. A clear explanation should be given so that the patient understands the recurrent nature of HSV infection and does not become overanxious. According to present knowledge, it is considered advisable for women with genital herpes to have cervical cytology performed more frequently, perhaps yearly.

A safe and effective vaccine for preventing HSV infections is not yet available (see also Chapter 12.2).

Anogenital herpes in immunocompromised patients

As HSV infection in immunocompromised patients, such as recipients of bone marrow transplants or those with HIV infection, tends to be very severe and prolonged, they may require intravenous antiviral therapy for up to 10 days. For less severe lesions, oral antiviral therapy is equally effective. Suppressive antiviral therapy on a long-term basis also needs to be considered. See Chapter 11.5 for the treatment of aciclovir-resistant infections.

Genital herpes in pregnancy and the neonate

There are few data on the prevalence of genital HSV infection during pregnancy and the incidence of neonatal herpes in the tropics (see also Chapter 1).

The majority of women with a history of genital herpes go through their pregnancies unaffected and deliver normal babies. However, pregnant women are at an increased risk of disseminated HSV infection. Genital herpes early in pregnancy has been reported to result in fetal death and abortion, and infection later in pregnancy may result in intrauterine growth retardation and premature labour. The infection of the fetus may occur transplacentally, which is extremely rare. More commonly, the neonate acquires the infection during labour by direct contact with infected maternal genital secretions with or without the presence of active lesions. These risks are approximately tenfold greater following primary infection than is the case with recurrent episodes.

Prevention of prenatal transmission of HSV

Pregnant women attending antenatal clinics should be asked if they or their sexual partners have had genital or oral herpes or recurrent genital or oral ulceration. If the woman's history is negative but that of the sexual partner is positive, then they should be advised to use condoms and also avoid orogenital contact throughout pregnancy to prevent primary genital herpes developing in the female partner. If the latter does develop symptoms of genital herpes, she should be advised to attend the clinic as soon as possible.

Management of HSV infection in pregnancy and labour

If a pregnant woman presents with herpetic lesions, the diagnosis should be confirmed and other STI screening tests performed if appropriate. There is limited experience on the use of aciclovir in pregnancy. Although no adverse effects have been reported so far, the drug is not yet licensed for use in pregnancy. The clinician therefore has to judge whether potential benefits outweigh the possibility of unknown risks, and the issue must be discussed fully with the patient. Thus, treatment with a course of aciclovir may be considered for a pregnant woman with primary or first attack of genital herpes during the last trimester, with a severe first attack at earlier gestation, or for disseminated infection. There is as yet inadequate information on the benefit of aciclovir for recurrent HSV infection in pregnancy.

Although abdominal delivery may not always prevent HSV infection in the neonate, an elective Caesarean section is recommended for women with a history of a first episode of genital herpes during third trimester. It is also recommended that women with herpetic lesions (primary or recurrent) in the genital area at the time of labour should be delivered by Caesarean section which should be performed before or within 4 h of rupture of membranes. The practice of obtaining weekly cultures from women at high risk, starting at 32 weeks gestation is now obsolete because antepartum maternal cultures do not always predict the state of viral shedding at the time of delivery. Invasive fetal procedures, such as fetal scalp electrodes, etc. should be avoided in all pregnant women with a history of genital herpes.

Clinical features of neonatal herpes

The clinical features of neonatal herpes include vesicular lesions of the skin, oral lesions, keratitis, choroidoretinitis, meningoencephalitis and involvement of other organs. Disseminated infection in the neonate carries a very high mortality (> 50%) and high morbidity with residual neurological damage.

Management of the neonate

Neonates born to a mother with herpetic lesions at the time of delivery should be managed, if possible, in collaboration with a paediatrician. Swabs from any skin lesions, mouth, and conjunctivae should be taken as soon as possible after birth and sent to the laboratory in the same container of transport medium for viral identification by electron microscopy, immunofluorescence, PCR or culture. CSF is also obtained for tests if indicated. Intravenous aciclovir, 10 mg kg^{-1} three times daily for 10 days should be prescribed as soon as possible if there is any evidence of neonatal infection. Treatment with aciclovir should also be considered if there was vaginal delivery in the presence of primary genital lesions or if in the latter patient Caesarean section was performed after membrane rupture. However, aciclovir may be discontinued, if the tests for HSV are negative and the baby has remained well. All infants suspected of having been exposed to risk of HSV infection should be kept under surveillance for at least 2 weeks.

CHAPTER 6.4
The other human herpesviruses

C.A. Hart

*Department of Medical Microbiology and Genitourinary Medicine,
University of Liverpool, Liverpool, UK*

The human herpesviruses are a ubiquitous group of eight DNA viruses (see Chapter 6.3; Table 6.3.1) with similar morphology and genomic structure but differing tissue tropism and disease manifestations. Some are transmitted sexually predominantly (e.g. HHV-2) or occasionally (e.g. HHV-4 and HHV-5) and some form part of the spectrum of infections in AIDS (e.g. HHV-1, HHV-3 and HHV-8). However, once infected, an individual will remain infected for life and continue to excrete the virus continuously or sporadically.

Herpes simplex type 1 (HHV-1)

HHV-1 can cause genital herpes but does so far less frequently than HHV-2. The primary infection with HHV-1 is usually acquired asymptomatically in the first 2 years of life, but up to 10% of cases may present with gingivo-stomatitis. The virus immediately travels up the sensory nerve (usually the mandibular division of the trigeminal nerve) and becomes latent in the trigeminal ganglion. It reactivates sporadically and usually asymptomatically (at any one time up to 5% of the population will have HHV-1 in saliva). However, if conditions are favourable (e.g. inflamed skin), the virus will grow to produce the secondary manifestation of herpes labialis or cold sores. In patients with AIDS, reactivation does not appear to be more frequent but, when lesions occur (recrudescence), they are more severe, more extensive or more widespread. Diagnosis is by culture, antigen detection, genome detection or electron microscopy. Treatment, when necessary, is with aciclovir, either orally (optimal) or topically, or valaciclovir orally. However, aciclovir-resistant mutants have emerged, that are missing the thymidine kinase gene (TK^- mutants).

Varicella zoster virus (HHV-3)

The primary infection with HHV-3 is the common childhood infectious disease chickenpox. Once in the skin, virus tracks back along the sensory nerves to remain latent in the dorsal root ganglia. Asymptomatic reactivation has not been described, but the secondary or recrudescent disease is shingles or herpes zoster. Shingles occurs within a dermatome with no more than ten vesicles outside the dermatome. AIDS patients are at increased risk of suffering severe and fatal chickenpox (if previously uninfected) and they are likely to suffer shingles which usually spreads beyond the affected dermatome. Electron microscopy will not distinguish between any of the herpesviruses. Culture, antigen detection or genome detection is needed for precise diagnosis. Treatment is with aciclovir, famciclovir or valaciclovir (see also Chapter 11.5).

Epstein–Barr virus (HHV-4)

HHV-4 is a cause of glandular fever or infectious mononucleosis (the other causes are cytomegalovirus and *Toxoplasma gondii*). In developed countries, the peak age of onset is in adolescence and early adulthood, when infection is more likely to be clinically expressed. However, in developing countries, most children are infected by 10 years of age and infection in young children is much more likely to be asymptomatic. It is spread by exchange of saliva and is sometimes called 'kissing disease'. Once infected, an individual will excrete virus in saliva continuously. HHV-4 is involved in the development of Burkitt's lymphoma, nasopharyngeal carcinoma and Hodgkin lymphoma, but there is no evidence that there is an inter-relationship with HIV/AIDS. In contrast, there is an increased incidence of HHV-4-positive cerebral lymphomata in patients with AIDS. Although some immunodeficiency disorders such as ataxia telangiectasia, are associated with more severe infection, there is no evidence of increased severity in AIDS. Diagnosis is by detection of specific anti-HHV-4 IgM or IgG. There is no specific antiviral chemotherapy, nor is there, as yet, a vaccine for prevention of infection.

Cytomegalovirus (HHV-5)

HHV-5 is prevalent throughout the world, and peak ages for acquisition are lower under conditions of crowding, poor hygiene and in extended families. In developing countries, 90% of children are seropositive by 5 years of age.

The virus

HHV-5 is a β-herpesvirus with a double-stranded linear DNA genome. It is 150–200 nm in diameter with a lipid envelope outside which is a fringe of glycoprotein spikes. The capsid is icosahedral, approximately 110 nm in diameter. The virus remains latent in cells of several tissues and is found in the white blood cells (monocytes and neutrophils). Sporadic excretion occurs throughout life, and infection with different strains of virus can occur through different portals (e.g. oropharynx and genitalia).

Transmission

Infection can be passed sexually or by non-sexual routes. The latter include transplacentally, via breast milk, by close contact and by blood (fresh) transfusion. The incubation period is 4–8 weeks.

Clinical features

The most frequent occurrence is asymptomatic infection. If a mother is infected with HHV-5 for the first time during pregnancy, there is approximately a 10% risk of congenital damage which ranges across a spectrum from school failure to hearing impairment to gross mental retardation. Worldwide, HHV-5 is the major infective cause of mental retardation. HHV-5 is also a cause of infectious mononucleosis but less frequently than HHV-4. However, it is particularly associated with post-transfusion mononucleosis, but only if the blood is fresh (i.e. the leukocytes are still viable). Rarer manifestations of HHV-5 infection in immunocompetent individuals include polyneuritis, cystitis, nephritis, hepatitis, pneumonia (< 1% of community-acquired pneumonias), encephalitis, thrombocytopenic purpura and haemolytic anaemia. These mostly occur as part of the mononucleosis syndrome but may occur as a single entity.

HHV-5 pneumonitis was one of the original AIDS-defining illnesses. The immune suppression of AIDS results in this mild-mannered virus assuming the mantle of a dangerous pathogen. The earliest manifestation of HHV-5 infection is of retinitis. This will present as blurred vision, scotomata and loss of visual acuity, which is usually unilateral but will progress to be bilateral. The distinctive appearance of HHV-5 retinitis includes scattered white dots or granular patches with sheathing of local blood vessels. This may then progress to scattered areas of haemorrhage. Eventually, as the inflammation decreases, these are replaced by grey–brown areas of retinal epithelial atrophy. It may begin focally but progresses to generalized involvement leading to blindness.

HHV-5 pneumonia may be asymptomatic but then progresses insidiously to present with fever, malaise, myalgia, arthralgia and a dry, hacking cough accompanied by high fever and tachypnoea. On examination, there may be diffuse rales and dullness in the lower lungs. On chest X-ray, there is a diffuse reticular or nodular pattern in both lungs.

Gastrointestinal infection occurs as part of a disseminated infection and may present as oesophagitis, gastritis, pancreatitis, enteritis, ulcerative colitis or proctitis. Encephalitis may also occur in AIDS patients (up to 50% of cases of encephalitis) which is most often diagnosed at postmortem.

Differential diagnosis

For mononucleosis, it must be distinguished from HHV-4 and *T. gondii*. HHV-5 retinitis can be distinguished from *T. gondii* retinitis in that in the former the retinal lesions have discrete edges. With HHV-5 pneumonia, all other causes of pneumonia must be considered; also the aetiology in AIDS can be polymicrobial. In children with AIDS, the differential diagnosis also includes lymphocytic interstitial pneumonia. HHV-5 must be included in the investigation of the multitude of causes of gastrointestinal infection.

Laboratory diagnosis

HHV-5 can be grown in MRC-5 or W1-38 cells but takes up to a week to produce a cytopathic effect. The time taken for diagnosis can be decreased by the DEAFF (direct early antigen fluorescent foci) test which uses immunofluorescence to detect HHV-5 early antigen 24–48 h after inoculation of sample into tissue culture cells. Even more rapid diagnosis (1–2 h) can be obtained by examining peripheral blood neutrophils for HHV-5 antigen (pp65) using immunofluorescence. Detection of the HHV-5 genome in serum or of its mRNA by RT-PCR are also useful.

Treatment

Antiviral drugs such as ganciclovir (5 mg kg^{-1} body weight) infused over 1 h every 12 h for 14–21 days, or foscarnet (40–200 mg kg^{-1} body weight per day depending on serum creatinine concentrations) infused either continuously or for 1 h every 8 h, are useful in treating HHV-5 infection in AIDS.

HHV-6 and HHV-7

These two lymphotrophic β-herpesviruses were first described in the last 10 years. Infection with either of these occurs most frequently in the first 2 years of life, mostly asymptomatically. In a proportion of cases, infection results in exanthem subitum or febrile convulsions. As yet there appear to be no proven links with these viruses and more severe infection in AIDS.

Human herpesvirus-8

This γ-herpesvirus was first described in 1994 in Kaposi's sarcoma cells. Its alternative name is Kaposi's sarcoma-associated herpesvirus (KSHV). It is associated with both endemic and AIDS-associated Kaposi's sarcoma (see Chapter 11.3).

CHAPTER 6.5
Anogenital warts and human papillomavirus infection

A.B. Alawattegama
Department of Genitourinary Medicine, Royal Liverpool University Hospital, Liverpool, UK

Anogenital warts are the most common of viral infections and perhaps the most common condition seen at STI clinics in developed countries. The propensity of the infection to remain latent as well as the recognition that some genotypes of the virus are oncogenic has aroused considerable concern, especially with regard to carcinoma of the cervix.

Aetiology

Anogenital warts are caused by human papillomavirus (HPV), often transmitted sexually. Papillomaviruses are small unenveloped icosahedral viruses approximately 55 nm in diameter. They have a circular double-stranded DNA genome of approximately 8 kb (8×10^6 Da). The viral capsid is made up of two structural proteins, a 53–59-kDa group antigen polypeptide (L1), and a 70-kDa type-specific antigen polypeptide (L2), arranged in 72 individual protein subunits in the overall ratio of 4:1.

The genomes of a number of human and animal papillomaviruses have been completely sequenced, and the genome organization of each appears similar (for HPV16 see Fig. 6.5.1). In HPV, all potential protein-coding sequences, or open reading frames (ORFs), are located on one DNA strand. Depending on the HPV type, up to ten ORFs have been identified to date. They are classified according to function as 'early' (E1–E8) or 'late' (L1 and L2) according to their sequence of expression in the viral replication cycle. Early ORFs encode proteins involved in transcription control (E2), viral DNA replication (E1), modification of immune response (E5) and oncogenic transformation (E6 and E7). Late ORFs L1 and L2 encode major and minor capsid proteins respectively. The other DNA strand is assumed to be non-coding, but evidence suggests it may have a regulatory role.

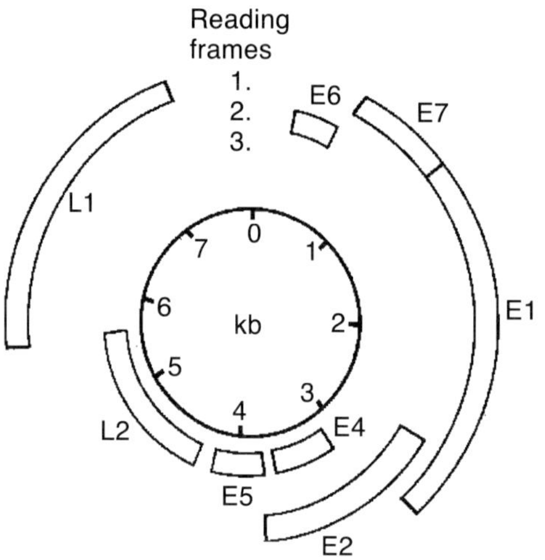

Functions of HPV16 proteins

Early proteins

E1 virus DNA replication

E2 transcription control

E4 binds cytokeratin

E5 activates growth factor receptor
? prevents class 1 antigen presentation

E6 binds p53

E7 binds retinoblastoma protein
? prevents apoptosis?

Late proteins

L1 major capsid protein

L2 minor capsid protein

Fig. 6.5.1. HPV16: genomic organization.

Classification of HPV

Based on DNA homologies, over 75 different HPV types have been characterized to date from mucosal and cutaneous sites. Each type usually has an affinity for a particular anatomical site producing a defined spectrum of pathological effects with distinctive histological features. Some HPV types have been shown to play an important aetiological role in head and neck tumours and in the development of malignant lesions of the skin, anogenital tract and oral mucosa.

The genital tract is the reservoir for all but two of the mucosal types, HPV13 and -32 restricted to the oral cavity, with some types exclusively found in the genital tract. Of the several anogenital human papillomavirus (GPV) types identified, types 6 and 11 are typically associated with exophytic warts whilst 16 and 18 are associated predominantly with either flat or dysplastic lesions, and 16, 18, 31, 33, 35 and others with cancers.

Epidemiology

Infection with HPV virus is ubiquitous. In some Western countries, the incidence of genital warts, commonly seen in young adults aged 16–25, has more than doubled in the last decade. Similarly, it is likely that there has been an increase in the detection of subclinical infection of the cervix, with a reported prevalence of up to 13% in those screened with cervical smears and colposcopy. Evidence based on clinical, morphological and molecular methods of detection indicates a high prevalence in the young sexually active population which rapidly declines with age beyond 55 years to less than 4%. Whereas accurate figures for anogenital warts in developing countries are largely unavailable, carcinoma of the cervix is the most common cancer among women in many of these countries (see also Chapters 1 and 11.3).

Mode of transmission

As a rule, GPV infections are acquired through breaches in the skin and mucosa during sexual contact and are considered to be sexually transmitted. Spread to other sites occurs in a similar manner. Nearly two-thirds of sexual partners of persons with genital warts will develop clinical warts within 2–3 months, although the incubation period may vary from a few weeks to months or even years.

Pathology and cytology

For centuries, the only recognized manifestation of GPV was the presence of the condylomatous wart. In the 1970s, the presence of subclinical infection became apparent on the evidence of specific morphological changes observed on exfoliative cytology, colposcopy or histology. More recently, following advances in molecular virological techniques (hybridization techniques and PCR), it is now evident that GPV can also be present as a latent infection in epithelium classified by all histological and cytological criteria as normal.

Having made the initial entry via skin abrasions, the virus enters the basal germinal cells, the only cells of the epithelium capable of dividing. Replication of the virus, which occurs exclusively in the nucleus, is dependent on the terminal differentiation of its host cell, the keratinocyte. Productive infection may influence the growth pattern of the host cell, resulting in disordered differentiation and proliferation, leading to wart formation, and is usually associated with a variety of nuclear changes. Histopathological changes (Fig. 6.5.2) include parabasal hyperplasia (acanthosis), hyperkeratosis, parakeratosis, dyskeratosis, cytoplasmic vacuolation (koilocytosis) and a range of other micromorphological changes. Cytological features (Plate 10) are characterized by koilocytosis, dyskeratosis and bi- or multinucleation. The nuclei vary in appearance and may show degenerative changes, usually in the form of pyknosis, borderline abnormalities or frank dyskaryosis. Koilocytosis may be identified in both histological and cytological material and is the specific cytopathic effect of HPV infection. Koilocytes are of superficial or intermediate squamous cell type and have a large perinuclear vacuole or halo which is sharply demarcated from the peripheral rim of condensed cytoplasm. Viral particles and capsid proteins are absent in the basal layer, as only the early genes of the virus are expressed in this layer. In contrast, both the early and late genes are expressed in the superficial differentiated layers of the epithelium, resulting in the presence of a large numbers of virus particles in

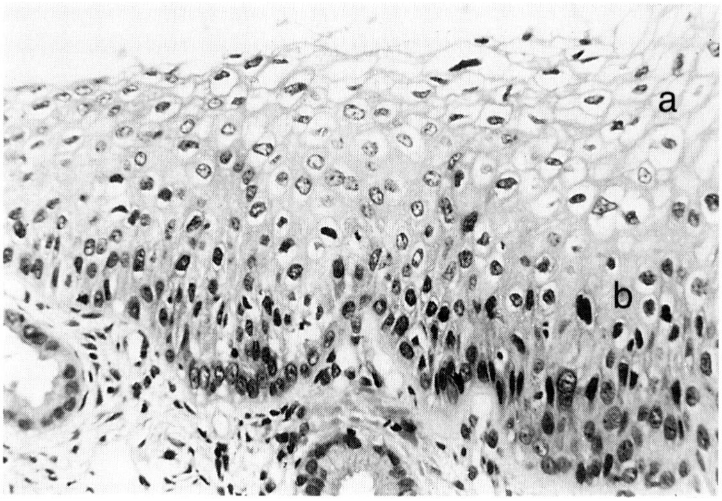

Fig. 6.5.2. HPV infection: histopathological changes showing koilocytosis (a) and CIN I (b).

the most superficial layers, a source for transmission to an unprotected contact.

Acuminate warts are characterized histopathologically by papillomatosis, an exophytic structure consisting of branching fibrovascular cores covered by thickened squamous epithelium, elongation and thickening of the rete ridges and accentuation of intracellular bridges. Within the epithelium, an array of microscopic epithelial features described above are seen. In the rare endophytic wart, the same histological findings are noted but with the branching extending down into the stroma. Clinically evident papular, macular and flat lesions have a similar histological pattern with less pronounced branching. Occasionally, warts may be pigmented, with melanin in basal cells and in some keratinocytes. Clinically these may be mistaken for pigmented intraepithelial neoplasia, seborrhoeic keratosis, or nevomelanocytic lesions.

The commonest type of subclinical lesion, invisible to the naked eye but evident on colposcopy, is variously described as 'flat wart', 'non-condylomatous wart virus infection' or 'subclinical wart virus infection'. Histologically, these lesions closely resemble condylomata acuminata without the papillomatous configuration and may show associated changes of cervical intraepithelial neoplasia (CIN) (see above).

Immunology

Although serum antibodies to papillomaviruses have been detected, humoral immunity has little or no influence in the natural history of infection. However, despite the latency of papillomaviruses, underlying its capacity for immune avoidance, the host's cellular immune response is widely assumed to be of key importance in the course and outcome of HPV infections. In the great majority of immunocompetent hosts, clinical infection is self-limiting, with spontaneous regression of warty lesions. The accompanying immune response, however, is usually transitory and not accompanied by clearance of the virus. Some form of tolerance or local immunosuppression rather than viral clearance seems the more probable response determining the course of anogenital HPV disease.

Clinical manifestations in men and women

Most GPV infections are asymptomatic. Patients present due to concern at discovering a growth or as contacts of partners with warts. In others, the condition is an incidental finding at clinical examination or on cervical cytology smears. However, some patients may have associated symptoms such as discomfort, pain and bleeding due to its location, size and extent, trauma or, rarely, malignant transformation.

Clinically apparent infection

Anogenital warts are polymorphic, varying considerably in size and in growth pattern, and may present as relatively flat and papular to markedly exophytic acuminate warts. Common warts occasionally appear in the genital area and may be associated with similar lesions in non-genital skin.

Acuminate warts

Condylomata acuminata (Plate 11) are soft, fleshy and vascular, with a pointed, irregular, fissured surface. The highly vascularized dermal core, often apparent to the naked eye, may, on magnification, show various capillary patterns (Plate 12) described as hair pin, corkscrew, hayfork or fan-like. They may bleed with trauma, for example during intercourse or wiping. Depending on the degree of keratinization, the colour may vary from pinkish red, through reddish white to greyish white. Acuminate warts may coalesce to form large cauliflower-like growths often seen in pregnancy and in more severely immunosuppressed individuals. They are found predominantly in moist and intertriginous areas, especially the sites liable to trauma during sexual intercourse. In the presence of poor hygiene, they may become macerated and malodorous.

In uncircumcized men, they often appear on the frenum, coronal sulcus, glans and inner lining of the prepuce (Plate 13). However, in circumcized men, the shaft of the penis is more frequently affected. They can also present on the scrotum and groin.

The male urethra is affected in about 10–25% of men, with nearly 80% involving the distal 2 cm (Plate 14). They are usually symptomless although some patients may complain of bleeding, discharge, dysuria or poor urine stream. Simple examination to ascertain the extent of the lesions may be difficult in men with a narrow meatus. However, extension beyond the fossa navicularis into the spongy urethra is rare and to the bladder is extremely rare. In the presence of persistent or recurrent meatal lesions or unexplained urinary symptoms, inspection of the proximal urethra may be necessary.

In women, the acuminate warts are the commonest clinical variety, and usually appear first in the vestibulum and on the posterior fourchette of the vulva. They may spread rapidly to involve other parts of the vulva, perineal and perianal areas. Involvement of the urethra is less likely than in men. The lesions may also appear on the vagina, and occasionally the entire vagina may be affected. The infection of the cervix is usually subclinical, but exophytic warts are not infrequent. The cervix is involved in about 6% of women with vulval warts and, rarely, may be the only site affected.

Perianal and anal warts (Fig. 6.5.3) occur in both sexes. Anal warts in men traditionally have been associated with practice of anal intercourse. However, anal warts are not uncommon in strictly heterosexual men, usually in coexistence with penile warts, although they may occur alone. The method of transmission of anal warts in heterosexual men is probably through self-inoculation from the penile lesions. In the homosexual population, anal warts are more frequent than penile warts. Over 70% of men with perianal warts practising receptive anal intercourse also have coexisting anal canal warts, usually confined to the area below the pectinate line. In women, concurrent occurrence of perineal warts is common, posterior spread being attributed to the close proximity to the vulva.

Although orogenital sex is a fairly common practice, condylomata acuminata of the mouth are infrequent. The lesions usually involve the tongue, lips, buccal mucosa, palate or alveolar ridge (Fig. 6.5.4). Laryngeal papillomatosis is discussed below.

Papular and clinically evident flat lesions

Warts tend to become more rounded or papular on fully keratinized drier genital areas such as the penile shaft, outer aspect of the foreskin, lateral parts

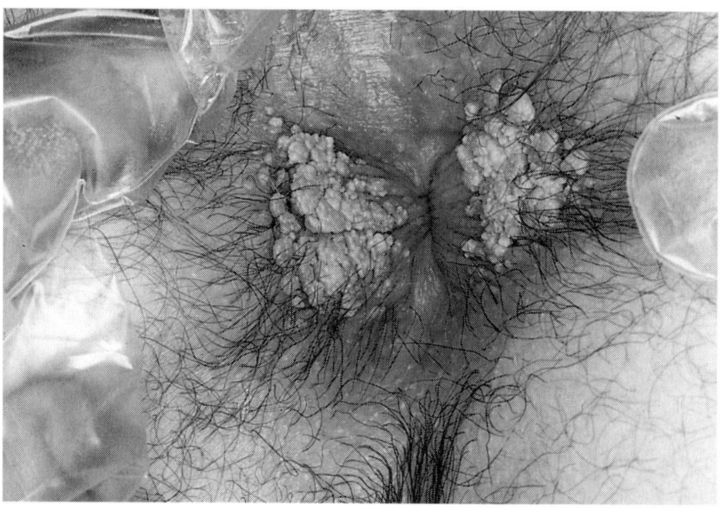

Fig. 6.5.3. Perianal condylomata acuminata.

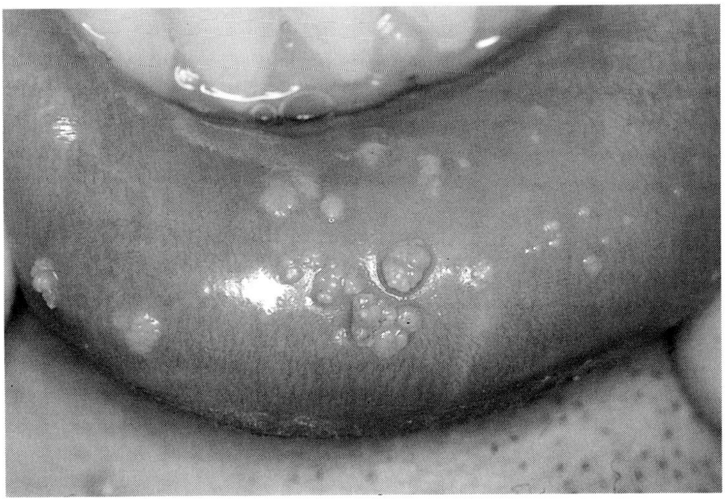

Fig. 6.5.4. Condylomas of the lip.

of the vulva, the perineum and the perianal area. Acuminate warts sometimes change into more papular types irrespective of anatomical site. The colour may be similar to acuminate warts, varying from pinkish red to greyish white, but often appears brownish when they grow on pigmented sites such as the penile shaft and the labia majora. The surface is smooth and velvety, unless covered by pronounced hyperkeratosis. They are often multiple, between 0.5 and 5 mm in diameter and tend to be dispersed rather than forming plaques.

Subclinical infection

Subclinical GPV infections are at least ten times as common as overt warts and are found coexisting in 60–70% of cases with overt warts. These lesions, frequently coexisting with and often indistinguishable from CIN, were first described on the cervix, observed under magnification with a colposcope, on application of 3–5% acetic acid (Plate 15). Identical lesions appear to be very common in the outer genitalia as well. In the female, the vulva and the perineal area are often covered with isolated macular lesions which are seen to coalesce on the medial aspect of the labia minora. Similar lesions are found commonly on the glans penis and the prepuce. Acetowhiting, however, is not a specific test and can be falsely positive. In both sexes, subclinical infection may be associated with superficial epithelial fissuring, especially in the posterior fourchette and perineal area in the female and the prepuce in the male. This may occur with symptoms, in the female, of severe superficial dyspareunia and vulvodynia and, in the male, itching, burning and discomfort at intercourse. Similar lesions may be noted in the perianal region of homosexual men practising receptive anal intercourse.

Clinical manifestations in special situations

Infants and children

Although rare, the occurrence of anogenital warts in prepubertal children is well documented, with a female to male ratio of 2.6 : 1. Whilst subclinical infection has not been described, a similar clinical spectrum to that found in adults could be expected. Demonstration of HPV2, -3, -6, -11 and -16 DNA sequences in wart material from children suggests different modes of acquisition. Manifestation of anogenital warts in infants several weeks after birth suggests transmission from the mother during delivery. Rarely they may be present at birth, indicating antenatal infection. When they occur in older children, this may be due to reactivation of latent infection acquired at birth or due to acquisition postnatally by non-sexual or sexual means. It is believed that they may follow close non-sexual contact with the family, or auto-inoculation or transfer of HPV types 2 and 3 from hand warts of the child or parent. However, sexual abuse must be considered, but utmost discretion should be used as the long incubation period, the existence of several possible routes of infection and poor correlation of HPV type with wart morphology cause problems in interpreting their significance.

Laryngeal papillomatosis

HPV types 6 and 11 have now been confirmed as the aetiological agents of benign papillomata occurring in the respiratory tract. These papillary lesions developing on the vocal cords may spread to other parts of the larynx and to the trachea, and cause obstructive symptoms. Juvenile laryngeal papillomata are closely associated with maternal genital warts, and cause symptoms in the neonatal, infant and preschool years. Whilst it is believed that transmission occurs at the time of delivery, the observed low rate of clinical laryngeal papillomata remains unexplained, with insufficient evidence to advocate delivery by Caesarean section for women with genital warts. It is unknown whether adult-onset laryngeal papillomatosis is acquired at birth or in later life via orogenital contact.

Pregnancy

Existing anogenital warts may enlarge considerably or they may appear for the first time in pregnancy due to reactivation of latent or subclinical GPV, probably facilitated by the natural immunosuppression of pregnancy. Although rarely causing obstruction to delivery, the increase in size and extent in pregnancy may result in physical discomfort, bleeding and poor healing of the episiotomy site. Spontaneous regression, partial or complete, often occurs in the puerperium. It is probably associated with immunostimulation induced by exposure of viral antigens by local trauma and inflammation at parturition.

GPV infection in immunosuppressed or immunodeficient patients

Individuals with chronic immunosuppression either associated with disease, inherited, acquired (e.g. AIDS) or due to immunosuppressive therapy, have a higher prevalence of and are prone to multiple and therapeutically intractable genital condylomata acuminata compared with immunocompetent persons. It is also not uncommon to observe substantial enlargement of condylomata acuminata, especially in women, in association with these conditions. Additionally, there is a 8- to 14-fold observed increased incidence over that expected for HPV-associated malignant and premalignant lesions of the cervix, vagina and vulva in female transplant recipients. An increased incidence of these lesions is also observed respectively, in the lower genital tract and the rectal mucosa in HIV-infected females and homosexual males. The need for close surveillance of immunosuppressed patients is emphasized by the heightened potential for malignant transformation of the premalignant lesions regardless of the HPV types.

HPV and genital neoplasia

Buschke Loewenstein tumour (giant condyloma)

Giant condyloma is a rare condition. Here, an initial wart-like lesion undergoes relentless enlargement to produce a foul-smelling, exudating or haemorrhagic exuberant cauliflower-like non-metastasizing growth. It is associated with extensive local destruction, with formation of multiple fistulae. Lesions are usually single and, although in most recorded cases the penis has been affected, they have been reported on the vulvovaginal and anorectal areas. Although papillomavirus particles have not been identified, its viral origin is suggested by the histological identity with condylomata acuminata and the presence of HPV6 and -11 DNA sequences in some specimens. An inherent feature, differentiating it from the common condylomata acuminata, is the simultaneous exophytic and endophytic growth patterns that result in penetration into the subcutaneous fat. However, deeper invasion, local lymph node involvement and distant metastases are absent, suggesting a benign nature, although malignant transformation into metastasizing squamous carcinoma has been reported.

GPV-associated premalignant and malignant lesions of the lower genital tract

The intraepithelial neoplastic changes are now well recognized not only in the cervix (CIN) but also in the vulva (VIN), vagina (VaIN), penis (PIN), perianal area and anal canal (AIN). Lesions are classified according to severity as grades 1, 2 and 3.

Cervix

Worldwide, cervical cancer is the second commonest cancer in women, with 460,000 cases reported per year, 77% occurring in non-industrialized countries where it is the leading cancer. It is assumed that most invasive cervical squamous cell cancers are preceded by CIN, occurring in the transformation zone. There is good epidemiological evidence to suggest a sexually transmitted aetiology, notably HPV, for CIN and cervical cancer. The postulated role of HHV-2 has been undermined by the failure consistently to detect HHV-2-specific DNA in cervical cancer biopsy samples.

HPV types 6 and 11 are associated mainly with genital warts and low-grade CIN lesions with polyploid nuclear DNA content. However, HPV types 16 and 18 are associated with lesions with aneuploid DNA content and are found consistently in higher grades of CIN, invasive cervical, vulval, penile and anal cancer. Whereas in the premalignant stage the viral DNA is predominantly episomal and remains circular and replicating free of cellular chromosomes, in over 90% of cervical cancers the virus is usually truncated, linear and integrated into host cellular DNA. The integration of HPV16 or -18 DNA into cellular DNA occurs in a specific manner at E1 or E2 ORFs of the HPV genome. The disruption of the circular viral genome in the course of integration removes the repressor activity of E1 and E2, resulting in deregulated expression of the transforming genes E6 and E7. This may result in inhibition of differentiation and immortalization of the host cell and, together with other factors such as oncogene activation, chromosomal rearrangements and external cofactors, may produce a cell with invasive properties. The exact role of HPV in malignant conversion is not yet clear.

Whilst 30–40% of untreated CIN 3 lesions progress to cancer, the majority of CIN 1 lesions have a low malignant potential and progression to cancer is unlikely. Since all CIN lesions do not proceed to malignant transformation, one agent alone is most unlikely to cause cervical cancer. It is believed that malignant transformation results from synergistic interactions with one or more external and internal cofactors, such as concurrent infection with HSV, smoking or immunological status.

Vulva, vagina and penis

Knowledge of the natural history of VIN, VaIN, AIN and PIN is limited, and it is believed that the malignant potential is far less than with CIN. The clinical presentation of VIN is quite variable, frequently being asymptomatic. When symptomatic, pruritus, burning and superficial dyspareunia are the commonest complaints. The clinical appearance of these lesions can also vary. They may present as solitary or multiple, partially pigmented, macular and papular lesions. Occasionally, colposcopic evaluation with application of 3–5% acetic acid may be necessary to identify subclinical lesions. Biopsy is mandatory if neoplastic change is suspected. HPV DNA has been demonstrated in 40–70% of VIN 3 and invasive squamous vulval cancer, with two-thirds positive for HPV16. VIN and vulval cancer with a non-viral aetiology are found in older women, whilst papillomavirus appears to be associated with neoplastic change in younger women. The latter may have multicentric intraepithelial neoplasia involving the cervical, vaginal and perianal sites. Malignant conversion of HPV-associated VIN is low, varying from 0 to 6%.

A range of clinical types of PIN, associated with HPV, similar to VIN have been described. The lack of a transformation zone on the penis compared with the cervix probably accounts for the low malignant potential of PIN and the relative rarity of penile cancer. Although HPV types (predominantly 16) have been found in up to 40% of penile cancers, their exact role is unclear.

VaIN is rare, occurring mainly multifocally in the upper third of the vagina and is usually seen in association with CIN. A high percentage of VaIN harbour HPV DNA. However, malignant transformation of VaIN is unusual, with primary vaginal squamous carcinoma being among the rarest malignancies of the female genital tract. A correlation between vaginal cancer and HPV16 and -18 has been reported.

Anus

The risk of anal cancer in homosexual men, especially in those practising receptive anal intercourse, has been recognized for some time. Many of the risk factors associated with cervical neoplasia are also associated with rectal cancer. HPV16 and HPV18 DNA have been identified in AIN and anal malignancies and are implicated in the aetiology of anal squamous cancer.

Differential diagnosis

Exophytic anogenital warts can usually be differentiated with confidence from other papular lesions in the area, including normal anatomical variants and infective and neoplastic conditions without the necessity of biopsy. In the male, prominent Tyson's glands, multiple yellow ectopic sebaceous cysts (Fordyce's spots – Plate 16) and prominent coronal papillae (Plate 17) may sometimes be confused with warts. Similarly, in females, small sebaceous glands and vestibular papillae (Plate 18) may pose diagnostic difficulties, needing colposcopic evaluation and biopsy. Warts must also be differentiated from hymenal and anal tags, fibroepithelial polyps, hidradenomata and other benign neoplasms.

Of the infective lesions, molluscum contagiosum (Chapter 6.6) is usually easily diagnosed by its characteristic smooth, umbilicated appearance. More importantly, the skin lesions of secondary syphilis [condylomata lata and papular skin eruptions (Chapter 7.1)], should be considered in the differential diagnosis. The lesions of granuloma inguinale (Donovanosis; Chapter 7.7) may superficially resemble anogenital warts.

Diagnosis and investigations

Genital warts are often associated with the presence of other STI. The patient should, therefore, be examined carefully and tests for full STI screen taken as described in Chapter 4. Anoscopy is required when there are perianal warts or a history of anal intercourse. Sexual partners should always be examined carefully for the presence of GPV infection and other STI. In children, the presence of another STI may be of medicolegal importance.

Biopsy of vulval, perineal and penile lesions is indicated, when the appearance is atypical or response to treatment is poor, to exclude neoplasia and other non-neoplastic conditions. The flat intraepithelial lesions of the vulva and penis may resemble or indeed coexist with genital warts. Although colposcopic criteria for distinguishing CIN from HPV have been described, it is often not possible to make a complete distinction between the lesions, and biopsy is mandatory. Similarly, exophytic lesions of the cervix must be biopsied as they might conceal significant CIN or even frank carcinoma (Plate 19).

Since women with genital warts have shown high rates of cytological abnormalities indicating underlying CIN, they should have cervical cytology with colposcopy reserved for those with cervical warts or dyskaryotic smears. In immunosuppressed women, surveillance with cervical cytology and colposcopy of the lower genital tract should, ideally, be carried out at 6-monthly intervals (see also Chapter 11.3).

Treatment

Treatment of clinical genital warts is advocated: (i) because the disease is worrying for the patients; (ii) to prevent or reduce transmission; and (iii) because of its association with neoplasia. However, in the absence of specific antiviral therapy, there is no evidence to suggest that conventional treatment of warts eradicates the viral infection and prevents transmission or neoplasia.

Of the many treatment methods, no one method has proved to be superior to the others. The choice of therapy depends on many factors, such as site, size, number, morphological appearance, immune status, pregnancy and cost, as well as the patient's preference. Recurrence of the disease is a major problem. The use of condoms and avoidance of oral sex should be advocated during treatment.

Treatment of clinical warts

Podophyllin and podophyllotoxin

Podophyllin resin is an impure extract of the roots of the plant *Podophyllum peltatum* or *P. emodi* composed of at least four cytotoxic chemicals, the most potent being podophyllotoxin. It is often the first line treatment of unkeratinized warts. Podophyllin, as a 15–25% solution in ethanol or tincture of benzoin is applied to warts, allowed to dry, and then covered with talcum powder, once or twice a week. In view of its local effects such as burn, ulceration and swelling, it should be applied under medical/nursing supervision and must be washed off 4–6 h later (1–2 h in the case of meatal warts). Not more than 0.5 ml of the solution should be applied at any one time, otherwise systemic toxicity, due to absorption, can be a serious problem. A variety of neurological, haematological and hepatic complications leading even to death have been recorded. When absorbed, it has a teratogenic effect and therefore should not be used in pregnancy. Similarly, because of its potential carcinogenic effect, it must not be used on the cervix and upper vagina. The preparation itself is relatively unstable, leading to crystallization with unpredictable therapeutic and toxic effects. If there is no improvement after 4 weeks, the treatment modality should be changed.

Podophyllotoxin, the purified active ingredient, is now available as a 0.5% solution and a paste. These preparations are pure, stable and standardized and much less toxic than the impure resin with minimal systemic absorption. If warts are easily accessible, this preparation can be used by the patient at home twice daily for 3 days followed by a 4-day interval to a maximum of four courses of treatment. The manufacturer's instructions should be followed regarding the amount to be used at any one time. It is not necessary to wash off the medication, unless unforeseen local reaction occurs. Most patients experience mild irritation. It is recommended for the treatment of anogenital warts in men and women, but contraindicated in pregnancy.

Trichloracetic acid

Trichloracetic acid (90%), a caustic agent, is considered to be effective for small warts. Since it has no systemic toxicity, it is the preferred treatment in pregnancy. As it can cause serious skin burns and pain, it should be applied carefully to the wart, and then covered with talcum powder, once a week. If there is no response after six applications, an alternative therapy should be considered.

5-Fluorouracil

5-Fluorouracil is a powerful cytotoxic drug and has been used as a 5% cream for the treatment of resistant genital warts and in particular urethral condylomata. In view of its unproven efficacy and side effects, such as ulceration and occasional intolerable pain, it is not in general use. It is potentially teratogenic and its use is contraindicated in pregnancy.

Cryotherapy

Cryodestruction of tissue can be achieved by the application of freezing agents to living tissue. Three main agents, liquid nitrogen, which is chemically inactive and non-toxic with a boiling point of –196°C, nitrous oxide (N_2O), a gas at –130°C, and carbon dioxide snow at –94°C are all used in the treatment of warts. All three agents can be delivered as a continuous flow in a closed system. Additionally, liquid nitrogen can be applied by a cotton wool-tipped swabstick. On application of the agent, the freezing temperature induces intracellular ice crystals and cellular dehydration. This will lead to tissue necrosis through mechanical and complex biochemical effects and a specific immunological response against autologous antigens of the frozen tissues. The best effect is obtained by double application of rapid freezing, with slow spontaneous thawing in between applications. Freezing should continue until an iceball 1–4 mm larger than the lesion is formed and, depending on the size of lesion, this may take 0.5–4 min. The area should be kept stretched during cryotherapy to avoid trauma to the unaffected parts. Treatment, although painful in most cases, can be achieved without local anaesthetic. The patient should be warned that the area may throb soon after treatment and may result in a blister within a few hours. Occasionally, pronounced oedema may follow but will usually respond to antihistamines, analgesics or cold compression. If performed properly, there should be no scarring. It is a safe method for use in pregnancy. Because of the possible risk of perforation and fistula formation, use of a cryoprobe in the vagina needs considerable care.

Surgical excision, cautery and laser

Most small filiform or papillomatous warts in the vulval, perineal and penile skin can be curetted easily with a Volkman's spoon of appropriate size using ethyl chloride spray or other appropriate local anaesthetic. They can also be removed under local anaesthetic by electrodesiccation with a 'Hyfrecator' or by burning with electrocautery. More extensive warts may need electrocautery or diathermy under general anaesthetic, but care must be taken to avoid scarring and anal stenosis. The scissor excision technique using local infiltrate to raise the lesions above the surrounding skin for the treatment of perianal and intraanal warts can achieve good results.

Originally used for treatment of CIN, the CO_2 laser increasingly is being used for treatment of genital warts under colposcopic vision, permitting precise control of the extent and depth of tissue destruction avoiding scarring. Healing is rapid with minimal inflammation. Small lesions can be treated under local anaesthetic, but extensive disease may need general anaesthesia.

Immunomodulating and other therapies

Systemic and intralesional injection of α-interferon has shown some effect against genital warts through immune stimulation of cell-mediated immunity. Treatment is associated with numerous hospital visits, frequent and painful injections and dose-related side effects including headache, fever, leukopenia, and elevation of liver enzymes. Its value in the management of anogenital warts has not been established. At present, there are no useful topical antiviral agents.

Treatment in pregnancy

Podophylline and podophyllotoxin are contraindicated in pregnancy. Although warts often regress during the puerperium, many specialists prefer to treat warts during pregnancy. Cryotherapy, electrocautery, trichloracetic acid or CO_2 laser may be used. Caesarean section is indicated rarely when the warts are so profuse and extensive as to interfere with vaginal delivery.

Treatment of children

In most children, warts disappear spontaneously over a period of months to 3 years. The treatment, if necessary, is with careful application of a cytotoxic agent or mechanical destruction.

Treatment of subclinical infection

Management of subclinical lesions depends on the presence and the degree of any associated intraepithelial neoplasia. Such lesions, especially on the cervix and vulva, should be assessed and managed by an expert colposcopist. Whilst lesions with grades up to VIN 2 and CIN 1 are generally managed conservatively, those lesions with VIN 3 or CIN 2 or greater should be treated. Recommended modalities for treatment of CIN, usually as an out-patient procedure under local anaesthetic, are laser, diathermy loop excision and cold coagulation.

Conclusion

GPV infection has become a major cause of morbidity and concern to health care professionals in view of the rising incidence and the close association with lower genital neoplasia. In the absence of any useful antiviral therapy and the not too bright prospects of an effective vaccine, prevention is based mainly on health education and behaviour modification to reduce or prevent transmission of GPV.

Further reading

Mindel, A. (1995) *Genital Warts Human Papillomavirus Infection*, 1st edn. Edward Arnold, London.

Munoz, N., Boshch, F.X., Shah, K.V. and Meheus, A. (1992) *The Epidemiology of Human Papillomavirus and Cervical Cancer*, 1st edn. International Agency for Research on Cancer, Lyon.

Stern, P.L. and Stanley, M.A. (1994) *Human Papillomaviruses and Cervical Cancer – Biology and Immunology*, 1st edn. Oxford University Press, Oxford.

CHAPTER 6.6.
Molluscum contagiosum

C.A. Hart
Department of Medical Microbiology and Genitourinary Medicine, University of Liverpool, Liverpool, UK

Molluscum contagiosum is a benign skin condition spread by contact. It can be transmitted sexually but more often non-venereally.

Epidemiology

Most often this is a mild disease which may not be reported to physicians. It occurs in all age groups and may be spread sexually and non-sexually. The sexual spread of molluscum contagiosum is inferred from its frequent occurrence in those with multiple sexual partners or who buy sex, and its co-occurrence with other STI. Sexually transmitted molluscum contagiosum tends to occur primarily on the lower abdomen, thighs, genitalia and buttocks. In the UK, in the decade from 1971, the number of cases recorded at STI clinics increased fourfold to represent 0.27% of cases attending the clinics. Since the advent of HIV and AIDS, the number of cases has increased further.

Surveys of non-sexual transmission have been limited largely to children, and prevalence rates of 6–22% have been reported from Fiji, Papua New Guinea and Japan. Attack rates in previously unexposed children range from 12 to 75%. No such data are available for sexually transmitted molluscum contagiosum.

The causative organism

The agent is a large DNA virus of the molluscipox family. On electron microscopy (Fig. 6.6.1) it has a typical poxviral brick shape (300 × 220 × 100 nm) and is sometimes described as looking like a ball of string. The virus has never been maintained successfully in artificial culture. However, using restriction endonuclease digestion of viral DNA obtained from lesions, two subtypes (MCV-I and II) have been delineated. MCV-I is the most prevalent type, but neither type is associated exclusively with sexual or non-sexual transmission. MCV-II has been found only rarely in children under 15 years.

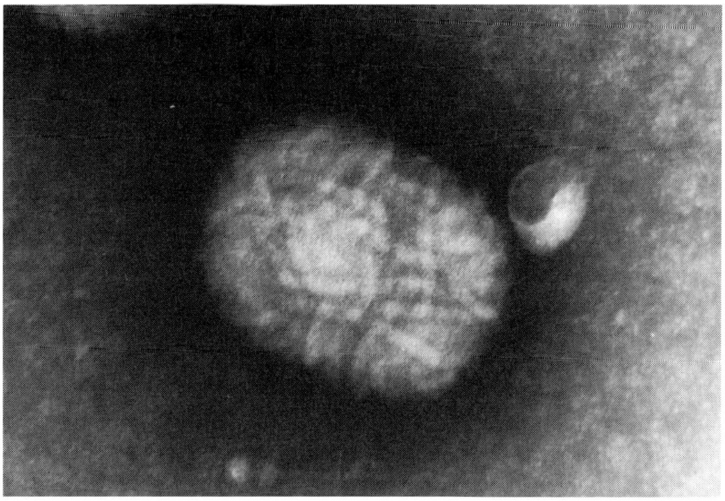

Fig. 6.6.1. Molluscum contagiosum virus: negative stain electron micrograph.

Transmission

Transmission occurs directly person to person by close skin contact such as when sexually acquired. It can also occur indirectly via fomites such as in swimming pools, towels, gymnasium equipment and benches.

Pathogenesis and immunity

Molluscum contagiosum lesions consist of focal areas of hyperplastic epidermis surrounding lobules filled with keratinized debris and degenerating molluscum bodies. They are usually confined to the epidermal layer. Anti-MCV antibodies can be detected during and after infection, but their role in immunity is unclear. The period prior to resolution of disease is often marked by an inflammatory response in the lesion. That infection is more common in children than adults suggests that immunity develops. That patients with AIDS and other T-cell deficiencies tend to have more widespread and florid infections suggests a role for T cell-mediated immunity.

Clinical features

The incubation period of molluscum contagiosum is on average 2–3 months. Most patients are asymptomatic but, in some, the lesions may itch or be tender. The lesions begin as small papules which grow to 3–10 mm in diameter over the next 3–4 weeks. The mature lesions are small, firm and dome-shaped, with central umbilication (Plate 20) expressing caseous material. They are usually flesh-coloured but may be pearl-grey, yellow or pink. In the immunocompetent host, there are on average 20–30 lesions (range 1–100), which in sexually acquired infection are in the genital region, lower abdomen and thighs. Approximately 10% of children will have genital lesions. More widespread infection occurs in eczematous skin or in patients with atopic dermatitis, especially if they are using corticosteroids. In patients with AIDS, T-cell deficiencies or immunosuppression, lesions are multiple, widespread and disfiguring. The distribution even in male homosexuals with AIDS tends to be on the face and trunk rather than on the genitalia (see also Chapter 11.5). The differential diagnosis includes cutaneous and genital warts, keratoacanthomas and cutaneous cryptococcosis in AIDS. The average duration of molluscum contagiosum is 2 years, but individual lesions may persist for 2-6 months. In AIDS patients, the lesions may persist for longer, continue to erupt and recur despite treatment.

The major complication of molluscum contagiosum is secondary bacterial infection which may occur in up to 40% of cases, especially if attempts are made by patients to remove the lesions. Molluscum dermatitis may occur in less than 8% of patients from 1 to 15 months after onset. This consists of eczematous halos around lesions with a radius of up to 5 cm, but not all the patient's lesions will necessarily show this.

Diagnosis

If necessary, molluscum bodies can be shelled out, or samples taken with a needle. These can be transported to the laboratory in a sterile dry container. Routine histopathological tests will show the characteristic features of molluscum contagiosum. However, for rapid diagnosis, negative stain electron microscopy of the material will show the characteristic molluscipox viral particles.

In most cases (except perhaps medicolegal and AIDS), the diagnosis is made clinically.

Treatment

None of the suggested treatments has undergone controlled trials. They range from squeezing lesions, applying a sharpened wooden stick dipped in phenol or tincture of iodine, to curettage, cautery and cryotherapy. In AIDS patients, no form of treatment (other than antiretroviral therapy) is highly effective. No vaccines are available nor is it likely that there will be in the near to medium future.

Chapter 6.7
Viral hepatitis

C.A. Hart
Department of Medical Microbiology and Genitourinary Medicine, University of Liverpool, Liverpool, UK

Hepatitis is not necessarily infective in nature, for example the inflammation can be caused by toxins (e.g. aphlatoxin), chemicals (e.g. carbon tetrachloride), drugs (e.g. paracetamol) or auto-immunity. Nevertheless, there is a large list of infectious causes of hepatitis (e.g. HHV-4, HHV-5, yellow fever, leptospirosis), but this chapter will concentrate on the known hepatitis viruses (Table 6.7.1).

Hepatitis A virus (HAV)

HAV is a small (28 nm) unenveloped virus with a single-stranded positive sense RNA genome (Table 6.7.1). It is a picornavirus in the genus *Hepatovirus*. It is solely a human pathogen and is spread predominantly by the faeco-oral route. In developing countries, HAV infection occurs early in childhood, with almost all having been infected by 10 years of age. In contrast, only 15–25% of those aged 20 years in developed countries are HAV seropositive. Most HAV infections are sporadic, but outbreaks can occur associated with food (e.g. shellfish), water or in day-care centres or crèches for children. As with other faecally excreted pathogens, sexual transmission of HAV can occur. This is much more apparent in developed countries when it is often homosexually acquired as a result of oroanal exposure.

The incubation period for HAV is 2–6 weeks (average 4 weeks). Infection in children is often asymptomatic (90% of those under 3 years), whereas infections in adults usually result in jaundice and may be severe. The onset of infection is abrupt, but may follow a short prodromal period of low-grade pyrexia, malaise and headache. Illness usually begins with anorexia, vomiting and, especially in children, diarrhoea, and is rapidly followed by jaundice. Recovery is rapid and liver enzymes return to normal within 6 weeks of onset. Chronic hepatitis following HAV has only ever been reported in one patient. HAV accounts for only 10% of cases of fulminant hepatitis. There are rare reports of encephalitis associated with HAV. There is apparently no interaction between HAV and HIV.

Specific diagnosis is by detection of anti-HAV IgM which will be positive at the time of onset of jaundice. There is no specific antiviral chemotherapy. Passive protection can be given by administration of immune globulin. Post-exposure prophylaxis (0.02 ml kg^{-1} intramuscularly) is 80–90% effective when

Table 6.7.1. Comparison of hepatitis viruses.

	Family	Size	Genome	Spread	Vaccine	Chemotherapy
Hepatitis A	Hepatovirus	28 nm unenveloped	Single-stranded positive sense RNA	Faeco-oral	Killed whole virus	No
Hepatitis B	Hepadnavirus	50 nm enveloped	Partially double-stranded DNA loop	Parenteral	Subunit (HBsAg)	Lamivudine, interferon
Hepatitis C	Hepacivirus	40 nm enveloped	Single-stranded positive sense RNA	Parenteral	No	Ribavirin, interferon
Hepatitis D	Unclassified	35 nm unenveloped	Single-stranded incomplete negative sense RNA loop	Parenteral	Hepatitis B vaccine	No
Hepatitis E	Calicivirus	32 nm unenveloped	Single-stranded positive sense RNA	Faeco-oral	No	No
Hepatitis G	Flavivirus	40 nm enveloped	Single-stranded positive sense RNA	Parenteral	No	No

given within 2 weeks of exposure. Pre-exposure prophylaxis (0.06 ml kg^{-1} intramuscularly every 5 months) can be given to travellers to endemic areas. However, it is far better to give active immunization. The current vaccine is formalin-killed whole HAV, which provides solid protection for at least 2–3 years.

Hepatitis B virus (HBV)

HBV is a small (42–50 nm) enveloped DNA virus. The genome is a partially (50–80% of its length) double-stranded DNA loop within an icosahedral capsid. The capsid carries the hepatitis B core antigen (HBcAg). Outside the nucleocapsid is a lipid envelope with glycoprotein spikes which form the hepatitis B surface antigen (HBsAg). The hepatitis B e-antigen (HBeAg) can be found on disruption of the virus but, more importantly, is secreted from infected hepatocytes and its presence is inferred as a marker of high infectivity. During either acute HBV infection or in persistently infected patients, virus is released into the bloodstream and three different particles can be seen (Fig. 6.7.1). The complete virion (sometimes called the Dane particle) carries HBsAg, HBcAg and viral DNA, and is infective. The other two are vesicular and tubular particles which are in essence the viral envelope. They express HBsAg but do not have HBcAg nor HBV DNA and are thus non-infective. During acute HBV infection, there are large numbers of Dane particles in the bloodstream. Chronic carriers will have varying ratios of Dane to tubular and vesicular particles, and the higher the ratio the more infectious the patient.

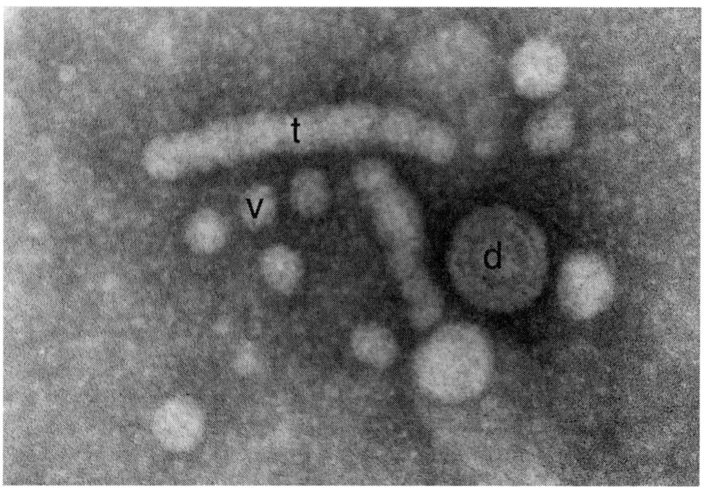

Fig. 6.7.1. Hepatitis B virus: negative stain electron micrograph of serum showing a complete virion (Dane particle d) and tubular (t) and vesicular (v) particles.

Epidemiology and transmission

HBV is solely a human pathogen and it is maintained by the 200–300 million persistently infected patients (carriers) worldwide. The prevalence of infection and chronic carriage are highest in China, Southeast Asia and sub-Saharan Africa, where 80–90% of the population have serological evidence of past or current infection and 20–30% are persistently infected. The Indian subcontinent, Middle East, Mediterranean Africa and Europe, Russia and South and Central America are areas of intermediate carriage rates, with 5–10% of adults being persistently infected. Northern Europe, North America and Australia (except for the Aborigines) have low infection (10%) and carriage (<0.1%) rates. HBV is spread by blood to blood contact. In developing countries, transmission of HBV occurs most frequently at delivery from carrier mother to neonate or in the first 5 years of life through cuts and grazes between family members. Infection at this time is more likely to be asymptomatic and result in persistent carriage. HBV is also transmitted by blood or blood products, organ transplantation and by needle-stick (there is up to a 25% risk if the donor is HBeAg positive). Transmission by large blood-sucking insects has also been suggested. HBsAg and HBeAg can be found in saliva and semen of chronic carriers. There is no doubt that HBV can be transmitted sexually, both homosexually and heterosexually. Risk factors for male homosexuals are rectal intercourse and multiplicity of partners. There is an increased prevalence of HBV seropositivity in prostitutes and attendees of STI clinics. In addition, sexual partners of HBV carriers have a higher incidence of HBV seropositivity than the general population.

Clinical features and diagnosis

The incubation period of HBV infection is 2–6 months (average 4 months). Approximately 30% of adults who become infected with HBV remain asymptomatic. However, HBV hepatitis is usually a much more severe infection than HAV. The onset is insidious, and 15–20% of patients develop erythematous macular, maculopapular or urticarial skin rashes, polyarthralgia and arthritis during the prodromal period. Some patients experience anorexia, abdominal discomfort, nausea, vomiting and may develop jaundice. Approximately 1% of adults with HBV will develop fulminant hepatitis and die. Recovery from HBV hepatitis is slower than for HAV, and approximately 10% of adults become chronic carriers. The risk of developing persistent infection is greater for intravenous drug users and for immune compromised patients. Up to a third of chronic carriers will develop chronic active hepatitis which may progress to cirrhosis. Hepatocellular carcinoma is another long-term result of persistent HBV infection and can occur in up to 50% of chronic carriers after an interval of, on average, 35 years. Some patients with persistent HBV infection develop immune complex disease manifested by necrotizing vasculitis, chronic glomerulonephritis and cryoglobulinaemia. HBV has the potential to promote HIV replication, but there is little clinical evidence to suggest that HBV speeds the progression to AIDS. HIV infection decreases response to HBV vaccine and increases HBV load but decreases liver damage (which is thought to be mediated by a cytotoxic T-lymphocyte response to HBV-infected hepatocytes). Diagnosis of acute HBV hepatitis is by detection of HBsAg, HBV DNA and anti-HBc IgM (Table 6.7.2). The last is measured to exclude the possibility that the episode is occurring due to another agent in a person persistently infected with HBV. In persistent HBV infection, the patient would also have detectable anti-HBc and anti-HBs IgG. Screening for asymptomatic chronic carriers is by detection of HBsAg or HBV DNA. Such carriers will also have detectable anti-HBc IgG. Detection of HBeAg in a carrier indicates that they are highly infective. A recently described exception is in patients with HBV pre-core mutants, which do not produce HbeAg, yet are highly infective.

Management and prevention

Treatment has been attempted using α-interferon and various nucleoside analogues alone or in combination. Interferon (very expensive) is useful in treating HIV-uninfected HBe antigenaemic carriers (10 million units thrice weekly for 12 weeks). A 40% success rate in clearing HBe antigenaemia and HBV DNA is reported. Lamivudine (3TC) has been used to treat HBV infection, but resistance develops rapidly. Famciclovir has been used with some success in treating HBV infection even though HBV does not possess thymidine kinase.

Prevention by passive or active immunization is possible. Passive protection is given as post-exposure prophylaxis in unimmunized recipients of needle-stick injuries involving HBV-infected persons, to babies born to HBsAg-positive mothers, and to sexual partners of patients with acute HBV

Table 6.7.2 Markers of hepatitis.

Markers	Nature	How measured	Significance
Antigens			
HBsAg	Envelope glycoprotein	ELISA	Indicates current, acute or chronic infection
HBcAg	Part of viral capsid	ELISA	Usually present in acute infection
HBeAg	Released by infected hepatocytes	ELISA	Presence indicates high infectivity
Genome			
HBV DNA	Viral genome	PCR, DNA hybridization	Presence indicates viral replication, high levels correlate with infectivity
Antibodies			
IgM anti-HBc		ELISA	Indicates recent infection
IgG anti-HBc		ELISA	Indicates infection at some time in past. Used for seroepidemiological studies
Anti-HBs		ELISA	Indicates infection or immunization at some time in past. Used to measure vaccine efficacy
Anti-HBe		ELISA	Marker of lower infectivity

infection. Hepatitis B immunoglobulin is given intramuscularly as soon as possible (within 48 h) after the incident or delivery, and no later than 1 week after exposure in the case of sexual partners who may be tested for susceptibility to HBV infection (anti-HBc, anti-HBs, HBsAg) to decide whether to continue with the vaccination schedule, the first dose already having been given. Neonates and children up to 4 years old should be given 200 units, children from 5 to 9 years 300 units and adults and children of 10 years and above 500 units (i.e. a 5-ml ampoule). The patient should be started on a course of active immunization at the same time, but injected into a different site.

HBV can only be grown with difficulty so the routes chosen to produce vaccine for active immunization are indirect. The first vaccine was made by plasmapheresing persistently infected patients, separating out the 22-nm vesicular HBsAg particles and inactivating any Dane particles with formalin. This vaccine is safe, immunogenic (95% of subjects become anti-HBs positive) and protective (89–91%) but no longer available in some countries (e.g. the UK). Serum anti-HBs levels seem to correlate with protection ($\geq$100 IU l^{-1}). If the anti-HBs level is less than 100 IU l^{-1}, a booster should be given and the level rechecked after 2 months. The vaccine should not be frozen or be given in the buttocks since this decreases the immune response.

The second approach uses genetic engineering. The gene encoding HBsAg was inserted into a yeast which then expressed a large amount of the non-glycosylated envelope protein. This was used (10 μg per dose for HB-Vax II and 20 μg per dose for Engerix B) as the vaccine. In children under 12 years, half the dose is used. It has a similar efficacy and safety profile to the plasma-derived vaccine. Each recombinant vaccine is given as three (1 ml per dose for adults) injections into the deltoid region (or anterolateral thigh in infants) at 0, 1 and 6 months. Anti-HBs levels should be checked 2–4 months after the final dose. A level of less than 10 IU l^{-1} indicates non-response, and the whole course should be repeated. Non-response after a further course could mean either a true non-responder or the patient is already infected with HBV. A level of over 100 IU l^{-1} indicates a protective response, and those with levels of 10–100 IU l^{-1} require a further booster dose. Boosters may be necessary every 3–5 years. For rapid immunization, e.g. for travellers or following exposure to the virus, an accelerated schedule may be used when the third dose is given at 2 months with a booster at 12 months. The best strategy in developing countries would be universal immunization in the neonatal period. In certain countries, this has already produced a decrease in HBV infection and in the incidence of hepatocellular carcinoma in children (see also Chapter 12.2).

Hepatitis C virus (HCV)

This virus has never been grown in artificial culture. Its nature was determined by transmission to monkeys and molecular cloning. It is an enveloped single-stranded positive sense RNA virus approximately 40 nm in diameter. It is a member of the *Flaviviridae* (genus *Hepacivirus*) although it is not transmitted by an insect vector. HCV shows tremendous genomic diversity and mutates to produce quasi-species within a patient. However, HCV can be subdivided into six genotypes with at least 40 subtypes based on variations in its 9000 ribonucleotide base sequence. Genotypes 1a, 1b, 2a, 2b and 3a are more common in Europe and the USA, genotype 3 is common in the Indian subcontinent, whereas genotype 4 is highly prevalent in Egypt, Yemen, Cameroon and other parts of Africa.

Epidemiology and transmission

The prevalence of HCV seropositivity and therefore of persistent infection varies according to geographic area. In northern Europe, the seroprevalence is 0.3–0.6%, in the USA and Japan it is approximately 1%, in the Middle East 5–10% and in sub-Saharan Africa 10–15%. In certain areas, especially where genotype 4 is present, rates of up to 30–40% have been recorded (e.g. Egypt and Cameroon). HCV accounts for 90% of non-A–non-B hepatitis. It is transmitted blood to blood via needle-stick (~ 10% risk), intravenous drug abuse, transfusion of blood or blood products and organ transplantation, but most infections are sporadic and it is not known how they have occurred. Sexual transmission and transmission from mother to baby is less efficient than for HBV. It is estimated that there is a 5–10% risk of acquiring infection from a sexual partner.

Clinical features and diagnosis

The incubation period is similar to that of HBV (6–7 weeks). The virus infects hepatocytes but there is also evidence that it can infect peripheral blood mononuclear cells. Infection can be asymptomatic and is so more often than HBV (only 10% of patients are jaundiced). It rarely causes fulminant hepatitis. Persistent infection is a common occurrence and this follows an indolent chronic course. HCV, unlike HBV, is directly cytopathic to hepatocytes, and in 20–30% of patients progresses to cirrhosis, taking on average 20–30 years. Hepatocellular carcinoma is another long-term effect of persistent infection. Because HCV is cytopathic to hepatocytes, immunosuppression as in AIDS can result in more rapid progression of HCV hepatitis. Maternal coinfection with HCV and HIV increases the risk of transmission of HCV to the baby, probably because HIV infection results in higher HCV loads.

Diagnosis is by detection of HCV antibody by ELISA, which is highly sensitive and specific. Viral genome can be detected by RT-PCR and genotype determined by serology or PCR. It is also possible to estimate HCV load, which is useful as a prognostic guide and for evaluating therapy.

Management and prevention

Treatment is with α-interferon (5 million units thrice weekly for 3 months followed by 3 million units thrice weekly for 9 months) which produces a sustained response in about 20% of patients. Currently, ribavirin with or without α-interferon is being evaluated in therapeutic trials. The main method for prevention is to screen the blood, blood products and organs for transplantation. There is no vaccine to prevent HCV infection and nothing in prospect.

Hepatitis D virus (HDV)

HDV is a small (35 nm) incomplete unenveloped RNA virus with a negative sense genome. It can only undergo full replication in the presence of HBV. This occurs either when HBV and HDV are acquired simultaneously or when a patient persistently infected with HBV is super-infected with HDV. Transmission is blood to blood, but there is an increased risk of being HDV seropositive with multiple sexual partners. Infection tends to result in more severe HBV hepatitis and can produce fulminant disease. Diagnosis is by detection of anti-HDV IgM or IgG by ELISA. There is no specific therapy, but HBV immunization will prevent HDV infection.

Hepatitis E virus (HEV)

HEV is a small (32 nm) unenveloped virus with a single-stranded positive sense RNA genome. It is closely related to the Caliciviridae. It is spread faeco-orally and infection can occur sporadically or as very large outbreaks often associated with contaminated water supplies. It is endemic in Asia, Africa, the Middle East and central America. Very large epidemics in India, Pakistan and China have affected tens of thousands of patients. Approximately 30% of cases are from intrafamilial spread. The incubation period (15–60 days) and clinical features are very similar to those of HAV. The major difference from HAV is that it is associated with a mortality rate of 25–30% in pregnant women if infection occurs in the last trimester. There is no evidence that it is sexually transmitted nor that it is affected by HIV coinfection.

Diagnosis is by detection of anti-HEV IgM or IgG by ELISA. RT-PCR is also available as a research tool. Treatment is supportive and prevention by hygienic precautions.

Hepatitis F virus (HFV)

Although a faeco-orally transmitted DNA virus was described in India, it has not been confirmed as HFV.

Hepatitis G virus (HGV)

This virus was obtained from a surgeon (G.B.) with hepatitis. His blood was used to infect tamarin monkeys which developed hepatitis. Confusingly, three viruses (GB-A, GB-B and GB-C) were obtained from the tamarins. GB-A and GB-B were shown to be endogenous tamarin viruses. GB-C is virtually the same as HGV which was also detected in Japan. HGV is also a flavivirus but distinct from HCV. It is transmitted blood to blood, and sexual transmission has not been described. Between 2 and 5% of the UK blood-donor population have HGV in the blood. There is some doubt over the role of HGV in producing hepatitis. It is probable that coinfection with HBV or HCV results in more severe disease. Diagnosis is by detection of viral genome by RT-PCR. Treatment is uncertain and may not be needed.

Appendix 6.A
HIV therapy

C.A. Hart
Department of Medical Microbiology and Genitourinary Medicine, University of Liverpool, Liverpool, UK

Available drugs

Nucleoside analogues	**Protease inhibitors**	**Other**
Zidovudine (ZDV, AZT)	Saquinavir	Nevirapine
Zalcitabine (ddC)	Ritonavir	Delavirdine
Didanosine (ddl)	Indinavir	Loviride
Stavudine (d4T)	Nelfinavir	
Lamivudine (3TC)		

In general, the nucleoside analogues exert their antiviral effect by inhibiting HIV reverse transcriptase and thus terminating development of the proviral DNA. Each must be phosphorylated intracellularly, and combinations of zidovudine and stavudine or lamivudine and zalcitabine should not be used since they inhibit each other's metabolism and are thus antagonistic. During the replication of HIV, the *gag* and *env* gene products are synthesized as polyproteins which must be cleaved by viral protease to produce the mature viral polypeptides. The protease inhibitors specifically inhibit the HIV protease and thus prevent viral maturation. Nevirapine, loviride and delavirdine are non-nucleoside reverse transcriptase inhibitors.

Combination therapy

The overall aim in the treatment of patients infected with HIV is to reduce viral replication, delay disease progression and prolong survival. Monotherapy of AIDS with zidovudine has resulted in the rapid emergence of zidovudine-resistant mutants thus limiting therapy. This has resulted in the concept of combination therapy, the aim of which is to prevent the emergence of mutants resistant to individual drugs and to provide optimal suppressive therapy. However, a strain of HIV has recently been detected that is resistant to six antiretrovirals, including the protease inhibitors. Since, as part of its replication cycle, HIV produces proviral DNA which becomes integrated into host chromosomal DNA, it is unlikely that any therapeutic regimen will completely eliminate HIV from a patient.

Sexually Transmitted Infections and AIDS in the Tropics (eds O.P. Arya and C.A. Hart)

The most recent trial data indicate that a combination of two nucleoside analogues and a protease inhibitor produces the best therapeutic effect even in patients who have received prior antiretroviral therapy. Examples of combination therapeutic regimens are:

1. Zidovudine (200 mg three times daily), lamivudine (150 mg twice daily) and indinavir (800 mg three times daily) by mouth. Stavudine (40 mg twice daily) can replace zidovudine if necessary.
2. Zidovudine (200 mg three times daily), didanosine (200 mg twice daily), nevirapine (200—400 mg once daily) by mouth.
3. Saquinavir (600 mg three times daily) and ritonavir (300 mg twice daily) by mouth.

Of the above, no. 2 is currently considered optimal, with best efficacy, least side effects and lowest chance of selecting resistant mutants.

When to treat

There are as yet no definitive data to determine whether it is better to start combination therapy in asymptomatic HIV infection or when patients are symptomatic. Under optimal conditions institution of therapy and assessment of response should be made by measuring CD4 levels and HIV load. Patients with $CD4^+$ cell counts above 300 μl^{-1} but a viral load above 50,000–100,000 copies per ml have rapid disease progression and should be treated early. It is considered prudent to treat patients when $CD4^+$ cell counts fall below 200–300 μl^{-1} or when they become symptomatic. Combination therapy will produce a 2 $\log_{10}$ or more fall in viral load, and prolonged therapy maintains low levels with, so far, little emergence of resistant mutants. Unfortunately, these combination therapies and their appropriate monitoring are very expensive. The combinations are also likely to produce more toxicity than the agents when used alone. All of these and compliance factors require careful consideration by both patient and physician. The treatment should, therefore, be initiated and supervised by a specialist or an appropriately trained physician.

Prophylaxis

Post-exposure prophylaxis

There is a risk that those managing HIV-infected patients could themselves become infected following exposure to infectious body fluids. The risk of transmission depends both on the nature of the body fluid and the mode of transfer. In decreasing order of importance, blood, CSF, seminal fluid, cervical secretions and other blood-stained secretions and excretions carry a risk of transmitting HIV. Needle-stick accidents involving hollow needles containing HIV-infected blood carry a 3–4 per 1000 risk of transmitting infection. Although HIV has been transmitted by cuts with solid needles or scalpels, and by mucous membrane or even skin exposure to HIV-infected blood, the level of risk is too low to be measurable. A recent meta-analysis has shown that post-exposure prophylaxis (PEP) with zidovudine following needle-stick accidents decreased the risk of transmission by about 60%. In deciding whether to give PEP, an assessment must be made of the likelihood of the donor being HIV-infected, the nature of the contaminating body fluid, the vehicle of transmission and if the donor has received prior antiretroviral therapy. If there is high risk of HIV transmission, then the recipient should be offered PEP. There are no data on how soon PEP should be administered, but it would seem logical to begin as soon as possible, ideally within 1–2 h after exposure. The information on efficacy of PEP relates only to zidovudine. However, there is increasing support for the use of three antiretrovirals for PEP, especially if the donor has received prior antiretroviral therapy. The combination regimens are described above, and the regimen for zidovudine alone is 1000 mg orally daily for 3–4 weeks. It must also be remembered that the needle-stick or other exposure incident could also result in transmission of other blood-borne viruses such as hepatitis B or hepatitis C, as well as syphilis (see Chapters 6.7 and 7.1).

Perinatal transmission (see also Chapter 6.2)

Between 15 and 45% of infants born to HIV-infected mothers will themselves become infected. Although transplacental transmission of HIV can occur early in pregnancy, most infections occur in the perinatal period or during breast feeding. The risk of transmission is related to high viral loads and low $CD4^+$ lymphocyte counts in maternal blood. Administration of zidovudine to HIV-infected mothers with $CD4^+$ counts above 200 μl^{-1} resulted in a decrease in HIV transmission from 22.6% in the placebo group to 7.6% in the treated group. The dosage regimen is zidovudine, 100 mg orally five times daily to women over 14 weeks gestation until the beginning of labour; then during labour and delivery until the cord is clamped, zidovudine, 2 mg kg^{-1} over 1 h followed by 1 mg kg^{-1} hourly intravenously. Starting within 12 h of delivery, the newborn is given zidovudine, 2 mg kg^{-1} every 6 h orally until 6 weeks of age. If the neonate is unable to take oral zidovudine, it should be given by intravenous infusion over 30 min (1.5 mg kg^{-1} every 6 h). There are no trial data available to demonstrate optimal duration of therapy in pregnancy or to infants postpartum, nor is there information on the value of combination antiretroviral chemotherapy. Although birth canal cleansing with chlorhexidine decreases transmission of some neonatal pathogens (group B streptococci, *E. coli*), its effect on preventing HIV transmission is at best marginal.

Further reading

BHIVA Guidelines Co-ordinating Committee (1997) British HIV Association Guidelines for Antiretroviral Treatment of HIV Seropositive Individuals. *Lancet* 349, 1086–1092.

US Department of Health and Human Services (1997) *Guidelines for the Use of Antiretroviral Agents in HIV Infected Adults and Adolescents.* USDHHS, Washington, DC.

APPENDIX 6.B

Diagnosis and management of AIDS-associated diseases

C.A. Hart

Department of Medical Microbiology and Genitourinary Medicine, University of Liverpool, Liverpool, UK

Patients with HIV/AIDS are, of course, susceptible to infection with the same pathogens responsible for disease in the non-HIV-infected. In HIV/AIDS patients, these primary pathogens tend to produce recurrent infections or, when normally localized, tend to be disseminated more frequently. This appendix will concentrate largely upon the common opportunist pathogens except when the infection is AIDS-defining or occurs with significant frequency (e.g. non-typhoidal *Salmonella* or pneumococcal bacteraemia). Appendix 6.B.1 tabulates the various AIDS-associated diseases by organ system; Appendix 6.B.2 lists their frequency, whether they occur early or late in AIDS, methods of diagnosis and their treatment and prophylaxis. The specimens needed for diagnosis will vary according to the site affected, but could include blood, CSF, pus, sputum, broncho-alveolar lavage, faeces and tissue biopsies as appropriate. Endoscopy, radiography and other imaging techniques are also valuable adjuncts to specific diagnosis.

Table 6.B.1. AIDS-associated pathogens and malignancies by organ system[a].

	Viruses	Bacteria	Fungi	Parasites	Other
Gastrointestinal tract					
Mouth	HHV-1 or -2 (herpes simplex)	*Porphyromonas gingivalis* (gingivitis)	*Candida albicans*	—	Hairy leukoplakia (?EBV) Aphthous ulcers Kaposi's sarcoma (HHV-8)
		Mixed bacteria including anaerobes (dental abcesses)	—	—	—
Oesophagus	HHV-1 or -2 CMV (HHV-5)	—	*C. albicans*	—	—
Intestine (non-inflammatory diarrhoea)	HIV, HHV-5 (CMV)	*Mycobacterium avium-intracellulare*	—	Microsporidia *Cryptosporidium parvum* *Isospora belli* *Giardia lamblia*	Lymphoma[b] Kaposi's sarcoma (HHV-8)
Intestine (inflammatory diarrhoea)	HHV-5 (CMV)	Non-typhi *Salmonella* *Shigella* spp *Campylobacter* spp. *Clostridium difficile*	—	*Entamoeba histolytica*	Kaposi's sarcoma (HHV-8)
Intestine (perforation)	HHV-5 (CMV)	—	*Histoplasma capsulatum*	—	Kaposi's sarcoma (HHV-8)
Rectum and anus	HHV-1 or -2 HHV-5 (CMV) HPV	*Chlamydia trachomatis* *Neisseria gonorrhoeae* *Treponema pallidum*	*C. albicans*	*E. histolytica*	Kaposi's sarcoma (HHV-8)
Liver	—	*Bartonella henselae* and *B. quintana* (peliosis hepatitis)	*H. capsulatum*	*C. parvum*	Kaposi's sarcoma (HHV-8) Sclerosing cholangitis

Respiratory tract					
Sinuses, middle ear	—	*Streptococcus pneumoniae* *Haemophilus influenzae* *Moraxella catarrhalis*	—	—	—
Lung	HHV-5 (CMV)	*S. pneumoniae* *H. influenzae* *Mycobacterium tuberculosis* *M. avium-intracellulare* *M. kansasii* *Nocardia asteroides* *Rhodococcus equi* *Legionella pneumophila*	*Pneumocystis carinii* *Aspergillus* spp. *Cryptococcus neoformans* *H. capsulatum* *C. albicans* *Coccidioides immitis*	*Strongyloides stercoralis*	Kaposi's ˜sarcoma (HHV-8) Lymphocytic interstitial pneumonitis (in children) Lymphoma[b] Non-specific interstitial pneumonitis (adults)
Nervous system					
Brain	JC virus HHV-5 (CMV) HHV-1 HHV-3 (VZV) HIV	*M. tuberculosis* (tuberculoma) *T. pallidum*	*C. neoformans* *Aspergillus* spp.	*Toxoplasma gondii*	Lymphoma[b] Kaposi's sarcoma (HHV-8)
Spinal cord	HHV-3 (VZV) HIV HHV-5 (CMV)	Non-typhi *Salmonella*	*C. neoformans*	—	Lymphoma[b]
Peripheral nerves	HHV-3 (VZV) HHV-5 (CMV) HIV	—	—	—	—

Continued

Table 6.B.1. Continued

	Viruses	Bacteria	Fungi	Parasites	Other
Eyes	HHV-5 (CMV)	*M. avium-intracellulare*	*C. neoformans*	*T. gondii*	Kaposi's sarcoma (HHV-8)
	HHV-3 (VZV) HIV		*C. albicans* *P. carinii*	Microsporidia (conjunctivitis)	Squamous carcinoma of conjunctiva
Skin and subcutaneous tissue	HIV (seroconversion illness)	*M. avium-intracellulare*	*C. albicans*	*Sarcoptes scabiei* (scabies)	Kaposi's sarcoma (HHV-8)
	HHV-1 HHV-3 (VZV) Molluscum contagiosum HPV	*M. marinum* *T. pallidum* *Staphylococcus aureus* *B. henselae* and *B. quintana* (bacillary angiomatosis)	*C. neoformans* *H. capsulatum* *P. marneffei* *Sporothrix schenckii* Dermatophytes		Squamous cell carcinoma Basal cell carcinoma Seborrhoeic dermatitis Drug reactions Papular eruption Psoriasis
Genital tract	HHV1 or 2 HPV	*T. pallidum* *N. gonorrhoeae* *C. trachomatis*	*C. albicans*	—	Cervical carcinoma
Disseminated infection	HHV-5 (CMV) HHV-1	Non-typhi *Salmonella* *S. pneumoniae* *M. tuberculosis* *M. avium-intracellulare* *M. kansasii*	*H. capsulatum* *C. immitis* *C. neoformans* *P. marneffei* *P. carinii*	*S. stercoralis* *T. gondii*	Lymphoma[b] Kaposi's sarcoma (HHV-8)
Generalized lymphadenopathy	HIV HHV-4 HHV-5	*M. tuberculosis* *M. avium-intracellulare* *T. pallidum*	*C. neoformans* *H. capsulatum*	*T. gondii*	Kaposi's sarcoma (HHV-8) Lymphoma[b]

[a] Many of the conditions have been described elsewhere in the book.
[b] Usually EBV-associated.

Table 6.B.2 Management and treatment of AIDS-associated diseases.

Agent or disease	Frequency	Early/late	Specific diagnosis	Treatment	Prophylaxis
Viruses					
HHV-1	Common	Early	Culture, IFAT, PCR	Aciclovir, famciclovir	Not recommended
HHV-2	Common	Early	Culture, IFAT, PCR	Aciclovir, famciclovir	Condom use
HHV-3	Common	Early	Culture, IFAT, PCR	Aciclovir, famciclovir	Zoster immune globulin for susceptible patients
HHV-5	Common	Early	Culture, IFAT, PCR	Ganciclovir, Foscarnet	Ganciclovir, Foscarnet
HPV	Common	Early	Clinical, Papanicolau stain histology, PCR	Curettage, cryotherapy diathermy, chemical	Condom use
JCV[b]	Rare	Late	EM, histology, PCR	Nil	Nil specific
Molluscum contagiosum	Common	Early	Clinical, EM, histology	Curettage, cryotherapy, chemical	Nil specific
Bacteria					
Bartonella henselae	Rare	Late	Culture, PCR, histology	Erythromycin, clarithromycin, doxycycline	Avoid cats and their fleas
B. quintana	Rare	Late	Culture, PCR, histology	Erythromycin, clarithromycin, doxycycline	Avoid rodent excreta
Campylobacter spp.	Common	Early	Culture	Erythromycin, ciprofloxacin	Nil specific
Chlamydia trachomatis	Moderate	Early or late	Culture, antigen detection, PCR, LCR	Erythromycin, tetracyclines, azithromycin	Condom use
Clostridium difficile	Rare	Late	Culture, detection of toxin	Metronidazole	Nil specific
Haemophilus influenzae	Rare	Early	Culture, antigen detection	Cotrimoxazole[a], cefuroxime, ciprofloxacin	Nil specific
Legionella pneumophila	Rare	Late	Culture, antigen detection, PCR	Erythromycin, rifampicin	Avoid exposure
Moraxella catarrhalis	Common	Early	Culture	Cefuroxime, augmentin[a]	Nil specific

Continued

Table 6.B.2. Continued.

Agent or disease	Frequency	Early or late	Specific diagnosis	Treatment	Prophylaxis
Mycobacterium tuberculosis	Common	Early	Z-N, culture, PCR	Rifampicin, isoniazid, pyrazinamide	Nil specific
M. avium-intracellulare	Common	Late	Z-N, culture, PCR	Rifabutin or clarithromycin	Clarithromycin
M. kansasii	Rare	Late	Z-N, culture, PCR	Rifampicin, isoniazid, ethambutol[a]	Nil specific
M. marinum	Rare	Late	Z-N, culture, PCR	Streptomycin, rifampicin, ethambutol[a]	Nil specific
Neisseria gonorrhoeae	Common	Early or late	Gram stain, culture	Ciprofloxacin[a], Ceftriaxone	Condom use
Nocardia asteroides	Rare	Late	Gram stain, culture	Penicillin	Nil specific
Non-typhi *Salmonella*	Common	Early	Culture	Ciprofloxacin, cotrimoxazole[a]	Nil specific
Shigella spp.	Common	Early	Culture	Quinolones	Nil specific
Rhodococcus equi	Rare	Late	Culture	Penicillin[a]	Nil specific
Staphylococcus aureus	Common	Late	Gram stain of pus, culture	Flucloxacillin, vancomycin[a]	Nil specific
Streptococcus pneumoniae	Common	Early	Culture, antigen detection	Penicillin, ceftriaxone[a]	Nil specific
Treponema pallidum	Moderate	Early or late	Dark ground microscopy, antibody detection	Penicillin	Condom use
Fungi					
Aspergillus spp.	Rare	Late	Culture	Itraconazole	Nil specific
Candida albicans	Common	Early	Gram stain, microscopy	Nystatin, amphotericin B, fluconazole, itraconazole	Nil specific
Coccidioides immitis	Rare	Late	Culture, antigen detection	Itraconazole, amphotericin B	Nil specific
Cryptococcus neoformans	Common	Early	India ink preparation, culture, antigen detection	Amphotericin B, fluconazole Itraconazole	Fluconazole, itraconazole
Histoplasma capsulatum	Rare	Late	Culture	Itraconazole, amphotericin B	Fluconazole, itraconazole
Penicillium marneffei	Rare	Late	Culture, microscopy	Amphotericin B,itraconazole	Fluconazole, itraconazole

Pneumocystis carinii	Common	Early	Silver stain, antigen detection, PCR	Cotrimoxazole, pentamidine	Cotrimoxazole, pentamidine
Sporothrix schenckii	Rare	Late	Microscopy, culture	Potassium iodide	Nil specific
Dermatophytes	Moderate	Late	Microscopy, culture	Clotrimazole, ketoconazole, griseofulvin	Avoid contact
Parasites					
Cryptosporidium parvum[b]	Common	Early	Microscopy of stained (safranin methylene blue (SMB) or auramine phenol) stool smear	Nil specific but paromomycin might give symptomatic improvement	Nil specific
Entamoeba histolytica	Rare	Early or late	Wet preparation of fresh stool by microscopy	Metronidazole, emetine	Nil specific
Giardia lamblia	Common	Early or late	Microscopy of stool or duodenal juice	Metronidazole	Nil specific
Isospora belli	Rare	Early or late	SMB stain of faecal smear	Cotrimoxazole	Nil specific
Microsporidia[b]	Moderate	Late	EM of intestinal biopsy, trichrome stain of faecal smear	Albendazole (?cotrimoxazole)	Nil specific
Sarcoptes scabiei	Common	Late	Demonstration of mite by microscopy	Lindane cream, malathion or permethrin	Nil specific
Strongyloides stercoralis	Rare	Late	Demonstration of larvae in lung or stool	Thiabendazole	Nil specific
Toxoplasma gondii	Common	Early or late	Serology, demonstration of organism by histology or PCR in biopsy	Pyrimethamine + sulphadiazine	Cotrimoxazole
Other					
Aphthous ulcers	Common	Early	Clinical and by exclusion	Thalidomide, corticosteroids	Nil specific
Basal cell carcinoma	Rare	Late	Histology	Surgery	Nil specific
Cervical carcinoma	Rare	Late	Papanicolau smear, histology	Surgery, radiotherapy	Condom use
Drug reaction	Common	Early	Clinical	Stop drug? corticosteroids	Avoid drug if possible

Continued

Table 6.B.2. Continued.

Agent or disease	Frequency	Early or late	Specific diagnosis	Treatment	Prophylaxis
Hairy leukoplakia	Common	Early	Clinical	Nil specific	Nil specific
Kaposi's sarcoma	Common	Late	Clinical, histology of biopsy	Surgery, cryotherapy, chemotherapy, radiotherapy	Nil specific
Lymphoma	Common	Late	Histology of biopsy	Surgery, chemotherapy, radiotherapy	Nil specific
Lymphocytic interstitial pneumonitis	Common (children)	Early	X-ray, histology of biopsy	?Corticosteroids	Nil specific
Pruritic papular eruption	Common	Early	Clinical	Corticosteroids, UVB	Nil specific
Psoriasis[b]	Common	Early	Clinical	Etretinate	Nil specific
Seborrhoeic dermatitis	Common	Early	Clinical	Topical ketokonazole, steroids	Nil specific
Squamous cell carcinoma	Rare	Late	Histology of biopsy	Surgery	Nil specific

[a]Sensitivities vary, local knowledge needed.
[b]Improved by antiretroviral therapy.
IFAT, immunofluorescent antibody test; EM, electron microscopy; ZN, Ziehl–Neelsen stain.

Appendix 6.C

Use of vaccines in HIV/AIDS patients

C.A. Hart
Department of Medical Microbiology and Genitourinary Medicine, University of Liverpool, Liverpool, UK

Vaccines in routine use

Toxoid	Subunit	Whole killed	Live attenuated
Diphtheria	Influenza[a]	Polio (Salk)	Polio (Sabin)
Tetanus	Hepatitis B[a]	Pertussis	Measles
	Haemophilus influenzae b (Hib)		Mumps
			Rubella[a]
	Pertussis[a]		Bacille Calmette–Guérin (BCG)[a]

[a]Not in routine use in all countries.

Vaccines for travel or special purposes

Toxoid	Subunit	Whole killed	Live attenuated
	Anthrax	Hepatitis A	Rotavirus
Nil	*Streptococcus pneumoniae* capsule	Rabies	Vaccinia
	*Neisseria meningitidis A,C,Y, W*135 capsule	Tick-borne encephalitis	Varicella-zoster (oka)
	Salmonella typhi Vi	Japanese B encephalitis	Yellow fever
		Salmonella typhi	*Salmonella typhi* (Ty21a)
		Vibrio cholerae	

The areas of concern for immunization in HIV/AIDS patients are firstly the potential for live attenuated vaccines to cause disease, secondly the decreased efficacy of vaccines, and, more theoretically, the effect of immunization on the progression of HIV infection to AIDS.

Live attenuated vaccines

No adverse effects have been described in HIV-infected individuals given measles, mumps, rubella or oral polio vaccines. It is advised that these vaccines should be given to symptomatically or asymptomatically HIV-infected individuals who are at increased risk from these diseases. However, there may not be a detectable antibody response in some of the vaccinees. It is possible that oral polio vaccine could be excreted for longer periods in HIV/AIDS patients, and those likely to be in contact with the vaccinees' excreta should be advised of this. This risk can be minimized by the use of inactivated polio vaccine (Salk). In developed countries, there is evidence of disseminated BCG infection in HIV-infected (symptomatic or asymptomatic) vaccinees and, in the UK, BCG is not given to HIV/AIDS patients. In developing countries, neonatal BCG immunization programmes should continue, and BCG is contraindicated only in those with symptomatic HIV infection. There are no data on the safety or efficacy of the yellow fever vaccine, and its use is discouraged in HIV-infected individuals.

Vaccine efficacy

There is evidence from developed countries that the antibody response to a number of vaccines in HIV-infected recipients is neither as high nor as prolonged as in the HIV-uninfected. Whether this reflects poorer immunity to the vaccine pathogens is unclear. However, it may be necessary to give the routine vaccines at more frequent intervals. There is also evidence that maternal HIV infection impairs the transplacental transfer of antibodies that normally provide passive protection to the neonate and infant. This may necessitate, for example, giving measles vaccine at an earlier age.

Effect of vaccines on AIDS

There is no evidence that the use of vaccines increases the risk of progression of HIV infection to AIDS. One study has shown that HIV-infected adults who were given the pneumococcal capsular vaccine had higher HIV loads immediately after vaccination.

Appendix 6.D
Infection control in HIV infection/AIDS

C.A. Hart
Department of Medical Microbiology and Genitourinary Medicine, University of Liverpool, Liverpool, UK

There is sometimes disquiet among the general public and even among some health professionals that HIV can be transmitted easily. There is no evidence that casual contact will spread HIV. The risk of transmission to household contacts or health workers is extremely low. For infection to spread there must be not only excretion of virus (in body fluids or blood) in sufficient quantities but also a portal of entry in the recipient. Although there are cases of HIV transmission via contamination of skin or mucous membranes by infected blood, they are so rare that it is not possible to quantify the risk. This risk can be minimized further by ensuring that cuts and abrasions are covered by waterproof plasters and that when exposure-prone procedures (e.g. phlebotomy) are undertaken, gloves are worn. Needles (which should not be resheathed) and other sharps should be disposed of in appropriate toughened containers (e.g. sharps bins) which should be placed out of reach of children (a recent case of acquisition of HIV by a child in a Danish hospital apparently resulted from the child putting her hand in the sharps bin). The risk of transmission by needle-stick is 0.3–0.4% and even less via solid needles or scalpels. Any spillages of blood or other body fluids should be cleaned as soon as possible using household bleach at home or hypochlorite powder (e.g. Titan sanitizer) in hospital. Cutlery, linen, towels, baths and sinks used by HIV-infected patients do not need any special washing procedure.

Although the risk of spread of HIV from patients to close contacts is extremely low, some of the pathogens infecting patients with AIDS do pose problems of cross-infection. These will include patients with tuberculosis, shigellosis and cryptosporidiosis, and appropriate infection control measures for respiratory and faecal containment are necessary.

CHAPTER 7
Bacterial infections

CHAPTER 7.1
Syphilis

O.P. Arya
Department of Medical Microbiology and Genitourinary Medicine, University of Liverpool, Liverpool, UK

Syphilis, one of the treponematoses, is caused by *Treponema pallidum* and is a multisystem chronic infectious disease. It can be passed from the pregnant woman to her unborn child. Its variety of manifestations, some very serious, may simulate many other medical conditions.

Epidemiology (see also Chapter 1)

To ascertain whether or not syphilis is being transmitted and is a public health problem requires incidence figures for infectious syphilis. These are not generally available in tropical countries. The reliance on concurrently positive rapid plasma reagin (RPR) tests and *T. pallidum* haemagglutination assays (TPHA) to diagnose active syphilis, as in several recent publications, can be misleading. Nevertheless, seroprevalence surveys published in the 1990s show alarmingly high positivity rates of 2–15% in pregnant women and other populations in sub-Saharan Africa.

The causative organism

T. pallidum (Fig. 7.1.1), the causative organism, is a thin spirochaete with tapering ends, 6–15 μm in length and about 0.2 μm in width, which is below the resolution of an ordinary microscope. It has 8–20 rigid coils with a distance of 1 μm between each coil. It is recognized under dark ground illumination by its shape and purposeful movements, which include slow forward and backward movement rotating on its long axis like a corkscrew, and compression, expansion and bending (flexuous) movements. Electron microscopy (Fig. 7.1.2) shows its structure to comprise an amorphous outer layer, an outer membrane containing a number of different proteins, a

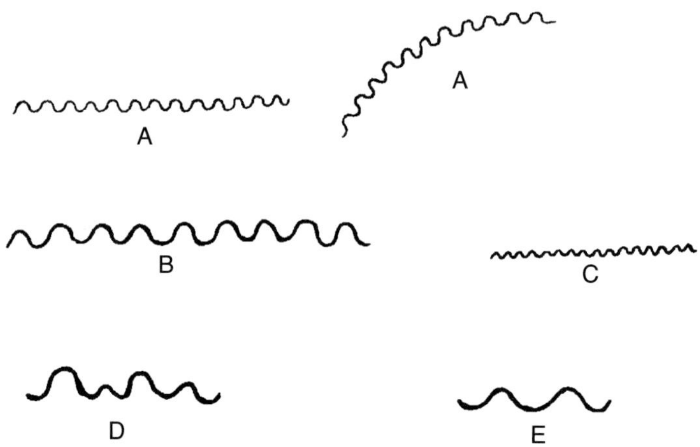

Fig. 7.1.1. *Treponema pallidum* and other spirochaetes: (A) *T. pallidum*, (B) *T. gracilis*, (C) *T. microdentium*, (D) *T. refringens*, (E) *T. balanitidis*.

peptidoglycan layer (site of action of penicillin) and axial filaments or flagella responsible for its motility.

It is susceptible to heat, drying, storage at refrigeration temperature and even the weakest antiseptics including soap. In a moist environment, it may remain alive outside the human body for a few hours, but may survive for up to 72 h in blood refrigerated at 4°C. It divides by binary fission every 30–33 h in early syphilis, but possibly more slowly in the later stages.

It stains poorly with the usual dyes, but in tissue sections the organism can be detected by silver impregnation or immunofluorescent techniques. No culture method is yet available to allow continuous growth of the organism.

Mode of transmission

Direct contact by sexual intercourse is the main mode of transmission in adults. Other direct methods include by needle-stick or blood transfusion, without the appearance of primary lesion (syphilis d'emblée), and kissing. Transmission by indirect contact, e.g. drinking from infected communal utensils, etc., is possible.

T. pallidum enters the body through the finest abrasion of the skin or mucous membrane. The infection then spreads by the lymphatics and the bloodstream and transplacentally in congenital syphilis.

Pathology and immunity

Polymorphonuclear leukocytes (PMN) are the first to appear at the infection site, replaced by T lymphocytes, plasma cells and macrophages within 48 h. The basic pathology is the same in all stages of syphilis, i.e. perivascular

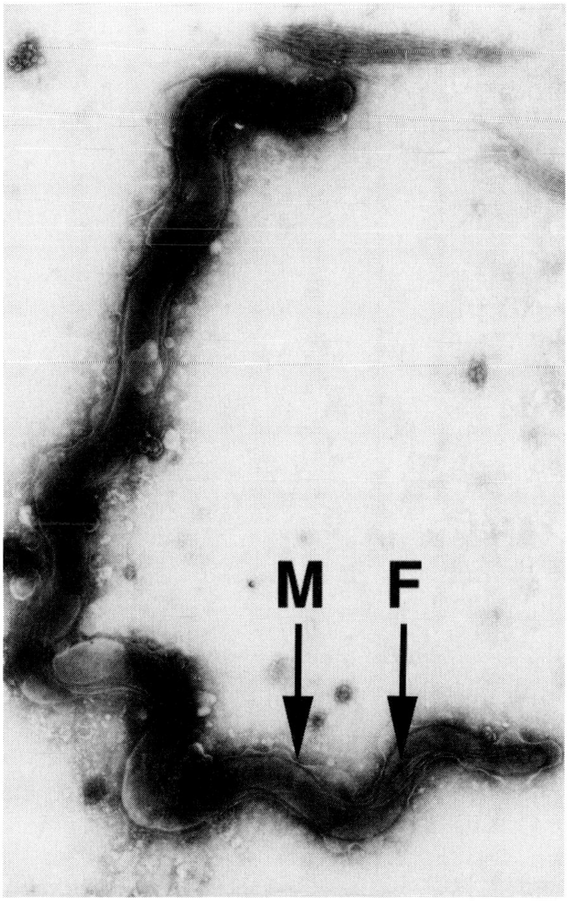

Fig. 7.1.2. *Treponema pallidum*: negative stain electron micrograph showing outer membrane (M), and axial flagella (F). (The material was obtained from the patient shown in Plate 25.)

infiltration with lymphocytes and plasma cells, and obliterative endarteritis associated with endothelial proliferation.

Primary and secondary syphilis

The endothelial proliferation may cause occlusion of the small blood vessels, resulting in impairment of blood supply to the area affected, necrosis and erosion as in the case of syphilitic ulcer in the primary stage, and mucocutaneous ulceration in secondary stage. The intensity of cellular and vascular response determines the induration and the type of skin rash which may be macular, roseolar, maculopapular, papular, papulosquamous, etc.

Benign late syphilis, cardiovascular syphilis and neurosyphilis are described in their respective sections later in this chapter.

The specific immunological and other mechanisms involved in the various stages of the natural history of syphilis (described below) remain largely unknown. Some of these might also explain the differences in the appearance of primary and secondary lesions; the tissue destruction in late syphilis, and the scarcity of treponemes in gummatous syphilis but their abundance in cardiovascular and neurosyphilis.

There is evidence of both humoral and cell-mediated immunity in syphilis. The humoral response is reflected in the serological tests (see also Chapter 5), but the exact role of these antibodies is unclear. The patient has both anticardiolipin as well as antitreponemal IgG and IgM antibodies in early syphilis. In later stages and after treatment, antitreponemal IgM antibody production may stop.

The healing of the primary lesion, which is preceded by the appearance of fibroblasts, involves destruction of treponemes by T cell-activated macrophages.

There is experimental evidence of local resistance to infection in the presence of chancre or untreated syphilis, but this does not alter the natural course of the infection. Although cell-mediated immunity is suppressed in early syphilis, there is evidence of delayed hypersensitivity to treponemal antigen, e.g. in the latent stage when the patient may develop a gummatous lesion.

Incubation period

The incubation period depends on the size of the inoculum, the virulence of organisms, the resistance of the host and recent medication. The average incubation period is 2–4 weeks and the range 10–90 days. The patient is, however, infectious during the incubation period, for example by blood transfusion.

Stages of syphilis

There are two broad stages: early syphilis and late syphilis. Early syphilis is infectious and includes primary syphilis, secondary syphilis and early latent syphilis within the first 2 years of infection. Late syphilis comprises late latent syphilis, benign late syphilis, cardiovascular syphilis and neurosyphilis.

Primary syphilis

Clinical features

General characteristics

Almost 90% of the primary lesions occur on the genitalia, and the rest are extragenital. The primary lesion, also called chancre, begins as a macule which progresses to a red papule. The surface of the papule becomes eroded, resulting in a shallow ulcer. The appearance of the lesion is determined by the site affected, any treatment received and secondary infection. A typical lesion (Plate 21) is single, well defined, round or oval, with a red smooth surface exuding clear serum, and painless. The lesion is also indurated because of the cellular infiltration of the base and surrounding tissue. In practice, however, over half of the primary lesions seen in the clinics are atypical, for example the lesions may be painful as a result of secondary infection and/or multiple (Plates 22–24) and/or non-indurated. Mixed infections with herpes and/or chancroid frequently are encountered, presenting as uncharacteristic single or multiple ulcers (Plates 25 and 26).

Genital lesions in males

The common sites affected in males include the coronal sulcus (the lesions usually very indurated), glans penis (lesions often shallow and infiltration not marked – Plate 27), fraenum, penile shaft (lesion often circular and scabbed – Plate 28), prepuce (lesion has button-like induration and flaps back in a characteristic fashion when retracted, phimosis if the mucous surface is involved) and meatus (patient may present with penile discharge, meatal oedema and stenosis). The primary lesion may be concealed in the urethra when the patient may complain of dysuria and/or urethral discharge mimicking non-gonococcal urethritis. A careful examination will reveal an indurated lump, usually in the distal urethra.

LYMPH NODES. In most cases, there is unilateral or bilateral inguinal lymphadenitis becoming obvious within a week after the appearance of the primary lesion.

In the absence of secondary or concurrent infection, the lymph nodes are neither painful nor tender. They are firm or rubbery, discrete, freely mobile and not attached to the skin or underlying structures. If the patient has concurrent chancroid, then the nodes may be painful and tender with or without bubo formation.

Occasionally, a patient may present with bubon d'emblé, i.e. inguinal adenitis without an ulcer, when the primary lesion may have remained concealed, e.g. in the distal urethra.

Genital lesions in females

The genital lesions in females are often invisible to the patient and, if painless, the patient remains unaware. Hence, female patients do not often present in the primary stage. However, the common sites affected include: the labia (indurated scabbed lesions on the outer aspect and kissing chancres on the inner aspects – Plate 29), clitoris, urethral orifice, fourchette (Plate 30), the walls of the vagina (Plate 31) and the cervix. A primary syphilitic infection of the cervix may manifest as focal congestion, induration, ulceration or an invisible endocervical lesion. A typical chancre of the cervix (Plate 32) is an extremely rare occurrence.

As the patient remains unaware of any cervical lesions, all female partners of patients with infectious syphilis should have a speculum examination, and cervical secretion should be subjected to darkfield examination even if clinical examination is normal.

LYMPH NODES. The inguinal lymph nodes will be enlarged only when the lesion is on the external genitalia or the lower third of the vagina (see Chapter 2 for lymphatic drainage of female genitalia).

Extragenital primary lesions

Up to about 10% of the primary syphilis lesions may occur on extragenital sites, such as the lips (lesions often scabbed with marked oedema – Plate 33), tongue, tonsils, nipples (Plate 34), fingers (accidental infection in medical personnel or as a result of curiosity, manifesting as painless or painful subungual swelling with or without ulceration and minimal pus formation – Plate 35), anus and rectum, especially in homosexuals (Plate 36).

LYMPH NODES. The regional lymph nodes draining the site(s) affected may be enlarged (see Chapter 2 for lymphatic drainage).

Differential diagnosis of primary syphilis

Whereas it is possible to make a fairly accurate diagnosis of primary syphilis on clinical grounds if the patient presents with a typical lesion, it is impossible to exclude syphilis in any case of genital ulceration, especially in areas where syphilis is common, without laboratory support. There are several causes of genital ulceration which may need to be considered in the differential diagnosis.

Chancroid (see Chapter 7.3 for details)

This is perhaps the most common condition to be considered in the differential diagnosis of genital ulcer in the tropics. The incubation period is much shorter. The lesions are usually multiple, painful, tender, the edges are undermined, the surface grey and the lesions may bleed easily. A bubo may also have formed. A good therapeutic response with ciprofloxacin or cotrimoxazole will exclude syphilis, but beware of a mixed infection as described above. Occasionally, a syphilitic chancre may appear after a chancroidal lesion has cleared with ciprofloxacin or sulphonamide treatment.

Anogenital herpes (Chapter 6.3)

If the patient presents with vesicles, the diagnosis is easy. A history of recurrent attacks with or without prodromal symptoms is also distinctive.

Lymphogranuloma venereum (Chapter 7.6)

The primary lesion is usually transient and has disappeared by the time the patient presents to the clinic with inguinal lymph node enlargement. Although the latter is painful and tender, the clinical differentiation from syphilis can be problematic.

Granuloma inguinale (Chapter 7.7)

The ulcer is well defined with raised edges. The pseudobubo may be mistaken for lymph node enlargement. The clinical diagnosis, therefore, can be difficult.

Genital trauma

Genital trauma during sexual intercourse usually involves the fraenum and the prepuce (Plate 37). Secondary infection may result in an ulcer which may be difficult to differentiate from an ulcerated chancre.

Erosive balanitis and pyoderma

These are described in Chapters 10.1 and 11.5.

Other conditions

Other conditions which may need to be considered in the differential diagnosis include: gumma which very rarely may occur, after some years, at the site of the primary lesion (pseudo-chancre redux), amoebiasis (Chapter 11.6), tuberculosis (Chapter 11.6), Reiter's syndrome (Chapter 7.5) and several of the dermatological conditions of the genitalia, such as, Behçet's syndrome, carcinoma of the penis, erythroplasia of Queyrat, fixed drug eruption, lichen planus, Zoon's balanitis (Chapter 11.5) and scabies (Chapter 9.2).

DIFFERENTIAL DIAGNOSIS OF EXTRAGENITAL PRIMARY LESIONS. The conditions include Bowen's disease, fissure, haemorrhoids, herpes and Crohn's disease in the case of anal lesion; aphthosis, Bechçet's syndrome, carcinoma, cheilosis due to vitamin deficiency, gumma, herpes and tuberculosis in the case of lesion of the lips and tongue; agranulocytosis, diphtheria, infectious mononucleosis, streptococcal infection and Vincent's angina for the tonsillar lesion; anthrax and epithelioma for a digital lesion; carcinoma and Paget's disease in the case presenting with lesion of the nipple; and filariasis, Hodgkin's disease, infectious mononucleosis, lymphatic leukaemia, lymphosarcoma, melanoma and septic lesions in the case of lymph node enlargement.

Diagnosis of primary syphilis

Darkfield examination

The diagnosis of primary syphilis is confirmed by demonstration of *T. pallidum* in the material obtained from the lesion. Wearing rubber gloves, any scab is removed and the ulcer is cleansed gently with gauze moistened in saline or water. This cleaning will help to rid the material of saprophytic spirochaetes which often inhabit the surfaces of dirty genital lesions. Clear serum from the ulcer is then allowed to ooze by squeezing the lesion, and any blood should be removed with a swab. The serum is then collected on a clean coverslip which in turn is placed on a microscopic slide. The two are then pressed firmly between two layers of blotting paper. If the slide cannot be examined under the darkfield microscope immediately, the edges of the coverslip should be sealed with petroleum jelly. If the laboratory is some distance away, the serum may be collected in a capillary tube, the ends of which are then sealed by wax before transporting the specimen. A capillary tube or bacteriological loop may be used to obtain specimens from sites not easily accessible, such as the cervix.

Considerable experience is required to differentiate *T. pallidum* from saprophytic genital and oral spirochaetes (Fig. 7.1.1). Genital spirochaetes include *T. refringens*, *T. balanitidis* (*T. phagedenis*) and *T. gracilis*. They vary in size, are thicker than *T. pallidum*, have fewer coils, and coarse movements. *T. balanitidis* has only three or four coils and has lashing eel-like movements. *T. gracilis* may resemble *T. pallidum*, but the former is thicker with more open coils and the movements not so characteristic. Oral treponemes such as *T. microdentium* and *T. macrodentium* have less regular coils and no rotation or bending movements, and yet may be difficult to differentiate from *T. pallidum*. Darkfield examination, therefore, is unreliable for oral lesions for which the direct fluorescent antibody (to *T. pallidum*) test is to be preferred. The latter test is likely to be available in only a few large teaching hospitals in the tropics.

It is not yet possible to differentiate *T. pallidum* from other human pathogenic species, namely, *T. pertenue*, *T. endemicum* and *T. carateum* (see also Chapter 7.2).

A negative darkfield examination does not exclude syphilis. Depending upon the strength of suspicion and if the patient has not already had an antibiotic, the examination should be repeated daily for 2–3 days. The patient should be instructed not to use soap or any topical medication other than saline. A short course of systemic treatment with a non-treponemicidal drug such as sulphonamides may be prescribed to clear secondary infection. Repeated failure to demonstrate *T. pallidum* necessitates consideration of darkfield microscopy of the material obtained by aspiration of the enlarged lymph node draining the lesion site, and/or reliance on serological tests for syphilis.

Lymph node puncture

In addition to the above indication, lymph node puncture may be considered if the ulcer has healed, the patient has applied antiseptics, the lesion is concealed, or if the lesion is in the mouth (saprophytic spirochaetes do not inhabit the lymph nodes). Wearing gloves, the skin over the enlarged lymph node is sterilized with an antiseptic and infiltrated with 1% lignocaine hydrochloride for local anaesthesia. The node is held firmly with the skin stretched. An intramuscular needle attached to a 2-ml syringe and containing 0.2 ml of sterile normal saline is plunged obliquely into the node and the saline injected. The node is then massaged gently, and fluid is aspirated and then expressed on to glass slides for darkfield microscopy for *T. pallidum*.

Serological tests

See Chapter 5 for classification and technical details of the serological tests for syphilis. The interpretation of the tests is covered later in this chapter.

The following points are relevant to primary syphilis: a positive serological test in a patient with genital ulcer does not mean that the ulcer is due to syphilis. The serological tests do not usually become positive until about 3–5 weeks after the infection or 1–2 weeks following the appearance of the chancre. It follows, therefore, that primary syphilis may be seronegative or seropositive. If the baseline tests are negative, the tests should be repeated weekly for 2–3 weeks and then, if necessary, monthly for 3 months before syphilis can finally be excluded. (The effect of HIV infection is dealt with later in this chapter.) An initial negative test subsequently becoming positive is significant and consistent with the diagnosis of primary syphilis. The fluorescent antibody absorption (FTA-ABS) test is usually the first to become positive, followed by RPR (or VDRL) and then the TPHA. However, as the FTA-ABS test is unlikely to be available in tropical countries except in the larger teaching hospitals, reliance will have to be placed on the RPR (or VDRL) test which will need to be repeated to allow comparison with the baseline result/titres.

Course of primary syphilis

Even without treatment, the chancre heals in 2–6 weeks, with or without a thin atrophic scar. The lymphadenopathy takes longer to resolve. There may then be a latent period of up to 6 months during which the patient remains infectious. Many patients, however, develop secondary syphilis within 8 weeks of the appearance of the primary lesion, and about a quarter enter the secondary stage while the chancre is still present.

Secondary syphilis

Clinical features

Secondary syphilis is characterized by widespread manifestations, those of skin and mucous membranes being the most obvious. However, any organ of the body may be involved. Patients may experience constitutional symptoms such as fever, malaise, headache, aches and pains, anorexia and loss of weight.

Skin lesions

Over 75% of the patients with secondary syphilis present with skin rashes, called syphilides. They are generalized (not necessarily profuse) and symmetrical, at least in the early stages. Several varieties have been described.

The initial rash is usually *macular*; the lesions, usually on the trunk and limbs, are pink in patients with fair complexions, and pale or difficult to see in dark-skinned people. *Papular* syphilis may emerge as such or develop from the macules, and may affect the whole body. Often the rash is *maculopapular* and polymorphic, with the papules at various stages of development. The rash tends to be more marked on the flanks, shoulders, back, arms, palms and soles (Plates 38–41). The papules, when grouped together on the forehead, have been termed 'corona veneris' (crown of Venus).

Later, scales may form on the papules when the lesion is called *papulosquamous* or *psoriasiform* syphilide (Plate 42). Annular lesions, more common on the face in dark-skinned people (Plate 43), and *corymbose* syphilides, formed by a central collection of papules surrounded by small satellite papules (Plate 44), are more common in relapsing secondary syphilis.

With increasing vascular damage, the centre of the papule may become necrotic, resulting in *acneiform* pustular lesions (Plate 45). Secretions from pustular lesions accumulate and, when dry, form layers of thick crust on the surface, and the lesion is called *rupial* syphilide (Plate 46).

At the mucocutaneous junctions as well as in other areas where there is excessive warmth, moisture and friction, the lesions become confluent, hypertrophic and flattened. They are called *condylomata lata* which commonly occur on the perianal region, vulva and scrotum (Plates 47–49), and less frequently on other sites such as nasolabial folds, angles of the mouth, behind the ears, axillae, under pendulous breasts, between the toes and in the umbilicus (Plates 50–53). The surface of these lesions, initially reddish, becomes greyish white due to necrosis. They have an abundance of organisms and hence are highly infectious.

The skin rash of secondary syphilis is usually not itchy. However, patients with condylomata lata, and psoriasiform or follicular syphilide (see below) may experience irritation.

The secondary syphilis rash is rather slow to evolve and may last for 4–12 weeks. Healing takes place without any scarring. However, patchy loss of pigmentation at the back of the neck, usually in brunettes, may occur (syphilitic leukoderma or collar of Venus). Hyperpigmenation may also occur (Plate 54).

Lesions of the hair and nails

Lesions of the hair follicles (*follicular syphilides*) may result in hair loss. Syphilitic alopecia is usually patchy (a moth-eaten appearance) especially on the sides and back of the head (Plate 55). The beard and eyebrows may also be affected.

The nails may be affected as a result of onychia or paronychia.

Mucous membrane lesions

Mucous membrane lesions, called mucous patches, are modified papules which become eroded, for example inside the mouth, to form oval or circular shallow erosions. They are covered with a greyish-white membrane and surrounded by a dull red areola. They may occur on the lips, cheeks, tongue (Plate 56), tonsils, pharynx, larynx, glans penis, prepuce, vagina, cervix and anal canal. They are painless unless secondarily infected. However, involvement of the pharynx and larynx may result in sore throat and hoarseness. The mucous patches on the soft palate and tonsillar region may, rarely, join together to form a snail-track ulcer.

Lymph nodes

Generalized enlargement of lymph nodes occurs in over half of the patients with secondary syphilis. The inguinal, epitrochlear, axillary, cervical and occipital nodes are those commonly involved. They are painless, discrete, firm and freely mobile. The enlargement may persist for several weeks.

Bones and joints

The patient may experience osteocopic pains or aching pains, worse at night, in one or more bones due to the tension caused by perivascular infiltration of the periosteum and the Haversian canals. The patient may present with tender elevation (periosteal nodes) of the anterior surface of the tibia. Radiological examination is usually normal. Other rare manifestations include osteitis (especially in immunocompromised patients), tenosynovitis and painless hydrarthrosis.

Other lesions

Other manifestations of secondary syphilis (or infectious relapse) include iritis, choroidoretinitis, hepatitis, gastritis, immune complex nephropathy, parotitis, anaemia and meningitis. Hepatitis may be associated with jaundice and elevation of serum bilirubin and alkaline phosphatase. The spleen may also be enlarged. The symptoms of gastric syphilis include abdominal pain, nausea and vomiting. Urinalysis may show albumin, casts and red cells due to nephritis. A patient with parotitis may present with a parotid swelling. Anaemia is not uncommon, and the erythrocyte sedimentation rate (ESR) may be elevated.

Neurological manifestations (see also the section on neurosyphilis below)

ASYMPTOMATIC NEUROSYPHILIS. In almost 30% of the patients with early syphilis, the cerebrospinal fluid (CSF) may show increased cells and proteins and reactive serological tests, but without any neurological symptoms or signs. Lumbar puncture is not usually indicated, and the changes in the CSF resolve with antisyphilitic treatment.

SYMPTOMATIC NEUROSYPHILIS. Symptomatic neurosyphilis is very infrequent in the first 2 years of infection. The most common form is meningitis, which may be focal or generalized. Acute meningitis is rare. The clinical features include persistent headache, neck stiffness, papilloedema, nausea, vomiting and clouding of consciousness. Involvement of the vertex may result in speech disturbances, monoplegia or hemiplegia. Basal meningitis may result in cranial nerve palsies, the third and sixth nerves being affected most frequently, resulting in pupillary abnormalities, ptosis, diplopia and squint. Eighth nerve involvement may be an isolated feature; the vestibular as well as cochlear branches may be affected, causing vertigo, tinnitus and deafness.

Differential diagnosis of secondary syphilis

Secondary syphilis should be suspected in the presence of a skin rash and/or mucous membrane lesions described above, and a generalized lymph-adenopathy as well as a history or evidence of primary chancre in a patient who generally looks well. However, secondary syphilis may resemble many conditions, and coexist with any of them. A detailed history and a thorough physical examination will help to exclude some of these conditions.

Skin lesions

Macular syphilides will need to be differentiated from seroconversion illness of HIV infection, measles, rubella, drug rashes, pityriasis rosea, pityriasis versicolor, infectious mononucleosis, leprosy, rose spots of typhoid and erythema multiforme. *Papular* lesions will include consideration of HIV infection, drug rashes, chickenpox, scabies, lichen planus and leprosy. *Papulosquamous* lesions should be distinguished from psoriasis and seborrhoeic dermatitis. *Pustular* lesions may mimic acne vulgaris, scabies, pyoderma, molluscum contagiosum and impetigo. *Annular* lesions may need to be differentiated from fungal infection, granuloma annulare, lichen planus, impetigo and erythema multiforme. Anal *condylomata lata* may be mistaken for anal tags, anal warts and haemorrhoids. Some of the above conditions are described in Chapter 11.5.

Mucous membrane lesions

Mucosal lesions in the mouth and throat may need to be differentiated from aphthous ulcers, herpes labialis, tonsillitis, diphtheria, Vincent's angina, infectious mononucleosis (which may be associated with biological false-positive reagin test), avitaminosis, agranulocytosis, Bechçet's syndrome, erythema multiforme, thrush and Reiter's syndrome. Persistent hoarseness, apart from being syphilitic, may necessitate investigations for tuberculosis and neoplasm. The lesions of the genital mucosa should be distinguished from genital herpes, balanitis circinata, lichen planus, psoriasis, erythroplasia of Queyrat and, in the female, from the vulval ulceration of Bechçet's syndrome. Some of the above conditions for the differential diagnosis are described in Chapter 11.5.

Other lesions

Syphilitic alopecia may be mistaken for alopecia areata and ringworm of the scalp. Lymphadenopathy may be due to HIV infection, Hodgkin's disease, infectious mononucleosis, lymphomas, trypanosomiasis and tuberculosis. The differential diagnosis of meningitis should include tuberculosis, cryptococcal infection, HIV-related neurological disease and other viral infections. The differential diagnosis of iritis is covered in the section on 'benign late syphilis'.

Diagnosis of secondary syphilis

The diagnosis of secondary syphilis is confirmed by the demonstration of *T. pallidum*, which is easier from the moist lesions such as those on the genitalia and condylomata lata. A search for the organism from the macular lesions is futile. Dry papules will need abrading to obtain serum. The demonstration of *T. pallidum* from oral lesions is described in the section on 'primary syphilis'. Serological tests for syphilis are almost always positive and the titres are high. Examination of the CSF is mandatory if there is an indication of neurological involvement. The CSF in syphilitic meningitis shows increase in cells (up to 1000 lymphocytes mm^{-3}), increase in proteins and elevated globulin level. VDRL and treponemal tests are always positive in blood and nearly always so in the CSF.

Natural course of untreated syphilis

The course of primary syphilis has already been described above. Many patients with secondary syphilis experience a single episode lasting for several weeks. The original knowledge on the natural progression of untreated early syphilis is based on the follow-up/review of the 1891–1910 Boeck–Bruusgaard patient material (Gjestland, 1955). Thus, about a quarter of the patients developed clinical secondary relapses mostly in the first year; 16% developed benign late syphilis usually during the first 15 years; 10.4% developed cardiovascular syphilis and 6.5% neurosyphilis. Over 60% of the untreated patients suffered minimal or no ill effects, the infection having remained latent; the serological tests remained positive in about half of these, and in the remainder the non-treponemal tests gradually became negative.

Relapsing early syphilis (see also the section on 'HIV infection and syphilis')

A relapse of early syphilis is usually due to inadequate or no treatment, and may be difficult to distinguish from re-infection. A history of further risk within the incubation period of a darkfield-positive primary lesion appearing at a different site in a seronegative individual, and evidence of infectious syphilis in the partner support the possibility of re-infection.

Clinical relapse

A primary chancre may reappear at the original site (chancre redux). The mucocutaneous lesions described above are the commonest form of recurrence, but the lesions are fewer and asymmetrical. Other rare manifestations include meningovascular neurorecurrence, periostitis, osteitis, iritis, choroidoretinitis, optic neuritis and hepatitis.

Serological relapse, seroresistance and other forms of relapse

In serological relapse, the reagin tests become positive after having been negative, or show a progressive rise in titres after a decline. Seroresistance implies persistently high reagin test titres at 6 months after treatment or less than a fourfold decrease in titres at 12 months. This serological scenario often precedes clinical relapse.

CSF should always be examined in cases of clinical or serological relapse which is also the only way to detect *asymptomatic neurorecurrence.*

Transplacental relapse means birth of a syphilitic child to an apparently cured mother. *Infection of a sex partner* also denotes relapse.

Prognosis of early syphilis

The prognosis of all manifestations of early syphilis is excellent with adequate treatment.

Latent syphilis

Latent syphilis is diagnosed when the blood tests for syphilis (confirmed by a specific test on a repeat specimen) are positive, but the patient has no symptoms and no abnormal physical signs on thorough physical examination, and radiological examination of the heart and aorta and the examination of the CSF are normal. The decision on lumbar puncture should be individualized. In the author's experience, if in a normally immune person, and especially if aged over 50 years, there are no symptoms and no signs suggestive of neurological or ophthalmic involvement and the reagin test titre is low (below 8), then the CSF is unlikely to be abnormal.

Latent syphilis is usually detected by routine screening, for example, in STI clinics, antenatal clinics and of blood donors.

Latent syphilis is divided into early latent and late latent syphilis. The early latent stage is confined to the first 2 years of infection (and hence is infectious) during which the patient may experience relapses (see above). Late latent syphilis (the infection is of more than 2 years' duration), is non-infectious sexually, but the infection can be transmitted by a pregnant woman to her fetus and, rarely, by blood transfusion for a few years. It is often difficult to determine the duration of the infection. Nevertheless, a careful history revealing the patient to be a contact of infectious syphilis, and a significant decline in the reagin test titres within a few months after treatment, point to early latency.

Although differentiation from yaws (if considered appropriate) is often impossible, a history or evidence of genital ulcer, positive treponemal serology in the partner, a history of miscarriages in the female patient, and a course of penicillin injections in the past, may suggest venereal syphilis. Differentiation from latent congenital syphilis will necessitate appropriate family history and examination of the relevant family members (see also the section on congenital syphilis).

Benign late syphilis

Benign late syphilis (or tertiary gummatous syphilis) becomes manifest about 3–10 years after the initial infection. The condition remains uncommon despite recent case reports associated with HIV infection.

Pathology

A gumma is mostly focal non-suppurative inflammatory tissue destruction. Histology shows an area of ischaemic central necrosis surrounded by lymphocytes, plasma cells, epithelioid cells and giant cells. The vascular changes are more pronounced than in early syphilis and there is a tendency to fibrosis and scarring. Despite a great deal of tissue destruction, the spirochaetes are difficult to find, suggesting a hypersensitivity reaction, possibly following reactivation of treponemes or superinfection in a sensitized host. Gummas vary in size from microscopic lesions to large swellings. There is no satellite adenopathy.

Clinical features

The majority of the lesions originate from the skin, subcutaneous tissue, mucous membranes, submucous tissue and bones. A fatal visceral lesion may, however, occur when the term 'benign late syphilis' would be inappropriate.

Skin lesions

The *cutaneous gummas* may occur on any part of the body, usually localized, as opposed to the generalized rash of secondary syphilis. They may be nodular or ulcerative (Plate 57), usually painless and occurring in groups in an arciform or serpiginous outline. They heal from the centre and spread peripherally. The scars, which are like tissue paper, retain the configuration of the original lesion and tend to have peripheral pigmentation. In some cases, the lesions develop surface scaling and may resemble psoriasis.

The *subcutaneous gummas*, which may be single or multiple, originate as painless lumps. They may take several months to increase in size when they merge with the skin which appears dull red in fair-skinned people. The tumour then softens and erodes to form a punched-out ulcer with a gummy discharge and the base covered with 'wash-leather' slough. The lesions heal very slowly leaving a 'tissue-paper' scar. Occasionally, a gummatous swelling may resolve without ulceration or scarring. The sites commonly involved are the legs, buttocks, sternoclavicular region, face and scalp.

Mucosal lesions

Common sites are the mouth, palate, pharynx, larynx and nasal septum. The lesions usually originate in the submucosa as painless swellings which gradually enlarge in size and encroach on the mucous membranes and deeper structures including bones. They subsequently may erode to form punched-out ulcers with wash-leather slough in the bases. Depending upon the site and extent of the gummatous process, the resulting deformities include perforation of the hard palate, destruction of the uvula, laryngeal stenosis (resulting in chronic hoarseness), nasal deformity and rhinopharyngitis with foul-smelling purulent discharge – the last being more common in yaws and endemic syphilis (Chapter 7.2).

Lesions on the tongue may start as a painless single circumscribed gumma or multiple gummata associated with diffuse interstitial glossitis. Later, the patient may experience pain with hot drinks, vinegar and condiments. Initially the tongue is swollen. As healing occurs, the scar tissue contracts and the tongue becomes fissured. In time, the impaired blood supply results in white areas of necrosis (*leukoplakia*) on the dorsum of the tongue and inner aspects of the cheeks and lips. These areas are well defined and may have a leathery consistency. The tongue may become smooth and glazed because of loss of papillae. This condition is prone to malignant change. Treatment with penicillin will not reverse the damage. Long-term follow-up is necessary. Use of tobacco should be avoided. Increased pain, bleeding and enlargement of lymph nodes are warning signs, and biopsy is indicated.

Lesions of bones and other supporting structures

Although any bone may be affected, those commonly involved are the clavicles, sternum, cranial and facial bones, and the tibiae. Trauma may be a predisposing factor.

Localized periostititis, which usually affects long bones, is the commonest manifestation. If a superficial bone is involved, the patient may present with a painful and tender swelling but no fever. The pain is deep seated and worse at night. There is subperiosteal thickening and formation of subperiosteal bone which can be seen radiologically. Diffuse periostitis of the tibia (and occasionally of the fibula – Fig. 7.1.3) and the deposit of new bone under the periosteum may result in bowing of the front of the tibia, called 'sabre tibia'. The gummatous process occasionally may involve deeper structures, resulting in osteitis/osteomyelitis, or superficial structures, resulting in subcutaneous gummata and cutaneous ulceration. In osteitis/osteomyelitis, there is bone destruction surrounded by sclerosis and invasion of the medullary cavity. In gummas of the nasal bone, there is pain, nasal discharge and perforation of the nasal septum which may result in collapse of the nasal bridge. Perforation of the hard palate will result in a nasal voice and regurgitation of fluid down the nose. X-ray of the skull may show a 'worm-eaten' appearance.

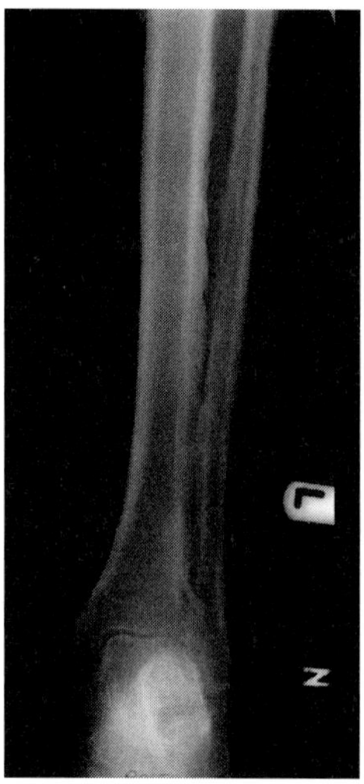

Fig. 7.1.3. Benign late syphilis: periostitis of tibia and fibula. (Courtesy of Dr J.H.E. Carmichael.)

Lesions of the other supporting structures including muscles, joints, tendon sheaths and bursae are extremely rare. The fibrous juxta-articular nodes in subcutaneous tissue or tendon sheaths near the joints, seen in an occasional patient, resolve with antisyphilitic treatment. A gumma of the vertebra is also rare and may cause compression of the spinal cord or a peripheral nerve.

Visceral lesions

EYES. Iritis and choroidoretinitis may occur in early as well as in late syphilis. The symptoms of iritis are pain in the eyes, photophobia, lachrymation and impairment of vision. The signs include circumcorneal injection, muddy oedematous iris, and later corneal opacities and irregular pupils due to adhesions of the iris. The symptoms of choroidoretinitis, which is more common in congenital syphilis, include flashes of light, distortion of objects and gradual loss of vision. Fundus examination will show yellow and grey–white retinal exudates and vitreous opacities in the acute phase, and white patches surrounded by black pigment when healing has taken place.

LIVER. Gummatous involvement of the internal viscera is very rare. The liver is the most common organ affected. Because the liver has considerable reserves, the patient may be asymptomatic. Gumma on the liver surface may present as a mass. Lesions within the liver, in time, may undergo fibrosis, scarring and lobulation (hepar lobatum). Depending upon the site of the gummata, the patient may develop symptoms and signs of pressure on the bile ducts and the blood vessels, and involvement of the liver parenchyma.

TESTES. A gumma of the testes may be localized but it may extend to the subcutaneous tissue and the scrotal skin, causing ulceration, usually of the anterior wall. The more common form is a diffuse painless interstitial orchitis presenting as a smooth hard swelling and loss of testicular sensation.

BRAIN AND SPINAL CORD. These lesions are described in the section on neurosyphilis.

Involvement of other organs, such as lungs, stomach, intestines, urinary tract and female genital organs is very rare.

Differential diagnosis

Mucocutaneous lesions

The most important consideration is to include the possibility of syphilis for any indolent lesion. Some of the common conditions to be considered include tuberculosis, leprosy, chronic eczema, psoriasis, seborrhoeic dermatitis, mycoses, dermatophytoses, Kaposi's sarcoma, epithelioma, sickle cell disease and varicose and tropical ulcers on the legs, rodent ulcer on the face, lichen planus and thrush of the mouth.

Bone lesions

Gummatous lesions may need to be differentiated from pyogenic osteomyelitis, endemic syphilis, yaws, tuberculosis, leprosy, malignancy, myeloma and Paget's disease.

Visceral lesions

The differential diagnosis of iritis and choroidoretinitis includes tuberculosis, leprosy, sarcoidosis, toxoplasmosis, rheumatoid arthritis, diabetes and Reiter's disease. Gummas of the testes should be distinguished from neoplasms (consider biopsy), chlamydial and gonococcal epididymitis and mumps orchitis (usually painful), and tuberculous epididymitis which produces a sinus posteriorly whereas gumma usually ulcerates on the anterior aspect. Syphilis of the liver may need to be differentiated from alcoholic cirrhosis, hepatoma, secondary carcinoma, amoebic abscess, hydatid disease, cholecystitis and carcinoma of the gall bladder.

Other differential diagnoses depending upon the site affected include gastric neoplasm, bronchial carcinoma, pulmonary tuberculosis and lymphogranuloma venereum of the rectum.

Paroxysmal cold haemoglobinuria

This rare haemolytic anaemia is due to the presence of a haemolysin in the blood of a few patients with late syphilis (acquired or congenital). This haemolysin combines with the erythrocytes on exposure to cold. The sensitized erythrocytes are haemolysed by complement in the plasma when the patient returns to a warm environment. The patient develops fever, headache, malaise and transient jaundice, and may experience a rigor. The urine becomes dark brown. The differential diagnosis is from march haemoglobinuria, blackwater fever and other causes of haemoglobinuria. Antisyphilitic treatment is curative.

Diagnosis of benign late syphilis

The diagnosis of benign late gummatous syphilis is based largely on the clinical features, the indolent nature of the lesions and serological tests. A past history of primary or secondary syphilis and/or evidence of syphilis elsewhere in the body may be helpful. The non-treponemal serological tests are positive in most, and the specific tests are positive in all patients. Darkfield examination for *T. pallidum* is futile in late syphilis. A therapeutic trial and biopsy may be necessary in some patients. A radiological examination of the heart and aorta and examination of the CSF should be considered to exclude cardiovascular syphilis and neurosyphilis.

Prognosis

The prognosis of benign late syphilis is generally excellent after treatment, except when permanent change has taken place. Thus antisyphilitic treatment will relieve the pain of glossitis but will have no effect on leukoplakia which requires continued careful observation.

Cardiovascular syphilis

Cardiovascular syphilis, involving mainly the thoracic aorta, aortic valves and the coronary ostia, occurs in about 10–15% of the patients with untreated syphilis. Although *T. pallidum* probably invades the aorta during the early stage of the infection, the condition does not usually become clinically manifest until 10–30 years later. Strenuous physical exertion may be a factor for why this complication is more common in men than in women.

A small proportion may concurrently have benign late syphilis or neurosyphilis which may be asymptomatic.

Pathology

The principal lesion is aortitis, the changes being more marked in the ascending aorta and aortic arch. All coats are involved. There is periarteritis and endarteritis of the vasa vasorum, resulting in degeneration, fibrosis and loss of elastic tissue, especially of the media. The intima, because of the contracted scar tissue, becomes wrinkled and may look like the bark of a tree. Later, atheromatous changes and calcification may supervene. The weakened vessel wall is liable to aneurysmal dilatations. The intimal pathology may involve the coronary ostia, resulting in their narrowing and thus ischaemia of myocardium. The aortitis may spread to involve the aortic valve ring and the cusps, resulting in dilatation of ring, separation, thickening and shortening of cusps and consequently regurgitation of blood into the left ventricle.

Other large and medium-sized arteries may also be affected, resulting in endarteritis, aneurysm and thrombosis.

Clinical features

Uncomplicated aortitis

Uncomplicated aortitis is usually asymptomatic, but some may complain of a localized substernal ache. A drum-like aortic second sound and/or a systolic murmur in the aortic area may be elicited (as also in hypertension). Radiological examination may show an irregular outline and calcification of the ascending aorta.

Aortic incompetence

Aortic incompetence may remain asymptomatic for several years until the onset of left ventricular failure. The symptoms include dyspnoea on exertion, nocturnal paroxysmal dyspnoea, headache, palpitation and later orthopnoea. Angina may also occur due to coronary ostial stenosis or due to the increased oxygen requirement of the dilated hypertrophied ventricle. The signs include a heaving impulse at the apex which is displaced downwards and outwards,

Corrigan's water hammer pulse as a result of high pulse pressure, a high-pitched blowing early diastolic murmur often louder at the left sternal edge accompanied by a systolic murmur at the base of the heart (thus resulting in a 'to and fro' murmur), pistol shot sounds over the larger vessels and, in severe disease, an apical mid-diastolic (Austin Flint) murmur with pre-systolic accentuation.

The chest X-ray (Fig 7.1.4) will show left ventricular enlargement, unfolding of the aorta and calcification. The echocardiogram shows aortic root dilatation and aortic valve disease. The electrocardiogram (ECG) shows left axis deviation, depression of the S–T segment and inversion of the T waves in leads over the left ventricle.

Coronary ostial stenosis

The anginal symptoms due to narrowing of coronary ostia are similar to those in a patient with coronary atheroma. Sudden death may occur. Aortic incompetence is also often present. The ECG may show depression of the S–T segment and inversion of the T wave.

Aortic aneurysm

Syphilitic aneurysms are usually confined to the thoracic aorta and may be fusiform or saccular. The symptoms and signs depend upon the site affected.

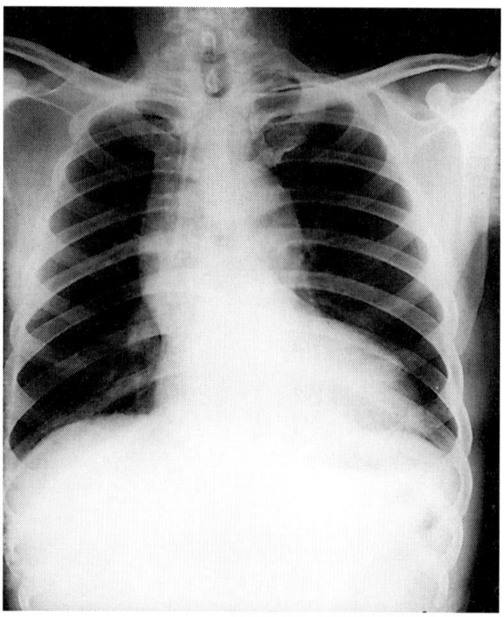

Fig. 7.1.4. Cardiovascular syphilis: marked unfolding of the aorta, and left ventricular enlargement due to aortic incompetence.

ANEURYSM OF THE ASCENDING AORTA. This is the commonest site involved and is associated with fewer symptoms than signs; hence it is called the aneurysm of signs. Symptoms include dull substernal pain and angina of effort. The signs include a pulsating mass in the second and third right interspaces, dullness on percussion in the same area due to pressure on the right lung, a systolic murmur in the aortic area and possibly aortic incompetence and displacement of the trachea and pulmonary artery.

ANEURYSMS OF THE AORTIC ARCH. These have been dubbed as aneurysms of symptoms. The clinical features include: a pulsating mass in the suprasternal notch; root pains due to pressure on the ribs and intercostal nerves; stridor and a brassy cough due to pressure on the trachea; dysphagia due to pressure on the oesophagus; hoarseness due to involvement of the left recurrent laryngeal nerve; tracheal tug and possibly collapse of the lung due to pressure on the left bronchus; Horner's syndrome due to involvement of the sympathetic chain; diaphragmatic palsy due to pressure on the phrenic nerve; and inequality of pulses and blood pressure in the arms as a result of distortion of, or pressure on, the ostia of the vessels arising from the aortic arch. In addition, compression of the superior vena cava may cause congestion of the veins of the head, neck and upper chest.

ANEURYSM OF THE DESCENDING AORTA. This is rare and often asymptomatic. With an enlarging aneurysm, the patient may, in due course, experience a piercing pain in the back as a result of pressure and later erosion of the corresponding thoracic vertebrae.

Gumma

Gummas of the heart are very rare. A gumma of the interventricular septum may result in heart block.

Differential diagnosis of cardiovascular syphilis

Other causes of aortic incompetence include rheumatic heart disease, bacterial endocarditis, atherosclerosis of the aorta, hypertension, congenital bicuspid valve, Marfan's syndrome and, more rarely, ankylosing spondylitis and Reiter's disease. Coronary atheroma should be considered in a patient with angina pectoris. Aortic aneurysms may be due to atherosclerosis, Marfan's syndrome and idiopathic cystic medial necrosis. They will also need to be differentiated from other causes of a mediastinal swelling, which include bronchial carcinoma, enlarged lymph nodes (lymphoma, tuberculosis, carcinomatous infiltration, sarcoidosis), retrosternal goitre, thymic tumours, fibroma, lipoma and congenital and other cysts.

Diagnosis of cardiovascular syphilis

The diagnosis of cardiovascular syphilis is made after all information is available comprising history, clinical features including evidence of syphilis elsewhere in the body, serological tests for syphilis and results of other routine and special investigations. The specific serological tests for syphilis will be positive in all cases and the non-treponemal tests in most cases. The other investigations and their results in aortitis and aortic incompetence have already been described. Coronary arteriography, when indicated, will differentiate coronary ostial stenosis from coronary artery disease due to atheroma. The diagnosis of aortic aneurysms will require plain chest X-rays and ultrasound, and occasionally special investigations such as barium swallow, computerized tomography and angiography (when surgery is contemplated) to assist differentiation from other mediastinal swellings. As some patients may also have neurosyphilis, lumbar puncture should be considered in all patients with cardiovascular syphilis.

Prognosis of cardiovascular syphilis

The prognosis of cardiovascular syphilis is variable, but is probably best in uncomplicated aortitis. Angina pectoris indicates poor prognosis. Aortic incompetence, when complicated by heart failure, deteriorates rapidly. Aortic aneurysms in some cases may enlarge rapidly, resulting in fatal rupture. Antisyphilitic treatment is unlikely to be of benefit once the anatomical damage has occurred. Appropriate surgical intervention may improve survival.

Neurosyphilis

Neurosyphilis may be divided into four categories: (i) asymptomatic neurosyphilis; (ii) meningovascular syphilis; (iii) parenchymatous neurosyphilis; and (iv) gummatous neurosyphilis.

The above categories are not mutually exclusive, and may overlap; they reflect the predominant clinical and pathological involvement.

Asymptomatic neurosyphilis

This is the most common form of neurosyphilis and has been defined in the section on secondary syphilis. The pathology is presumably confined to the meninges. Some of the 30% of the patients who show evidence of asymptomatic neurosyphilis in the early stages will continue to be asymptomatic (i.e. latent neurosyphilis) in the later stages. If left untreated, about a third (10% overall) will go on to develop late clinical neurosyphilis. The prognosis of asymptomatic neurosyphilis with adequate treatment is excellent.

Meningovascular syphilis

Pathology

Both the meninges and blood vessels are involved, although the clinical features may be predominantly meningeal or vascular. There is periarteritis and proliferative endarteritis of the blood vessels of the meninges, brain and spinal cord, basically in all types of neurosyphilis. There is infiltration of the pia-arachnoid with lymphocytes, plasma cells and fibroblasts around the meningeal vessels. The vascular changes may result in thrombosis and arterial occlusion, resulting in infarction of the brain or spinal cord. Miliary gummas may form in association with a diffuse inflammatory infiltrate, usually most marked at the base of the brain. The meninges are thickened and may interfere with the CSF flow, resulting in increased intracranial pressure and hydrocephalus.

Clinical features

Clinical manifestations of meningovascular syphilis may occur in early or late stages of the disease.

BRAIN. *Meningitis* is described in the section on secondary syphilis. A *vascular occlusion* may involve any artery of the brain. However, the arteries most commonly affected are the middle cerebral, posterior cerebral and their branches. The symptoms include headache, dizziness, transient paresis of a limb and the face, or sudden onset of monoplegia, hemiplegia, hemianaesthesia, homonymous hemianopia, dysphasia and seizures or other manifestations depending upon the site of the vascular accident. Occasionally a persistent headache may be the only symptom.

SPINAL CORD. *Meningomyelitis* has a gradual onset and, depending on the site affected, may manifest as spastic weakness of the legs, impairment of bladder sphincter control, sensory changes, root pains and lower motor neurone lesions or paraesthesiae in the upper limbs. A *vascular* lesion such as thrombosis of the anterior spinal artery (acute transverse myelitis) may result in rapidly progressive paralysis of both legs (later replaced by spastic paraplegia), sensory loss below the lesion and disturbance of bladder and rectal sphincter control.

Differential diagnosis of meningovascular syphilis

For the differential diagnosis of cerebral meningitis, see the section on secondary syphilis. Cerebrovascular syphilis will need to be differentiated mainly from cerebrovascular accidents associated with atheroma, hypertension or cerebral emboli. Spinal meningeal syphilis should be distinguished from tuberculosis, disseminated sclerosis, motor neurone disease, neoplasm and disc lesions, and spinal vascular lesions from other causes of transverse myelitis and space-occupying lesions.

Diagnosis of meningovascular syphilis

Specific blood tests for syphilis (TPHA, FTA-ABS) are always, and non-treponemal tests (RPR, VDRL) almost always positive. CSF changes (increase in lymphocytes and proteins and positive VDRL) are more prominent in cases of meningitis than in patients with predominantly vascular lesions in whom the CSF may even be normal in some cases.

Prognosis of meningovascular syphilis

With early and adequate treatment, the prognosis of meningovascular syphilis is generally good. Any structural damage as a result of vascular occlusion may be permanent.

Parenchymatous neurosyphilis

Parenchymatous neurosyphilis includes general paralysis of the insane (GPI) and tabes dorsalis. Both may occur together (taboparesis).

Pathology of GPI

GPI is a chronic progressive meningoencephalitis. There are meningovascular changes and parenchymal degeneration, most marked in the anterior two-thirds of the brain. At necropsy, the meninges are thickened, the dura mater adherent to the skull and the pia to the cortex. The brain surface is atrophied, sulci widened, ependyma granular and the ventricles dilated. There is diffuse perivascular infiltration of the meninges and the cortical blood vessels with lymphocytes and plasma cells, loss of neurones, gliosis and deposition of iron pigment in the microglia. *T. pallidum* may be demonstrated in the brain substance by special staining methods.

Evidence of tabes dorsalis and/or syphilitic aortitis may also be found.

Clinical features of GPI

GPI is more common in men and becomes manifest about 10–20 years after infection.

SYMPTOMS. The earliest symptoms include subtle personality changes, lack of concentration and intellect, irritability, headache and impaired memory. In due course, there is increasing carelessness about personal appearance, defective judgement, lack of insight, alcohol excesses, sexual aberrations, manic symptoms with paranoid features, confusion, euphoria and delusions of grandeur and wealth. Any of these may bring the patient into conflict with the law. The patient may become depressed and develop epileptiform attacks, transient hemiparesis and aphasia at any stage. Later the patient becomes more severely demented, confined to bed, paralysed and incontinent.

SIGNS. The signs include flat expression, disorientation, small and irregular pupils with sluggish reaction to light, tremors of the lips, tongue and hands, slurred and repetitive speech, nominal aphasia, shaky handwriting with words misspelt or omitted in a sentence, exaggerated tendon reflexes and extensor plantar responses followed by spastic weakness (tendon reflexes in lower limbs absent and posterior column involvement in tabo-paresis). Syphilitic aortitis may coexist.

Differential diagnosis of GPI

GPI will need to be differentiated from HIV infection, various psychiatric illnesses, chronic alcoholism, hepatic failure, drug addiction, pre-senile and senile dementia, cerebral atheroma, miliary tuberculosis, trypanosomiasis, lead encephalopathy, Parkinson's disease, Huntington's chorea, disseminated sclerosis, subdural haematoma, cerebral cysticercosis and other space-occupying lesions.

Diagnosis of GPI

Careful history and clinical examination may suggest the diagnosis. CSF in all untreated patients will show increases in lymphocytes up to 100 mm^{-3}, total protein above 50 mg 100 ml^{-1} with an excess of globulin and positive VDRL. Blood tests for syphilis will be positive in all cases. Chest X-ray may show evidence of aortitis.

Prognosis of GPI

Without treatment, the patient may die within 5 years. With early adequate treatment, one-third of the patients may return to their former job and another third to an alternative occupation. In the remainder and in late cases, the neurological damage is permanent. The patient continues to deteriorate and remains bed-ridden until death from a convulsive state or intercurrent infection.

Pathology of tabes dorsalis

The main feature is atrophy of the posterior nerve roots in the lower thoracic lumbosacral region and ascending degeneration of the posterior columns. There may be meningovascular changes elsewhere, and other areas involved include the mid-brain, the ciliary ganglion, the optic nerve, sensory fibres of the trigeminal and glossopharyngeal nerves, other cranial nerves (3rd, 4th, 6th and 8th) and the autonomic nervous system.

Symptoms of tabes dorsalis

The disease is more common in men. The symptoms appear 10–30 years after infection. The onset is usually insidious. A variety of symptoms may occur in any order. They include: episodes of lightning or stabbing pains (often the earliest symptom) of varying severity, usually in the legs, occasionally in the arms or in the distribution of trigeminal nerve, lasting for up to a few minutes, and may be repeated over several days followed by pain-free intervals of weeks or months; paraesthesiae including numbness of feet, 'things' crawling under the skin, a feeling of walking on cotton wool, a girdle sensation of tight constricting bands around the trunk; unsteady gait especially in the dark; visceral crises (gastric crisis – sudden onset of epigastrial pain, anorexia, vomiting; rectal crisis – rectal pain and tenesmus; renal crisis simulating renal colic; laryngeal crisis – cough, dyspnoea and stridor); bladder disturbances (overdistension, difficulty in starting micturition, retention with overflow); constipation, faecal incontinence; impotence; loss of testicular sensation; failing vision; loss of smell; loss of taste; deafness with or without vestibular symptoms; painless swellings usually of weight-bearing joints with increased mobility in chronic cases and painless indolent ulcers especially under the big toe.

Signs of tabes dorsalis

The patient may present with any one or more of the signs.

EYES AND INTRACRANIAL NERVES. The patient may have a characteristic expression ('tabetic facies') as a result of ptosis, compensatory wrinkling of the forehead and flabbiness of facial muscles. Pupillary changes, which may be unilateral in the early stages, are common, but not always typical Argyll–Robertson type in which the pupils are small, irregular and unequal, reacting normally to accommodation but not to light and a mydriatic. Other signs include optic atrophy with concentric constriction of visual fields and pale and well-defined discs, other ophthalmoplegias and sensorineural hearing loss.

SENSORY DISTURBANCES, TONE AND ATAXIA. The signs include: impairment of appreciation of pin-prick and cotton wool on the centre of the face, over the sternum, ulnar borders of the forearms, lateral aspects of the legs, the perianal area and occasionally over 'stocking' areas; a patchy hyperaesthesia in the areas just mentioned; loss of deep pain and hence absence of response to compression of the Achilles tendon or testis: loss of vibration sense in the lower limbs and of position sense in the toes; ataxia (a wide-based high stamping tabetic gait, worse with eyes closed or in the dark; a positive Romberg's test; a positive heel–shin test and, later, a positive finger–nose test); distension of atonic bladder; hard impacted faeces in rectum due to colonic hypotonia.

REFLEXES. Ankle jerks and later knee jerks are diminished and finally absent. Plantar reflexes remain flexor (may be extensor in a patient with tabo-paresis). Upper limbs may be affected later.

CHARCOT'S JOINTS. Charcot's joints are the outcome of the cumulative effects of muscular hypotonia, repeated trauma to the articular cartilage and loss of protective pain sense. There is destruction of the cartilage, and osteoarthritic changes. The joints are swollen, hypermobile and painless. The weight-bearing joints are especially involved, including the knees (Figs 7.1.5 and 7.1.6), spine (Fig. 7.1.7), hip, ankles and feet. X-ray will show destructive changes, exostoses, loose bodies due to avascular necrosis, dislocation and, occasionally, pathological fractures.

TROPHIC ULCER. Chronic indolent trophic ulcers, usually under the big toe, are the result of repeated trauma at pressure points combined with loss of pain sense. The underlying bone may be involved. Secondary infection and osteomyelitis may follow.

Differential diagnosis of tabes dorsalis

Tabes dorsalis will need to be differentiated from peripheral neuropathies associated with alcoholism, vitamin deficiencies, diabetes mellitus, infective polyneuritis, leprosy and heavy metal poisoning, Other neurological conditions include multiple sclerosis, subacute combined degeneration,

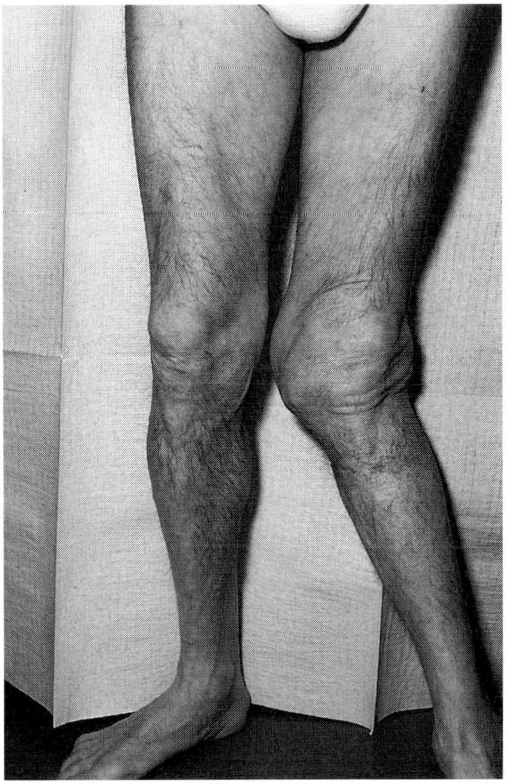

Fig. 7.1.5. Tabes dorsalis: Charcot knee joint; the left knee has large effusion and valgus deformity.

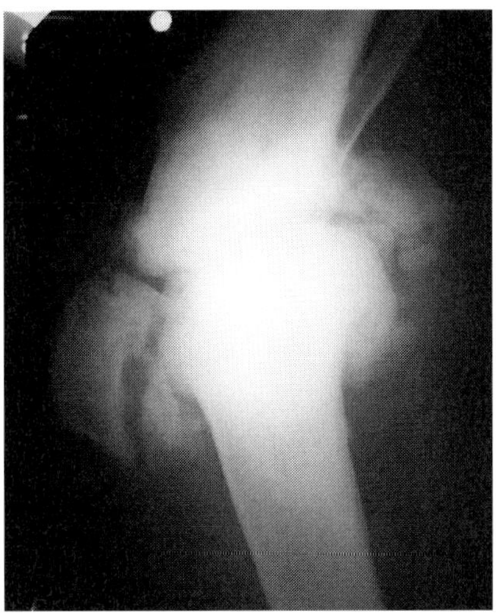

Fig. 7.1.6. Tabes dorsalis: X-ray of Charcot knee joint showing destructive changes, new bone formation and loose bodies. (Courtesy of Dr R.W. Galloway.)

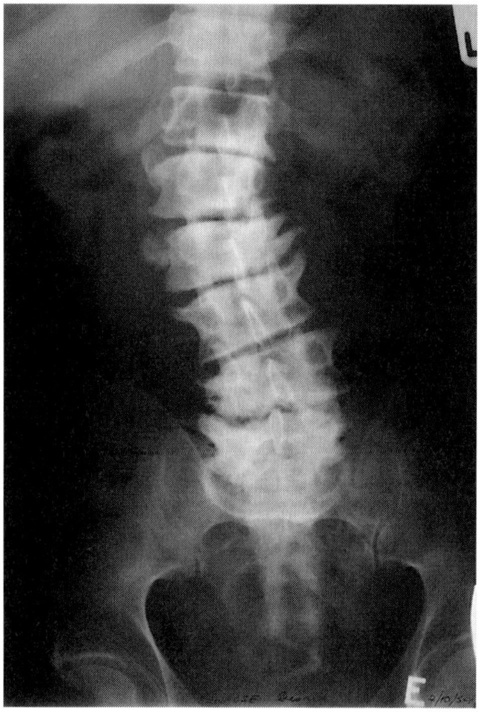

Fig. 7.1.7. Tabes dorsalis: Charcot's arthropathy of lumbar spine showing scoliosis, osteophytes and bone destruction. (Courtesy of Dr J.H.E. Carmichael.)

Friedreich's ataxia, cord injury and neoplasm. In addition, the Argyll–Robertson pupils may need to be distinguished from the myotonic pupil of Adie's syndrome; optic atrophy from pituitary tumours; lightning pains from rheumatism; visceral crises from an abdominal surgical emergency; distended bladder from that due to urethral strictures and prostate disease; Charcot's joints from syringomyelia and osteoarthritis; and trophic ulcer from diabetic neuropathy.

Diagnosis of tabes dorsalis

The clinical features elicited after a detailed history and thorough physical examination will provide a clue to the diagnosis of tabes dorsalis in the majority of patients. The CSF may be normal in an old burnt-out case of tabes dorsalis. In others, either cells or proteins or both may be elevated. In about a quarter of the patients, non-treponemal tests may be negative in the blood as well as in the CSF. Treponemal tests are almost always positive in the blood and, in most cases, in the CSF. However, a reactive treponemal test as the only abnormal finding in the CSF does not necessarily indicate neurosyphilis as it may be due to contamination of a CSF specimen with treponemal antibody-positive blood or diffusion of the specific immunoglobulins from serum into the CSF.

Prognosis of tabes dorsalis

Prognosis is variable and response to treatment unpredictable. Lightning pains, ataxia, optic atrophy, deafness and Charcot's arthropathy may continue to progress. In some cases, any further worsening of these and other manifestations may stop either spontaneously or after treatment. Administration of adequate treatment is, therefore, essential. Most cases eventually become dependent and succumb to urinary or other complications or other conditions.

Gummatous neurosyphilis

Gummas of the brain and spinal cord are extremely rare. The pathological process starts in the meninges. Because of similarities in the symptoms and signs, the clinical differentiation from other causes of space-occupying lesions is difficult. Thus the diagnosis is often made by biopsy in the course of investigations or after surgical intervention. Nevertheless, if blood tests for syphilis are positive and the CSF shows changes consistent with syphilis, a therapeutic test with antisyphilitic treatment in collaboration with a neurologist may be appropriate.

HIV infection and syphilis

The immunological impairment in HIV infection may alter the natural history of a concurrent infection. With regard to the effect of HIV infection on syphilis, the current knowledge (some based on only anecdotal reports) can be summarized as follows.

1. In the majority of patients with HIV infection, the clinical presentation of syphilis, and the response of serological tests for diagnosis and following treatment, are no different from those in persons not infected with HIV.
2. The healing of primary syphilis ulcer may be delayed, thus prolonging the infectivity.
3. The secondary syphilis rash may be very severe, with ulcers and nodules (lues maligna).
4. The syphilitic patient may fail to produce antitreponemal antibodies. In such patients, especially those with suspected secondary syphilis, the serological tests should be repeated and attempts made to demonstrate *T. pallidum* in the lesion material by darkfield examination or by direct fluorescent monoclonal antibody staining. In addition, histopathology may help.
5. Because of polyclonal B-cell stimulation, the non-treponemal tests may show high titres whether or not the patient has syphilis. The large amounts of antibody may result in prozone phenomena.
6. Syphilis may run a more aggressive course and neurological manifestations may occur early.
7. The patient treated for early syphilis may suffer a clinical and/or serological

relapse/seroresistance, especially if the treatment was with benzathine penicillin.

8. In a treated patient, the specific tests may become negative, thus masking any evidence of syphilis.

Because of certain similarities in the clinical features and CSF findings, HIV infection should be considered in the differential diagnosis of some forms of neurosyphilis. Because HIV infection may, possibly, accelerate progression of syphilis, it is advisable that all patients with syphilis should, after informed consent, be tested for HIV infection and vice versa.

Congenital syphilis

Epidemiology

Although pregnancy does not seem to have any effect on symptoms and signs of syphilis, syphilis remains an important cause of fetal and infant loss in some tropical countries, notably in sub-Saharan Africa (see Chapter 1).

Mode of infection

Although syphilis is not infectious sexually after the first 2 years of infection, an infected mother can transmit the infection to the fetus for 5 years, possibly longer. The treponemes present in the maternal circulation reach the fetal circulation via the placenta. The organisms may cross the placenta throughout pregnancy, but the pathogenic changes in the fetus do not take place until after 4 months of gestation, i.e. when the fetus becomes immunocompetent. A miscarriage during the first 4 months, therefore, is not due to syphilis.

The outcome of pregnancy in untreated syphilis

The outcome of pregnancy in untreated syphilis depends on the stage of infection in the mother. The risk of congenital syphilis is greater and the effects more likely to be more severe in the early stages of active syphilitic infection, with a much larger number of circulating treponemes available to cross the placenta than in the later years. Consequently the possible outcomes include: mid-trimester abortion; premature or term stillbirth; delivery of a syphilitic infant; delivery of an apparently healthy infant who develops symptoms and signs of congenital syphilis within weeks or months, later in childhood or in later life; or delivery of a healthy child remaining normal throughout life with or without positive serological tests. The above sequence, however, is uncommon. Thus, a healthy child may be born between two unfavourable outcomes; this is probably because the treponemes, which are fewer in number in the later stages of infection and perhaps present in a deep focus in the mother, may be released intermittently.

Pathology

The treponemes have disseminated throughout the body. The basic pathology is the same in all affected areas, as described earlier, i.e. perivascular infiltration with lymphocytes and plasma cells and obliterative endarteritis resulting in necrosis, fibrosis and formation of gummas.

The placenta

There is perivascular infiltration with lymphocytes and plasma cells and endarteritis of the villous vessels, diminished vascularity, hyperplasia of chorionic villi and diffuse fibrosis which may result in a bulky, firm and pale placenta. Nevertheless, the placenta may look completely normal. Treponemes are scanty and hard to find.

Syphilis of the fetus

If the mother with early stage syphilis is not treated, about one-third of the fetuses may die *in utero*, resulting in miscarriage (after 4 months) or stillbirth. An older fetus may show characteristic changes which include bullous eruptions containing haemorrhagic fluid, a collapsed skull, a protuberant abdomen due to hepatosplenomegaly, diffuse interstitial inflammation of the lungs which may appear pale grey (white pneumonia), changes in kidneys and pancreas and at metaphyseal–epiphyseal junctions of the long bones, and an abundance of treponemes in skin lesions, liver, spleen and lungs.

Clinical features

Congenital syphilis may be divided into early infectious stage during the first 2 years of life and late non-infectious stage including stigmata.

Early congenital syphilis

The symptoms and signs do not usually appear until about 2–8 weeks after birth. Infants born with physical signs carry a poor prognosis.

GENERAL SYMPTOMS AND SIGNS. Failure to thrive and gain weight may be the first signs to be noticed. The child may become marasmic and develop an 'old man look'. Other features include anaemia and thrombocytopaenia associated with bleeding disorder. The child so affected is very ill and may succumb to pneumonia, gastroenteritis and possibly also pancreatitis.

Many of the features in congenital syphilis are similar to those in acquired secondary syphilis.

SKIN LESIONS. These include: bullous eruptions (not seen in acquired syphilis) which may be present at birth ('syphilitic pemphigus'), mainly on the palms and soles, containing seropurulent or haemorrhagic fluid with many treponemes; a generalized rash which may be macular, papular or papulo-squamous (Plates 58–60) with shiny erythema especially on the palms and soles (Plate 61); 'eczematous' lesions and condylomata lata on mucocutaneous and other moist areas; radiating fissures which after secondary infection may heal and become linear scars (rhagades) at the angles of the mouth and around the nose and anus; patchy alopecia on the sides and back of the head; occasionally plentiful coarser hair ('syphilitic wig'); paronychia, onychia and deformed nails.

MUCOUS MEMBRANE LESIONS. Mucous patches may occur in the mouth, nose, pharynx and larynx (hoarse cry). Rhinitis (snuffles) may occur early. The nasal discharge, which is teeming with treponemes, may be mucoid, mucopurulent or blood stained. It may block the nose, causing breathing and suckling difficulties and hence weight loss. The lesion may progress to involve supporting structures, resulting, later, in septal perforation and saddle nose deformity.

LYMPH NODES. There may be a generalized lymphadenopathy, the lymph nodes being rubbery, discrete and not tender.

BONE LESIONS. These include osteochondritis and periostitis which may be present at birth but usually manifest some weeks later. Osteochondritis, which is due to invasion of the growing ends of the bones by *T. pallidum*, causes painful swelling which often may be the presenting feature of congenital syphilis. The bones chiefly affected are the distal ends of the radius and ulna and the upper end of the tibia (Plate 62). Other bones may be involved. Because of pain, the affected limb is kept immobile (Parrot's pseudoparalysis). X-ray of the long bones shows irregular thickening of the temporary zone of calcification in the distal metaphysis, giving it a saw-toothed appearance, rarefaction of the submetaphyseal zone, and periostitis with subperiosteal deposits of new bone encircling the shaft, i.e. periosteal cloaking (Fig. 7.1.8). While osteochondritis may resolve spontaneously after 6 months, periostitis may persist and continue to progress. Bilateral erosion of the inner aspects of the upper ends of the tibiae (Wimberger's sign) is considered to be pathognomonic (Fig. 7.1.9). Osteoperiostitis of the proximal phalanges (dactylitis) may occur.

OTHER LESIONS. Other manifestations include: hepatosplenomegaly – protuberant abdomen (see Plate 60); jaundice (low serum proteins and reversed albumin/globulin ratio); meningitis (convulsions, vomiting, bulging fontanelles, neck rigidity, positive Kernig's sign and hydrocephalus, CSF shows increase in cells and proteins and positive VDRL) and other forms of meningovascular syphilis (asymptomatic neurosyphilis is more common); choroidoretinitis; uveitis; and nephrotic syndrome due to deposition of immune complexes in the glomeruli (oedema, ascites, proteinuria) and orchitis.

DIFFERENTIAL DIAGNOSIS OF EARLY CONGENITAL SYPHILIS. Hepatosplenomegaly, lymphadenopathy and intrauterine growth retardation may be due to other intrauterine infections such as rubella, cytomegalovirus infection and toxoplasmosis. Skin lesions may need to be differentiated from infantile

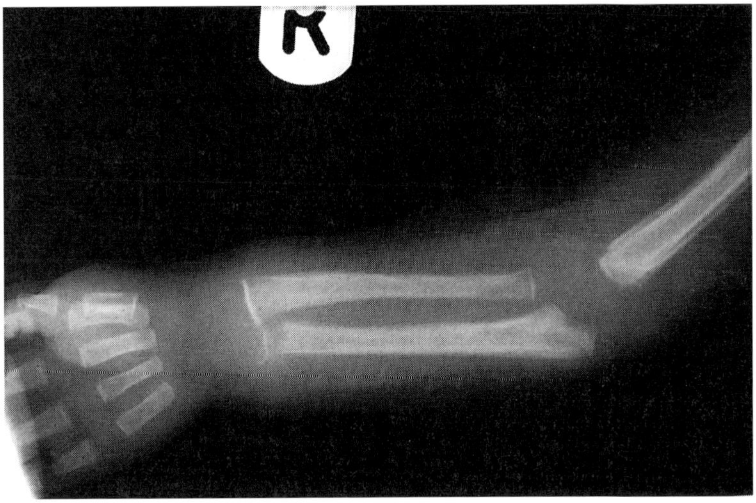

Fig. 7.1.8. Early congenital syphilis: rarefaction of the submetaphyseal zones of the distal radius and ulna, and periosteal cloaking. (As osteochondritis requires 5–6 weeks and periostitis over 14 weeks to appear on X-ray, this baby was probably infected during the second trimester.)

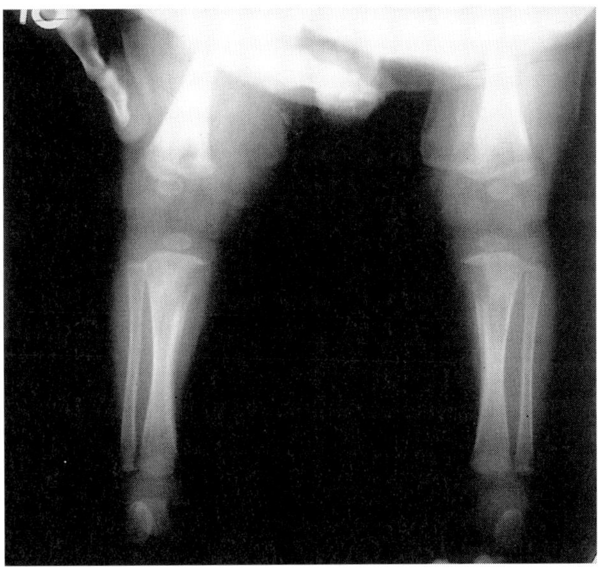

Fig. 7.1.9. Early congenital syphilis: metaphyseal defects on the medial sides of the upper ends of the tibiae (Wimberger's sign). (Courtesy of Dr J.H.E. Carmichael.)

eczema, impetigo, pemphigus, napkin rash, insect bites, scabies and ringworm infection; snuffles from coryza (suspect syphilis if discharge is haemorrhagic); pseudoparalysis from birth injury to brachial plexus, bacteraemia, sickle cell disease, poliomyelitis and infantile scurvy (the last three are uncommon in neonates); and dactylitis from sickle cell anaemia and tuberculosis.

DIAGNOSIS OF EARLY CONGENITAL SYPHILIS. The diagnosis of early congenital syphilis is confirmed by the demonstration of *T. pallidum* in the serum, from the skin and mucous membrane lesions and from nasal discharge (saprophytic treponemes do not appear in the mouth until about 6 weeks after birth). Radiological examination of the long bones may indicate osteochondritis and periostitis, and may need to be repeated after 2–3 weeks for evidence of progression to a more characteristic picture.

In all cases of maternal syphilis, the infant, even if clinically normal, must be followed up. The serological tests must be interpreted with caution. A positive serological test at birth may be due to passive transfer of maternal IgG antibodies, in which case the titre should fall fourfold within 2 months and the non-treponemal tests (RPR, VDRL) become negative by 3–6 months. Treponemal tests, especially TPHA, may remain weakly reactive for up to 15 months. If the mother was infected late in pregnancy, serological tests at birth of an infected baby may be negative. The serological tests should, therefore, be repeated at 3, 6, 9, 12 and 24 weeks. If by 24 weeks there are no clinical signs and the serological tests are negative or the titres of maternal antibodies in the infant have been falling, syphilis can be excluded. If the infant's VDRL or RPR titre is higher than the mother's, or seen to be rising or the test has become positive after having been negative, then the infant is infected. The detection of specific IgM antibody in the neonate, i.e. a positive FTA-ABS (IgM) test, in the absence of placental leakage, may indicate congenital syphilis. However, it may be falsely positive due to toxoplasmosis, HHV-5 infection and rubella, and falsely negative in those with delayed onset of disease or suppression of neonatal synthesis of IgM by the excessive maternal IgG.

The CSF should be examined before commencing treatment.

Late congenital syphilis

There are many similarities between late congenital and late acquired syphilis.

LATE LATENT CONGENITAL SYPHILIS. Over half of the patients are diagnosed and remain in the latent stage, with positive serology as the only abnormal finding. With time, the titres decline and the non-treponemal tests may become negative.

BENIGN LATE CONGENITAL SYPHILIS. Benign late lesions, which may involve the skin, mucous membranes, subcutaneous and submucous tissues, viscera, bones and joints, are rare before the age of 5. Nasal and palatal gummata are more common than in acquired syphilis. The former may result in septal perforation and collapse of the lower part of the nose, resulting in 'saddle nose' deformity, and the latter may cause perforation of the palate, resulting in nasal voice and regurgitation of food.

Osteoperiostitis of the tibia may produce anterior thickening of the bone and the appearance of bowing of the legs, i.e. sabre tibia. Other bone lesions include osteoperiostitis of frontal and parietal areas of the skull and dactylitis.

CLUTTON'S JOINTS. This is a chronic painless bilateral hydrarthrosis of the knees appearing around the age of 10 years. There may be a history of trauma. Radiological examination shows widening of the joint space but no bony change. The condition is thought to be a hypersensitivity reaction and resolves spontaneously after some months without any residual disability.

INTERSTITIAL KERATITIS. Interstitial keratitis is a common manifestation of late congenital syphilis. The age of onset is between 4 and 40 years. It is almost always bilateral, but one eye is affected initially. It is thought to be a hypersensitivity reaction. The symptoms are supraorbital pain, photophobia, lachrymation and blurred vision. On examination, there is circumcorneal congestion and later the cornea may look pink due to invasion of its deeper layers by small blood vessels from the surrounding sclera. The cornea subsequently develops a ground glass appearance due to cellular infiltration. Without topical corticosteroids, the condition may last for several weeks and relapse repeatedly after intervals of up to a year or longer. The patient is left with corneal opacities which may be large and dense in poorly managed cases, and interfere with vision, if in the centre of the cornea. The prognosis is good in well-managed cases, although nebular opacities and ghost vessels may be seen with a slit lamp. The prognosis with regard to vision is worse if choroidoretinitis is also present. Iritis may also coexist.

CARDIOVASCULAR SYPHILIS. Cardiovascular manifestations are very rare in congenital syphilis.

NEUROSYPHILIS. Neurological involvement in congenital syphilis may be asymptomatic or symptomatic. The symptomatic involvement may be meningeal (e.g. cranial nerve palsies), vascular (e.g. hemiplegia, monoplegia) or parenchymatous, resulting in juvenile tabes dorsalis or GPI, manifesting earlier or around the age of 10 years. Urinary incontinence or visual impairment may be the first symptoms of tabes dorsalis. GPI may begin with epileptiform seizures or mental deterioration. In general, the pattern and the CSF findings are similar to those in acquired neurosyphilis.

EIGHTH NERVE DEAFNESS. The age of onset is 3–50 years, usually 6–15 years. The pathological mechanisms include temporal osteitis leading to cochlear degeneration, membranous labyrinthitis or gummatous lesion in the nerve itself. The deafness is preceded by tinnitus and vertigo and is almost always bilateral, one ear being affected first. There is impairment of both air and bone conduction. Conversation loss is preceded by the loss of higher frequencies. Speech discrimination is affected disproportionately. The CSF may be normal. The prognosis is unpredictable even with treatment.

STIGMATA OF CONGENITAL SYPHILIS. The stigmata of congenital syphilis are permanent deformities or scars as a result of the pathological changes, most of which have been described earlier. The stigmata include: frontal and parietal bossing; saddle nose; perforation of the palate (Plate 63) and nasal septum; bulldog jaw (poorly developed maxilla making the mandible look prominent); Hutchinson's teeth (widely spaced permanent central incisors, usually upper, with anteroposterior thickening and narrow notched cutting edges as a result of invasion of the central tooth buds by *T. pallidum*); Moon's mulberry molars (defective enamel and imperfectly formed cusps packed in the centre, liable to caries and hence not seen in adult life); corneal opacities and ghost vessels; 'salt and pepper' fundus (black pigment and white atrophic patches as a result of choroidoretinitis); optic atrophy; 8th nerve deafness; rhagades (Plate 64); and sabre tibia (Plate 65).

PAROXYSMAL COLD HAEMOGLOBINURIA. This is described in the section on benign late syphilis.

DIFFERENTIAL DIAGNOSIS OF LATE CONGENITAL SYPHILIS. The differential diagnosis of the manifestations of late congenital syphilis is from among the various conditions listed under acquired benign late syphilis and neurosyphilis. However, deafness may be due to non-syphilitic middle ear disease, drug ototoxicity, acoustic injury, tumours and Menière's disease. Interstitial keratitis is seldom due to another cause and, when present in conjunction with nerve deafness and Hutchinson's teeth (Hutchinson's triad), almost certainly indicates congenital syphilis.

DIAGNOSIS OF LATE CONGENITAL SYPHILIS. The diagnosis is usually established by history, clinical features, including stigmata, and blood tests. The pattern of blood tests is similar to that in acquired late syphilis. Differentiation from the latter may be aided by examination of the mother and siblings. The mother will have evidence of treated or untreated syphilis. The CSF should be examined if neurological involvement is a possibility.

THIRD GENERATION SYPHILIS. Transmission of infection from an untreated congenital syphilitic mother to her fetus is extremely rare. The conditions of proof include exclusion of acquired syphilis, proven congenital syphilis in mother and infection-free father.

Interpretation and use of serological tests for syphilis

A positive serological test for syphilis may be due to a clerical or technical error, a biological false-positive reaction or past or present treponemal infection. In the absence of any evidence of syphilis, a positive test must always be repeated on a different specimen to exclude mistakes in labelling or technical error. (See Chapter 5 for classification and technical details of the tests.)

Non-treponemal tests

Non-treponemal tests (RPR or VDRL) are usually used as screening tests. When reactive, they should be repeated and at the same time confirmed by a treponemal test. If the latter is negative, then the non-treponemal test is said to be biological false positive (BFP – see below). A positive treponemal test confirms treponemal infection which may be treated or untreated syphilis or a non-venereal treponematosis such as yaws.

The non-treponemal test must be quantitated to serve as a baseline and also to monitor the adequacy of treatment. The same test must always be used in the follow-up of a patient.

The non-treponemal tests become positive about 3–5 weeks after the infection. The titre peaks when secondary syphilis makes its appearance and persists at the same level for about 2 years, and then may gradually decline even without treatment. The non-treponemal tests, in the large majority of patients, become negative within 6 months after adequate therapy of primary syphilis and in 12–18 months after the treatment of secondary syphilis. In the later stages of syphilis, the decline in titres to seronegativity is slow and variable.

Low-titred reactive non-treponemal test

In many tropical countries, non-treponemal tests in low titres (1:8 or below) are frequently encountered and antibiotics frequently consumed. A careful history and thorough clinical examination should be undertaken, especially for any evidence of acquired syphilis, stigmata of congenital syphilis or a non-venereal treponematosis such as yaws in childhood. If a repeat test within a few weeks shows a rising titre in two or more dilutions, the possibility of active syphilis is very high. If the repeat test is negative or shows a falling titre, syphilis is unlikely and a BFP reaction should be suspected. If there is no change in titre, the condition may be untreated syphilis, serological fastness following treated syphilis, yaws in childhood or a chronic BFP reaction. Attempts must be made for a treponemal test to be carried out to exclude a BFP reaction.

Biological false-positive (BFP) reactions

A reactive non-treponemal test in the serum of a patient who has never had a treponemal infection and has a negative treponemal test is termed a BFP reaction. The antibodies responsible for false-positive reactions can cross the placenta during pregnancy causing a false-positive reaction in the neonate's serum. The titres of BFP reaction are usually not higher than 1 : 8.

BFP reaction may be acute or chronic, the cut-off point being 6 months' duration. Conditions which may give rise to acute BFP reaction include infective hepatitis, infectious mononucleosis, viral pneumonia, chickenpox, measles, immunization, lymphogranuloma venereum, malaria, trypanosomiasis, pregnancy, etc. Chronic BFP reaction may be encountered in autoimmune diseases such as systemic lupus erythematosus, thyroiditis, rheumatoid arthritis, chronic infections such as tuberculosis and lepromatous leprosy, and other conditions including ageing, narcotic addiction and malignancy.

When a BFP reaction is confirmed, the patient should be fully assessed and given an appropriate explanation including the need for further investigations and follow-up.

Treponemal tests

These tests (FTA-ABS and TPHA) are used mainly as confirmatory tests or to distinguish true non-treponemal reactivity from BFP reaction, and also to obtain serological evidence in cases of late-stage syphilis when non-treponemal tests may be negative. In a patient with genital ulcer, the FTA-ABS test may be requested, usually being the first test to become positive in primary syphilis.

These tests tend to remain positive for long periods or indefinitely, especially if treatment has been delayed until later stages. Consequently, they play no part in assessing the outcome of treatment. Nevertheless, the TPHA titres usually fall significantly and fairly rapidly after treatment of secondary syphilis. A significant rise in TPHA titre may indicate re-infection, and in relapsing syphilis a rise in TPHA titre may precede that of VDRL.

False-positive treponemal tests

These are very rare and occur in diseases associated with chronic BFP reactions, notably in the presence of antinuclear and rheumatoid factors, lepromatous leprosy as well as in acute genital herpes. Infectious mononucleosis may give a false-positive TPHA test due to elevated heterophile antibody.

Management of syphilis

After the diagnosis has been explained to the patient, the importance of treatment compliance and follow-up and partner notification should be emphasized, and sexual contact forbidden until 2 weeks after the treatment has been completed.

Antitreponemal treatment

Penicillin, in the absence of allergy to it, remains the drug of choice in all stages of syphilis. A minimum serum treponemicidal level of 0.018 $\mu g\ ml^{-1}$ maintained for 7–10 days is required in early syphilis. There is no universal agreement on the optimum treatment regimens for the various stages of syphilis. Table 7.1.1 shows the recommended penicillin regimens as well as the alternative regimens for patients allergic to penicillin. Most specialists now agree that the drug regimens for neurosyphilis should achieve treponemicidal concentrations in the CSF. The penicillin regimens shown in Table 7.1.1 to treat neurosyphilis would satisfy that criterion in the large majority of patients.

Table 7.1.1. Antitreponemal treatment regimens for acquired syphilis.

	Penicillin regimens[a]	Alternative regimens if allergic to penicillin[b]
Early syphilis		
Primary syphilis	Aqueous procaine penicillin G, 900 mg (1.2 g for patient >80 kg) i.m., daily for 10 days	Tetracycline, 500 mg by mouth, four times daily, on an empty stomach, 1 h before or 2 h after meals for 15 days or Doxycycline, 100 mg by mouth, twice daily for 15 days
Secondary and early latent syphilis	Aqueous procaine penicillin G, dose as above, for 15 days	As above
Late syphilis		
Late latent and late benign syphilis	Aqueous procaine penicillin G, dose as above, for 15 days	Tetracycline dose as above, for 30 days or Doxycycline dose as above, for 21 days
Cardiovascular syphilis	Aqueous procaine penicillin G, dose as above, for 20 days	Tetracycline or Doxycycline as above for late syphilis
Neurosyphilis	Crystalline penicillin G, 1.2–2.4 g i.v., every 4 h, for 15 days or Aqueous procaine penicillin G, 1.2–1.8 g i.m. once daily *plus* probenecid 0.5 g by mouth every 6 h, both for 15–20 days	Tetracycline dose as above for 30 days or Doxycycline dose as above for 30 days

[a]Benzathine penicillin: see text.
[b]See also text.

The penicillin regimens recommended for the other stages of syphilis will produce serum levels much higher than the minimum required and, although not achieving treponemicidal levels in the CSF, do seem to prevent the development of neurosyphilis, perhaps by working in synergy with the host's immune responses.

BENZATHINE PENICILLIN. An injection of benzathine penicillin may provide an effective blood level for over 10 days. Thus it has the advantage of single session treatment. However, it does not penetrate into the CSF and its serum levels have also been reported to be erratic. There have been several reports of neurosyphilis developing after treatment of early syphilis with benzathine penicillin even before the advent of HIV infection. Therefore, its use is not recommended in cardiovascular and neurosyphilis. In the author's opinion, it should be avoided in any stage of syphilis unless none of the other options in Table 7.1.1 is feasible. The dose is 1.8 g (0.9 g intramuscularly into each buttock) at a single session for early syphilis and a similar dose once a week for 3 weeks for late latent and late benign syphilis.

Experience with the alternative regimens using tetracycline and doxycycline is limited. The patients so treated should, therefore, be followed up carefully for several years. Erythromycin (dosage regimen similar to tetracycline) has given high failure rates; it diffuses into the CSF poorly and should, therefore, be used as a last resort (see also 'Treatment in pregnancy'; some experts suggest desensitization of patients who are allergic to penicillin). Azithromycin, which is a long-acting azalide macrolide derived from erythromycin, has a high tissue penetration and is acid stable. At the time of writing, a dosage regimen of 500 mg orally once daily for 10 days had been reported to be promising in early syphilis. However, this drug is very expensive, and recently a macrolide-resistant *T. pallidum* has been reported. Another option for treatment of patients with a history of non-anaphylaxis type allergy to penicillin is to use ceftriaxone, 250 mg intramuscularly daily for 10 days in early syphilis and 1 g intramuscularly daily for 14 days in late syphilis. As these regimens are based on insufficient data, the patients will need to be followed up carefully.

Other measures

Iritis

The additional treatment includes topical atropine and corticosteroids. The patient should be managed in collaboration with an ophthalmologist.

Benign late syphilis

The additional measures include plastic surgery after the gummatous lesions have healed, a dental plate to cover the perforation of the palate and surgical intervention in the case of vertebral collapse causing compression of the spinal cord.

Cardiovascular syphilis

The patient should be managed jointly with a cardiologist. The supportive measures include: advice on diet, alcohol, smoking, exercise and occupation; symptomatic treatment for angina pectoris with glyceryl trinitrate, and digitalis and diuretics for heart failure; a cardiothoracic surgeon's opinion with regard to surgery for aortic incompetence (valve replacement), saccular aneurysm (excision, replacement with graft) and coronary ostial stenosis (endarterectomy, coronary artery bypass).

Neurosyphilis

A neurologist may be consulted. Therapeutic options for lightning pains include soluble aspirin, paracetamol, carbamazepine 200 mg, phenytoin 100 mg, sodium valproate 200 mg (any of these by mouth three times daily), hydroxocobalamin, 1000 µg intramuscularly weekly for 10 weeks. Other measures include: rest; analgesics including an intramuscular injection of 100 mg pethidine hydrochloride for tabetic crises; physiotherapy for muscle weakness; callipers to protect and stabilize Charcot's joints; cleanliness, avoidance of pressure, appropriate footwear and treatment of secondary infection in the case of trophic ulcer; bladder drill and initially carbachol, 0.25 mg by subcutaneous injection for atonic bladder (avoid catheterization, although it eventually may become necessary); appropriate therapy for urinary infection; and manual evacuation for faecal incontinence.

Optic neuritis, optic atrophy and 8th nerve deafness

The treatment of these conditions is described below.

Contact tracing (partner notification)

The patient's cooperation should be solicited to trace all contacts within the last 3 months in the case of primary syphilis, 6–12 months for secondary syphilis and 2 years for early latent syphilis. Those found infected should be treated. Those found uninfected but exposed to infectious syphilis in the preceding 3 months should be kept under observation (contact holding) until syphilis is proved or excluded.

Contact tracing in late syphilis is usually limited to regular (including marital) partners. If the patient is female, then her children if any, should also be examined.

Epidemiologic treatment

Epidemiologic treatment, i.e. treatment after exposure but before the diagnosis is confirmed, is not to be undertaken lightly. Only in exceptional circumstances should this be offered; for example if 'contact holding' is impossible or diagnostic facilities are poor, or if the female partner of infectious syphilis is pregnant. The partner should, nevertheless, be examined, and screened, if possible, for other STI, and given full antitreponemal and other appropriate treatment. Surveillance of these patients is similar to that for the rest of the patients.

Surveillance after treatment of early syphilis

The frequency of follow-up visits will be determined by the type of treatment regimen used (benzathine penicillin and non-penicillin regimens require more intensive follow-up) and the resources available. All patients should be advised, at the minimum, to attend after 3, 6 and 12 months, but ideally at the end of 6 weeks, 3 months, every 3 months for 18 months and then at the end of 2 years. At each visit, the patient should be clinically examined and blood taken for tests for syphilis. The darkfield examination for *T. pallidum* becomes negative within 24–48 h after starting treatment. The mucocutaneous lesions resolve in a few weeks. In a successfully treated case, the titres of quantitative tests, i.e. RPR or VDRL (not to be used interchangeably), progressively fall, becoming negative within 6 months in the majority of patients and within 2 years in most of the remainder. In those in whom RPR or VDRL remains positive at the end of 2 years, the titres are usually low. Unless the treatment was given at a very early stage, the specific tests, i.e. FTA-ABS and TPHA, will remain positive for several years.

If the non-treponemal tests have become negative, the patient can be discharged at the end of 2 years, or earlier if the seronegativity has been maintained over a period of 12 months. Others will need longer follow-up and CSF examination before final discharge.

Retreatment

A relapse, whether clinical, serological or in any other form, is an indication for retreatment. The CSF should be examined in every case. The dosage regimen should be that recommended for late syphilis (Table 7.1.1). Surveillance should begin from the time of re-treatment.

Surveillance after treatment of late syphilis

Surveillance of patients following the treatment of late syphilis initially is similar to that in early syphilis (see above). However, serological tests which measure the outcome of treatment in early syphilis are often not so helpful in late syphilis. Their results and titres may remain unchanged for long periods. The specific tests will remain positive for life. A further course of antimicrobial therapy should be considered if clinical signs and symptoms persist or if the titres of quantitative non-treponemal tests are rising or persistently high. In many patients, these tests will continue to remain positive at low stable titres (<1 : 8) which will not be affected by repeated courses of treatment.

After the initial 2 years' follow-up, most patients with late syphilis will need to remain under surveillance for many years, probably for life. The frequency of visits should be individualized such that the patient does not become overanxious. The surveillance comprises thorough clinical examination, blood tests for syphilis, occasional radiological checks and CSF examination and other tests when indicated. All patients with latent syphilis should be assessed thoroughly every 2–3 years, those with cardiovascular syphilis and neurosyphilis more frequently, and those with syphilitic leukoplakia every 3 months.

Any improvement following treatment of neurosyphilis is apparent within 6 months, after which little further improvement is likely. The CSF examination, if abnormal in the initial test, should be repeated after 3 months and then every 6 months for 2 years, or longer if necessary, until two negative specimens. The cell count may be expected to become normal and protein levels to decrease by 6 months after treatment, especially if the patient was treated with penicillin. Re-treatment is indicated if the cell count is abnormal at the end of 6 months or protein levels persistently high in the later tests. Such patients should receive intravenous penicillin (see Table 7.1.1) if not allergic to penicillin. If the patient is allergic to penicillin, some experts suggest desensitization to complete the treatment with penicillin.

Treatment of syphilis in patients with HIV infection

The CSF examination should be considered in all these patients. The treatment regimens shown in Table 7.1.1 are expected to be adequate. The surveillance plans are similar to those described above.

Management of syphilis in pregnancy and of congenital syphilis

Prevention of congenital syphilis

The overall strategy must include control of infectious syphilis in the general population. Congenital syphilis is easily prevented by testing all pregnant women for syphilis and treating those found to be infected. This is one of the most cost-effective procedures in preventive medicine, especially in areas with a high incidence of infectious syphilis. Treatment in the first 16 weeks of pregnancy will prevent congenital syphilis and even as late as in the 8th month will ensure the birth of a healthy baby. Blood tests (RPR or VDRL) may be carried out on two occasions (especially if the patient or partner is suspected of being at 'high risk') in early pregnancy and again around the 7th or 8th month. Alternatively, or in addition, both the mother and her infant may be tested at the time of delivery. If possible, a specific test (e.g. TPHA) should be done, especially in low prevalence areas (<1% prevalence) to exclude false-positive RPR or VDRL. The differential diagnosis from yaws may be difficult. A rising titre of RPR or VDRL if repeated after 3–4 weeks is suggestive of syphilis. However, no change in titre does not exclude syphilis. A history of genital ulcer, miscarriage and stillbirths may indicate syphilis.

Treatment in pregnancy

Penicillin is the treatment of choice. The dosage regimen depends upon the stage of syphilis (Table 7.1.1). Tetracycline is contraindicated in pregnancy because of the risk of maternal hepatotoxicity and enamel defect and discoloration of the infant's teeth. If the patient is allergic to penicillin, the usually suggested alternative is erythromycin, 500 mg orally, four times daily for 15 days in early syphilis and for 30 days in late syphilis. However, fetal blood levels of erythromycin have been reported to be low and hence the efficacy of erythromycin in the prevention of congenital syphilis is unreliable. Several failures have been reported. (There is no information on the use of azithromycin in these patients.) Some experts suggest desensitization of such patients to allow completion of treatment with penicillin. The other option is to use one of the third generation cephalosporins provided that there was no history of anaphylactic reaction to penicillin (see the section on anti-treponemal treatment for the dosage regimens).

Sexual partner(s) should be examined and treated. The patient should be followed up and serological tests repeated once monthly until delivery. Retreatment is indicated if there is clinical or serological relapse or evidence of re-infection. The surveillance plan as described earlier is then put into effect. If the patient becomes pregnant again and there is no evidence of serological relapse and the patient is known to have had adequate treatment, there is no need for further therapy.

Treatment of congenital syphilis

ABORTIVE TREATMENT. If the syphilitic mother was untreated, or treated with a drug other than penicillin, or the treatment (and/or response to it) was inadequate or unknown, or the follow-up of the infant is not ensured, the newborn should be given a course of penicillin as recommended below.

EARLY CONGENITAL SYPHILIS. The child is often ill and should be admitted into a medical centre, and precautions taken against transfer of infection from skin and mucous membrane lesions. The recommended treatment regimens are as follows:

- if CSF is normal: aqueous procaine penicillin G, 50 mg kg^{-1} of body weight intramuscularly daily for 10 days, or benzathine penicillin G, 37.5 mg kg^{-1} of body weight intramuscularly in one session (to be used only if the above regimen is not possible).
- if CSF is abnormal: crystalline penicillin G, 30 mg kg^{-1} of body weight every 12 h intramuscularly or intravenously daily for 10–15 days, or aqueous procaine penicillin G, 50 mg kg^{-1} of body weight intramuscularly daily for 10–15 days.

If the child is allergic to penicillin (i.e. after the neonatal period), use erythromycin, 30–50 mg kg^{-1} of body weight in four divided doses by mouth daily for 15 days.

LATE CONGENITAL SYPHILIS. The antibiotic dose will depend on the age and weight of the child. Adult doses should be used for those over the age of 15 years. The duration of treatment is the same as in acquired syphilis. Because of their effect on bones and teeth, tetracyclines should not be given to children under the age of 12 years.

INTERSTITIAL KERATITIS. Interstitial keratitis may continue to progress despite adequate treatment with penicillin, presumably because the condition is a hypersensitivity reaction. Nevertheless, treatment as intensive as for neurosyphilis has been suggested, including consideration of the use of amoxycillin (plus probenecid: see below for dosage regimen) which would give higher concentrations than penicillin in the ocular compartments. That said, the topical corticosteroids (e.g. 0.5% prednisolone eye drops to be instilled initially every 2–4 h), although not curative, suppress the condition and are the mainstay of treatment. Corneal graft may be helpful in a case with extensive scarring. An ophthalmologist must always be consulted.

NERVE DEAFNESS, CHOROIDORETINITIS, OPTIC NEURITIS AND OPTIC ATROPHY. Although the prognosis of these conditions, whether as a result of acquired or congenital syphilis, is unpredictable, the patient must be offered a course of intensive therapy at the earliest opportunity. This should be either with an intravenous crystalline penicillin regimen (Table 7.1.1) *or* a high dose amoxycillin–probenecid combination because of amoxycillin's greater penetration into the eye and inner ear than penicillin's; the adult dose is amoxycillin, 1 g plus probenecid, 0.5 g by mouth four times daily for 15–20 days (one should be aware of the side effects including pseudomembranous colitis). Even a slight improvement, for example in the vision or speech discrimination, will be a bonus. Prednisolone is always prescribed to prevent Jarisch–Herxheimer reactions (see below for the dose), but whether or not corticosteroids have any role in clearing these conditions is uncertain. The regimen for the latter is prednisolone, 30 mg by mouth daily in divided doses for 1 week and then 20 mg by mouth daily in divided doses, initially for 4 weeks. If there is no improvement by then, prednisolone should be tailed off and discontinued; otherwise it may be continued for another 3 months, after which the patient should be reviewed. The patient should be managed in conjunction with an ophthalmologist and/or an ENT specialist.

Surveillance after treatment of congenital syphilis

The surveillance plan after treatment of early congenital syphilis is similar to that of early acquired syphilis as are also the clinical and serological responses and the re-treatment criteria. Radiological healing of the bony lesions is usually achieved 3–4 months after treatment. Hepatosplenomegaly may take longer to resolve. If the CSF is normal and the non-treponemal blood tests are negative at the end of 2 years, the child can be discharged.

The post-treatment surveillance of late congenital syphilis is also similar to that of late acquired syphilis. Retreatment will depend on the clinical and serological progress as well as the physician's experience. Some patients may develop interstitial keratitis (or relapses) or deafness in the late teens or adulthood.

CONTACTS. The mother will need to be examined and treated. The spouse and other siblings should be investigated, and treated if necessary.

Treatment reactions

Jarisch–Herxheimer (JH) reaction

The mechanism of this reaction is not entirely clear, and may have an immunological basis. It is more common in early syphilis, occurring in about

70% of the cases, than in late syphilis. It consists of local and generalized reactions beginning about 6–8 h after the first dose of antitreponemal therapy. The patient experiences general malaise, bone and joint pains, shivering, headache, fever and tachycardia. The local component consists of cellular infiltration and oedema. Thus a preputial primary lesion may become more oedematous, resulting in phimosis and the prepuce becoming irretractable. A secondary rash initially barely visible may become quite obvious. Slight hoarseness may worsen to almost complete loss of voice. JH reaction in a pregnant woman treated in the second half of pregnancy may result in premature labour and/or fetal distress.

The patient must be warned about this reaction to prevent undue anxiety. The reaction is usually harmless in early syphilis and often all that is required is bed rest and aspirin or paracetamol. It is not a drug reaction, from which it must be differentiated so that the patient can continue and complete the course of antisyphilitic treatment. A pregnant woman beyond 20 weeks' gestation may be hospitalized at the start of treatment.

In late syphilis, the patient may become febrile, but the local component occasionally can be life threatening, for example coronary ostial occlusion resulting in sudden death, rupture of aortic aneurysms or occlusion of a cerebral artery, or laryngeal stenosis in the case of laryngeal gumma. Other possibilities include epileptiform convulsions, acute mania, delusions and hallucinations after initiating treatment of GPI, cranial nerve palsies in other forms of neurosyphilis, and blindness in a case of optic neuritis.

PREVENTION OF JH REACTION. Most specialists now prescribe steroids, although of unproven efficacy, for patients with cardiovascular involvement, neurosyphilis and laryngeal gumma, in the hope of suppressing the JH reaction. The dose is prednisolone, 5 mg four times daily for 24 h before starting antisyphilitic treatment, then continued for 2 days along with the antisyphilitic treatment and then tailed off by 5 mg per day. In a patient with GPI, sedation prior to antisyphilitic therapy may prevent seizures. All such patients should be treated under observation in the hospital at least for the first few days.

Penicillin reactions

Penicillin is virtually non-toxic in therapeutic doses. Penicillin reactions are due to hypersensitivity which may be immediate (type 1) and delayed. The *immediate* reactions include urticaria, facial flushing, generalized pruritus, palpitation, tightness in the chest, wheezing, laryngeal oedema and anaphylactic shock. Anaphylactic shock is the most serious, i.e. severe hypotension and rapid death within seconds or minutes after giving a penicillin injection. The *delayed* reactions, which may appear up to several days after penicillin administration, include various skin rashes, arthralgia with effusions into joints, fever, proteinuria and, in some cases, redness, urticaria and pruritus around the injection site.

TREATMENT OF PENICILLIN REACTIONS. All patients may be advised to wait in the clinic for 20 min after the penicillin injection. If an anaphylactic reaction is suspected, proceed as follows:

1. The patient should lie down, head down and feet raised.
2. Establish an airway.
3. Give 0.5 ml of 1 : 1000 adrenaline intramuscularly, repeat if no improvement in 10 min.
4. If angio-oedema is present, give chlorpheniramine, 10 mg intravenously.
5. Treat bronchospasm with aminophylline, 250 mg in 10 ml of sterile water intravenously, slowly.
6. If there is no response, give hydrocortisone sodium succinate, 100 mg intravenously.
7. Additional measures include an intravenous drip to facilitate treatment and combat hypotension, administration of oxygen, artificial respiration, tracheostomy and external cardiac massage, summoning of the cardiac arrest team and admission into an intensive care unit.

Successful management of anaphylactic shock requires medical and nursing staff with training in handling such cases. An emergency pack containing the above medications, syringes and needles should be readily available.

Most patients with delayed reactions will respond to an oral antihistamine such as chlorpheniramine, 4 mg three times daily until the reaction subsides. In addition, more severe cases may be treated with prednisolone, 10 mg four times daily, to be tailed off gradually after a few days.

PREVENTION OF PENICILLIN REACTIONS. The most important preventive measure is a carefully taken reliable history of penicillin allergy. If the answer is yes, then penicillin is contraindicated. Some suggest desensitization to permit completion of treatment with penicillin for syphilis in pregnancy and neurosyphilis.

Procaine reaction

There are two types of procaine reaction. Soon after the intramuscular administration of procaine penicillin, the patient experiences mental disturbance manifested by a fear of impending death, auditory and visual hallucinations, shouting and hysterical symptoms, sometimes seizures. The blood pressure is normal. This type of reaction is thought to be due to the procaine toxicity of the central nervous system, the procaine blood level having increased due to a low level of procaine esterase in these patients. In the second type of reaction, the patient, in addition to the above symptoms, experiences pulmonary and cardiovascular symptoms. This reaction is thought to be due to accidental intravenous administration of procaine penicillin, resulting in direct procaine toxicity as well as micro-embolization of the lungs and brain. Cardiovascular collapse is very rare when the differential diagnosis is from anaphylactic shock.

TREATMENT AND PREVENTION OF PROCAINE REACTIONS. Treatment is with rest and maintenance of airway. The patient may need to be restrained. The symptoms usually subside within a few minutes. More severe cases may need oxygen. Convulsions may be controlled by a small dose of Diazepam given intravenously. Intravenous injection of procaine is prevented by aspirating, before injecting, to ensure the needle has not entered a blood vessel.

Vaso-vagal attack

Some patients feel faint or, more rarely, go stiff or exhibit jerky movements, when given an injection or when a blood specimen is being collected. There is a risk of injury if the patient falls. The condition is more common in men. Recovery is usually quick after the patient is made to lie down or put the head between the knees. It would be advisable to perform the above procedures, i.e. giving an injection or taking a blood specimen, with the patient lying down.

Further reading

Gjestland, T. (1955) The Oslo study of untreated syphilis: an epidemiologic investigation of the natural course of syphilitic infection based on a restudy of the Boeck–Bruusgaard material. *Acta Dermato Venereologica* 35 (Suppl. 34), 1–368.

Goldmeier, D. and Hay, P. (1993) A review and update on adult syphilis, with particular reference to its treatment. *International Journal of STD and AIDS* 4, 70–82.

Hira, S.K. (1991) *Guidelines for Prevention of Adverse Outcomes of Pregnancy due to Syphilis.* World Health Organization, WHO.VDT/91.455.

Meyer, M.P., Roditi, D. and Louw, S. (1992) IgM rheumatoid factor removal and performance of the FTA-ABS (IgM) test in congenital syphilis. *Genitourinary Medicine* 68, 249–253.

van der Sluis, J.J. (1992) Laboratory techniques in the diagnosis of syphilis: a review. *Genitourinary Medicine* 68, 4413–4419.

Young, H. (1992) Syphilis: new diagnostic directions. *International Journal of STD and AIDS* 3, 391–413.

Chapter 7.2
Endemic treponematoses

O.P. Arya
Department of Medical Microbiology and Genitourinary Medicine, University of Liverpool, Liverpool, UK

Endemic treponematoses are non-venereally acquired conditions and comprise yaws, bejel and pinta. Their causative organisms, respectively *Treponema pertenue*, *T. endemicum* and *T. carateum*, cannot yet be distinguished from *T. pallidum* which causes venereal syphilis described in the previous chapter. The significance of a one-base difference between the DNA sequences of *T. pallidum* and *T. pertenue* remains to be clarified. There are similarities too in serology and response to penicillin. These similarities pose problems in differentiating the treponematoses from one another. This difficulty is of particular concern in distinguishing non-venereal treponematoses from venereal syphilis because of the social stigma attached to the latter diagnosis. This diagnostic dilemma necessitates a brief description of the non-venereal treponematoses. Indeed, there are epidemiological and clinical differences which may help, though not always, in making an appropriate diagnosis.

Epidemiology, historical perspective and transmission

Half a century ago, endemic treponematoses were among the most prevalent diseases worldwide. After the availability of long-acting penicillin, cheap, safe and curative in one intramuscular injection, a global control programme was established in 1948 under the auspices of the World Health Organization. Over 50 million individuals were treated in 46 countries. The diseases were brought under control. However, the lack of proper surveillance resulted in resurgence of these conditions in many areas towards the end of the 1970s.

There are no reliable data on the incidence of these conditions. Yaws, which is the most common, is encountered in warm, humid, remote rural areas of Africa, the Caribbean, South America, the Pacific islands and Southeast Asia. Bejel is endemic in the arid Sahelian areas of Africa and among the nomadic people in the Arabian peninsula. Pinta is confined to the rural areas of Central and South America.

These diseases are contracted in childhood or early adolescence among communities living in poor, overcrowded and insanitary conditions. Yaws and pinta are transmitted from one person to another by direct skin lesion–skin contact, transmission being facilitated by a breach in the recipient's skin. In the case of bejel, the initial lesion being on the oral mucosa, transmission is by direct contact through kissing as well as by indirect contact through shared eating and drinking utensils. Congenital transmission is assumed not to occur.

Clinical features

The incubation period is 10–90 days.

Yaws (buba, framboesia, pian)

The clinical course of yaws may be divided into an early infectious stage (up to 5 years or longer) and a late non-infectious stage. (The lesions may, possibly, be more severe in a patient with HIV infection.) The primary lesion, which is itchy, appears at the site of inoculation on an exposed part of the body as a localized maculopapular rash or a papule which develops into a large exudative papilloma, 2–5 cm in diameter. It lasts for 3–6 months and heals with or without scarring. Haematogenous and lymphatic spread of the organisms produces lesions elsewhere on the body. These secondary lesions become manifest a few weeks to 2 years after the primary lesion. They are multiple excrescences or papillomata (Plates 66 and 67) covered with yellow crust, which when removed gives the lesions the appearance of raspberry granulomata (framboesides). The lesions on the moist areas may look like condylomata lata of secondary syphilis. These lesions may last for up to 6 months and heal with or without scarring. Infectious relapses with lesions in polymorphic forms (Plate 68) may appear during the next 5 years. The other early lesions include generalized enlargement of lymph nodes, palmar and plantar fissuring, plantar papillomas (resulting in painful crab-like gait), and osteoperiostitis of the long bones (causing nocturnal bone pain) or of proximal phalanges of the fingers (Plate 69). The patient may then enter latency, which may persist with serological tests remaining positive, usually in low titres. Others may develop late lesions which include gummatous lesions of the skin, further progression of osteoperiostitis (e.g. sabre tibia – Plate 70) of the long bones, osteitis of the maxillae (goundou – Plate 71), destructive ulceration of the nasopharynx (gangosa), hyperkeratosis of palms and soles (Plate 72), juxta-articular nodes, scarring and cicatricial contractures.

Bejel (dichuchwa, endemic syphilis, firzal)

Apart from the initial lesions which occur on the mouth and lips, the clinical features of bejel are largely similar to those of yaws.

Pinta (azul, carate, mal de pinto)

Pinta is the mildest of all treponematoses and its manifestations are confined to the skin. The primary lesion appears at the site of entry of the organisms, on an exposed part of the body such as an arm, leg or the face. It starts as an itchy erythematous papule which develops into an erythematosquamous patch with satellite lesions. The regional lymph nodes may be enlarged and painless. The secondary lesions (pintids) develop several months later and are widespread itchy erythematosquamous plaques. These lesions harbouring treponemes may persist and remain infectious for many years. Thus, in pinta, there is virtually no latent non-infectious stage, unlike in the other treponematoses. Eventually the pintids undergo a variety of colour changes with shades of red, grey and bluish black, followed by depigmentation. Varying degrees of these changes may be encountered simultaneously.

Diagnosis and differential diagnosis

Clinical diagnosis of the various endemic treponematoses in the presence of classical lesions is usually straightforward in the endemic areas. However, milder forms frequently being encountered may pose problems. Nevertheless, the diagnosis is confirmed by the demonstration of typical treponemes by darkfield microscopy of the material from early lesions. Serological tests behave as in venereal syphilis, and radiography will show bone lesions in late cases of yaws and bejel.

Several conditions may need to be considered in the differential diagnosis, and the reader is referred to the Further reading list at the end of this chapter. However, the most important and most difficult is the differential diagnosis from venereal syphilis, which has social implications. A detailed history should include place of birth, residence and history of yaws in childhood and any treatment received, history of genital lesions, miscarriages in the female, and congenital syphilis in the offspring. All of the clinical features of endemic treponematoses may also be encountered in venereal syphilis. However, any evidence of cardiovascular or neurological involvement will point to venereal syphilis. The interpretation of serological tests is described in Chapter 7.1. If, after carefully considering all the facts available, it is not possible to arrive at a clear cut diagnosis, then the patient should be treated as for venereal syphilis.

Treatment

At the time of writing, there is no proof of the existence of penicillin-resistant treponemes. However, clinical resistance to penicillin among cases of yaws has been encountered recently in Ecuador. This calls for continued vigilance. For the present, the treatment of choice remains benzathine penicillin G intramuscularly in a single session. The dose is 600,000 units (0.45 g) for children under the age of 6 years; 1.2 mega units (0.9 g) for those aged 6–15 years, and 2.4 mega units (1.8 g) for those over 15 years. The dose may be divided so that half is given into each buttock.

For those allergic to penicillin, the options are tetracycline or erythromycin, 500 mg orally four times daily for 15 days, *or* doxycycline, 100 mg orally twice daily for 15 days. Children between 12 and 15 years of age should receive half that dose. Tetracyclines should be avoided in pregnancy and for children under the age of 12.

Close contacts should be examined and treated.

Other details

For further details of the above and other aspects of endemic treponematoses, the reader may refer to the Further reading list.

Further reading

Anselmi, M., Araujo, E., Narváez, A., Cooper, P.J. and Guderian, R.H. (1995) Yaws in Ecuador: impact of control measures on the disease in the Province of Esmeraldas. *Genitourinary Medicine* 71, 343–346.

Arya, O.P. (1995) Endemic treponematoses. In: Cook, G.C. (ed.) *Manson's Tropical Diseases*, 20th edn. Saunders, London, pp. 940–950.

Hacket, C.J. and Loewenthal, L.J.A. (1960) *The Differential Diagnosis of Yaws.* World Health Organization, Monograph No. 36, Geneva.

Meheus, A. and Tikhomirov, E. (1998) Endemic treponematoses. In: Holmes, K.K. *et al.* (eds) *Sexually Transmitted Diseases.* McGraw-Hill, New York, in press.

Noordhoek, G.T., Hermans, B.W.M., Paul, A.M. *et al.* (1989) *Treponema pallidum* subspecies *pallidum* (Nichols) and *T. pallidum* subspecies *pertenue* (CDC 2575) differ in at least one nucleotide, comparison of two homologous antigens. *Microbial Pathogenesis* 6, 29–42.

Perine, P.L., Hopkins, D.R., Niemal, P.L.A. St. John, R.K., Causse, G. and Antal, G.M. (1984) *Handbook of Endemic Treponematoses.* World Health Organization, Geneva.

CHAPTER 7.3
Chancroid

O.P. Arya
Department of Medical Microbiology and Genitourinary Medicine, University of Liverpool, Liverpool, UK

Chancroid is an STI characterized by painful genital ulceration and suppurative inguinal buboes. It is a prominent cause of genital ulceration in many tropical areas. The facilitating effect of genital ulcers in the transmission of HIV infection has added urgency to the control of chancroid.

Epidemiology

Chancroid is common in Africa, Asia, Central and South America. Promiscuity, prostitution and poor hygiene contribute to its spread. The prevalence and significance of asymptomatic carriage of the causative organism are unclear. See Chapter 1 for further details.

Aetiology

The causative organism *Haemophilus ducreyi* is a short, non-motile, non-sporing, Gram-negative facultative anaerobic bacterium requiring haemin for growth.

Transmission and pathogenesis

Transmission is by sexual contact. The pathogenesis is not entirely clear. After penetrating the skin through a minor abrasion, the organism attaches to and possibly invades the epithelial cells before causing a cytopathic effect. Whether or not a toxin is involved in this effect remains to be clarified.

Histology

Histology shows necrosis and a large number of neutrophils in the surface zone, newly formed blood vessels perpendicular to the ulcer surface and endothelial proliferation in the mid-zone, and, infiltration by plasma cells, lymphocytes and fibroblasts in the deepest zone.

Clinical features

The incubation period is short, usually not longer than 10 days. The lesion begins as a tender papule, which develops into a pustule which breaks down to form an ulcer. The lesion may remain single (Plate 73) but more often multiple lesions develop as a result of auto-inoculation. Vesicles are not encountered in chancroid. The ulcers are non-indurated, shallow, with undermined ragged edges (Plate 74). The base is formed of irregular vascular granulation tissue covered with dirty slough. The ulcers are very painful and tender and bleed easily. However, pain may be absent in some, especially in females who may be unaware of the presence of ulcers. The sites affected in the male are usually the prepuce, the fraenum and the coronal sulcus, occasionally the glans penis and, rarely, the urethra and other areas (Plates 75 and 76). In the female, the labia are the usual sites (Plate 77) and, less frequently, the other areas.

Occasionally, a lesion may not progress beyond the pustular stage and is then termed a dwarf chancroid.

In over half of the patients, the inguinal lymph nodes become enlarged on one or both sides within 1 week. They are painful and tender. In some, the inguinal adenitis may progress to abscess formation – a bubo (Plate 78).

Extragenital lesions, as a result of direct inoculation, are rare. Systemic spread does not occur. HIV-infected patients with chancroid may develop extensive genital ulceration.

Course and sequelae

Without treatment, the ulcers and inguinal abscess may persist for months or years. In some cases, the ulcers may extend rapidly and merge to form an ulcus molle serpiginosum or a giant chancroid. Secondary infection with *Bacteroides* sp. or fusospirochaetal organisms may cause foul-smelling discharge and destructive or phagedenic ulceration (Plates 79 and 80). The preputial lesions may result in phimosis and those of the fraenum may lead to perforation (Plate 81). The skin over the bubo may become hot, red and shiny, along with the formation of a fluctuant unilocular abscess. The latter may eventually burst open, resulting in sinus formation and a spreading ulcer (Plate 82). The complications in females include a rectovaginal fistula.

Differential diagnosis

Chancroidal lesions have to be differentiated from other causes of genital ulceration and septic adenitis. The differential diagnosis of genital ulcer disease has been covered in the section on the differential diagnosis of primary syphilis (Chapter 7.1). In addition, the typical presentations of the various conditions have been described elsewhere in this book. Whereas a careful history and thorough physical examination may help to make a fairly accurate diagnosis in some cases, the sensitivity and specificity of the clinical diagnosis of genital ulcer disease are rather poor. In many of the patients, clinical differentiation from genital herpes is almost impossible; others may have mixed infections, e.g. chancroid, primary syphilis and genital herpes in any combination [Plate 83 (see also Plates 25 and 26)].

Depending upon the laboratory facilities available, the tests include repeated darkfield examinations for *T. pallidum*, syphilis serology and swabs for other STI as considered appropriate. Ciprofloxacin or suphonamides may then be administered, but penicillin and other treponemicidal drugs should be avoided until syphilis has been confirmed or excluded.

Diagnosis

Direct smear

Due to a variety of bacteria in the ulcer material, demonstration of *H. ducreyi* by direct smear is unreliable. Both the sensitivity and specificity of a Gram-stained smear are less than 50%. A monoclonal antibody test applied directly on a clinical specimen with a high specificity is not yet available.

Culture

Culture (of material from ulcer or bubo aspirate) is essential for a definitive diagnosis (Chapter 5). Culture media, however, are expensive and have a limited shelf life, and, therefore, may not be available at the site. Amie's transport medium may maintain the viability of *H. ducreyi* for up to 3 days at 4°C (not longer than 24 h at room temperature). Newer transport media being evaluated may maintain the viability of *H. ducreyi* for longer than 3 days. Sensitivity of culture is about 80%.

Polymerase chain reaction

DNA amplification using a PCR is expected to be a highly sensitive and specific test. A multiplex PCR assay for the simultaneous detection of herpes simplex virus, *H. ducreyi* and *T. pallidum* from genital ulcer material has been shown to be more sensitive than the standard diagnostic tests for the detection of these organisms.

Serology

There is no widely available serological test for the diagnosis of chancroid. Enzyme immunoassays for the detection of circulating anti-*H. ducreyi* serum antibodies have been used for epidemiological studies.

Histology

Histology of the ulcer biopsy material may be used as an aid to the diagnosis (see above).

Prognosis

The prognosis of chancroid is excellent with appropriate treatment. However, repeated infections may occur on subsequent exposure to the organism.

Treatment

There is a considerable geographical variation in the sensitivity of *H. ducreyi* to antimicrobials. Many of the strains are β-lactamase producers. Plasmid-mediated resistance to sulphonamides, ampicillin, streptomycin, chloramphenicol and tetracycline has been observed. A single organism may contain multiple resistant plasmids. Information on chromosomally mediated resistance is scarce and probably accounts for the decreased susceptibility to trimethoprim and some quinolones. An appropriate choice of treatment may be made from the regimens listed in Box 7.3.1. Single dose regimens may be ineffective in patients with HIV infection. With effective treatment, epithelialization commences on about the third day after treatment, and ulceration usually resolves within 7 days.

The fluctuating bubo should be aspirated, using a wide bore needle, through the surrounding healthy skin to prevent sinus formation. Incision and

Box 7.3.1. Treatment of chancroid.

Single dose regimens
- Azithromycin, 1 g orally[a]
- *or*
- Ciprofloxacin, 500 mg orally[b]
- *or*
- Norfloxacin, 800 mg orally[b]
- *or*
- Ofloxacin, 400 mg orally[b]
- *or*
- Ceftriaxone, 250 mg by i.m. injection (high failure rate reported from Kenya)
- *or*
- Spectinomycin, 2 g by i.m. injection

Multiple dose regimens
- Erythromycin, 500 mg orally, four times daily for 7 days
- *or*
- Ciprofloxacin, 500 mg orally, twice daily for 3 days[b]
- *or*
- Cotrimoxazole (80 mg trimethoprim and 400 mg sulphamethoxazole), two tablets orally, twice daily for 7 days (high failure rates reported from several countries).[c]

[a]Safety in pregnancy and lactating women not established.
[b]Avoid in pregnancy and adolescents.
[c]Avoid in pregnancy.

drainage, and excision of nodes will delay healing. Circumcision or dorsal slit, if indicated, should be delayed until after appropriate treatment and after the ulcer has healed in order to avoid secondary chancroidal lesions developing on the site of incision.

Contacts

Sexual partners should be traced, examined, investigated and epidemiological treatment with a similar drug regimen considered.

Management of genital ulcer disease at primary health care level

See Chapter 10.1 for details of this.

Prevention

Preventive measures include use of condom, washing the genitalia with soap and water immediately after sexual exposure, prompt treatment of the patient and examination and treatment of sexual partners.

Further reading

Dangor, Y., Radebe, F. and Ballard, R.C. (1993) Transport media for *Haemophilus ducreyi*. *Sexually Transmitted Diseases* 20, 5–9.

Hawkes, S., West, B., Wilson, S., Whittle, H. and Mabey, D. (1995) Asymptomatic carriage of *H. ducreyi* confirmed by polymerase chain reaction. *Genitourinary Medicine* 71, 224–227.

Roggen, E.L., Hoofd, G., Van Dyck, E. and Piot, P. (1994) Enzyme immunoassays (EIAs) for the detection of anti-*Haemophilus ducreyi* serum IgA, IgG and IgM antibodies. *Sexually Transmitted Diseases* 21, 36–42.

Trees, D.L. and Morse, S.A. (1995) Chancroid and *Haemophilus ducreyi*: an update. *Clinical Microbiology Reviews* 8, 357–375.

Van Dyck, E. and Piot, P. (1992) Laboratory techniques in the investigation of chancroid, lymphogranuloma venereum and donovanosis. *Genitourinary Medicine* 68, 130–133.

CHAPTER 7.4
Gonorrhoea

O.P. Arya
Department of Medical Microbiology and Genitourinary Medicine, University of Liverpool, Liverpool, UK

Gonorrhoea is an infectious disease affecting the genital tract and other structures of the body such as the conjunctiva, the pharynx, the rectum, the skin, the joints and internal organs. Its main importance is due to its ability to cause pelvic infection, infertility and neonatal blindness.

Epidemiology

The incidence of gonorrhoea has declined in many developed countries, largely because of a change in sexual behaviour mainly directed against the risk of HIV infection. In England and Wales, however, rather unexpectedly, the number of new cases between 1995 and 1996 rose by over 13%, calling for continued efforts towards control measures. (See Chapter 1 for epidemiology in the tropical countries.)

The causative organism

Gonorrhoea is caused by *Neisseria gonorrhoeae*, commonly known as the gonococcus. The organisms are small, Gram-negative, non-motile, aerobic or facultative anaerobic cocci, usually arranged in pairs with their adjacent surfaces flattened, giving them a bean-shaped appearance. When outside the body, they are easily killed by drying and simple disinfectants including soap.

Four colonial forms of the gonococcus have been described. Colonies of types T_1 and T_2 are small and virulent and possess pili (protein spikes that attach the bacteria to mucosa). The larger types T_3 and T_4 are avirulent and lack pili.

The fermentation characteristics permit its differentiation from other *Neisseria*. The gonococcus ferments only glucose, while the meningococcus (*N. meningitidis*, the other pathogenic member of the group) ferments both maltose and glucose. Of the others frequently found in the respiratory tract and occasionally in the genital region, *N. sicca* ferments all three, i.e. glucose, maltose and sucrose.

Gonococcal strains and their differentiation

There is a considerable antigenic heterogeneity among gonococci. It is now possible to differentiate the gonococcal strains from one another. The methods include *auxotyping* based on the nutritional requirement for the growth of the organism, e.g. proline- or arginine-requiring or AHU (arginine, hypoxanthine, uracil) strains, etc.; *serotyping* using monoclonal antibody against the serogroups P.1A and P.1B (the two distinct classes of the outer membrane protein 1); and *molecular typing* using plasmid analysis, opa typing, por typing, etc.

Molecular typing gives greater differentiation between strains than the other methods. Thus opa typing, which is highly discriminatory, is reported to be able to differentiate between isolates of the same auxotype/serovar class. Typing based on molecular methods, i.e. molecular epidemiology, has uses in monitoring temporal changes, antimicrobial resistance, forensic problems (e.g. child abuse, rape) and sexual networks.

Antimicrobial resistance

Antimicrobial resistance among gonococci is common. It may be chromosomally mediated (e.g. to penicillin, tetracycline, spectinomycin and, more recently, to fluoroquinolones) or plasmid mediated [e.g. tetracyline-resistant *N. gonorrhoeae* (TRNG) and penicillinase-producing *N. gonorrhoeae* (PPNG)]. See Chapter 1 for epidemiology of these strains.

Laboratory aspects

Various aspects, including staining methods, culture and antimicrobial susceptibility and other methods for the detection of *N. gonorrhoeae* and transporting specimens, are described in Chapter 5.

Immunity

Protective immunity does not develop to any significant level during the course of gonococcal infection. Repeated infections do occur. The possible explanation/mechanisms include antigenic heterogeneity and variability, blocking antibodies, antibody cleavage by IgA protease and intracellular growth.

Transmission

Transmission in adults is mainly by physical contact with an infected person's mucosal surfaces, as may happen during vaginal, rectal and oral sex. Non-sexual transmission occurs in gonococcal infection of the eyes, and vulvovaginitis in children (see below for extragenital infections and for gonococcal infections in infants and children).

Pathogenesis

The gonococcus has a predilection for columnar and transitional epithelium, readily available after the gonococcus has gained entry at any of the body's main orifices, such as the urethra, rectum, pharynx, conjunctiva, endocervix and Bartholin's ducts. The gonococci multiply on the mucosal surface in these areas. The infection subsequently can spread to the other structures lined with susceptible epithelium, such as Littre's glands, Cowper's glands, the prostate gland, seminal vesicles and epididymes in the male, and Skene's glands and the fallopian tubes in the female.

The gonococci, with the help of pili, attach themselves to the epithelial cells and the secretory surface of the mucous cells of the host. They may become embedded within the epithelial cells and multiply intracellularly. However, once the gonococci are taken up by neutrophils, they may undergo lysis, especially after appropriate treatment.

Initially there is a neutrophil response in the submucosa, later replaced by mononuclear cells. The inflammatory response coupled with the patchy destruction of the epithelium results in a mucopurulent discharge. In many females, however, the tissue response, and hence the production of pus, is minimal. If left untreated, the inflammatory process, notably in the urethra, the epididymes and the fallopian tubes, may resolve by fibrosis.

Primary cutaneous infection with *N. gonorrhoeae* has been reported, manifesting as 'localized ulcer' on or around the genitalia. This is probably secondary colonization of a pre-existing ulcer which may be a herpetic or chancroidal lesion.

See below for the pathogenesis of disseminated gonococcal infection.

Clinical features of urogenital gonococcal infections in males

Urethritis

Incubation period

The incubation period in the majority of symptomatic patients is 2–7 days, and in about 90% of cases it is less than 15 days. Concurrent infection with *Chlamydia trachomatis* does not seem to make any difference to the incubation period. The infection can be transmitted during the incubation period.

Symptoms

If history is taken diligently, less than 10% of the patients are asymptomatic. A careful examination (Chapter 4) will reveal a scanty urethral discharge in almost all of these patients, especially after urine has been held overnight. Most of such cases are discovered through screening or contact tracing. In my experience, among those with symptoms, over 75% complain of urethral discharge as well as dysuria, less than 5% of dysuria alone and the remainder of only urethral discharge. Dysuria may be severe if the infection has reached the posterior urethra, when the additional symptoms will include urgency, frequency and occasionally terminal haematuria.

Signs

The urinary meatus may be reddened and oedematous. The urethral discharge is often creamy yellow pus (Plate 84). The amount may vary with the interval since the patient last urinated. In about 20% of the patients, the discharge may be scanty, not so purulent and may be cloudy mucoid or clear, i.e. the type frequently encountered in non-gonococcal urethritis. Occasionally, no discharge may be seen, especially if the patient has urinated just before attending the clinic. In most of such patients, the discharge is readily demonstrable if he is re-examined after urine has been held overnight or for several hours. The two-glass urine test will show haze and threads in the first glass and clear urine in the second. Haze in the second glass may be suggestive of posterior urethritis.

In about 5% of patients, especially in those with frankly purulent urethral discharge, the inguinal lymph glands on one or both sides are slightly enlarged and tender.

Rarely, there may be preputial oedema and balanitis. In these patients or in those with a long phimotic prepuce which cannot be retracted, it is often impossible to tell whether the discharge is subpreputial or urethral. Such cases should be re-examined after subpreputial irrigation with plain water or saline. Appearance of fresh pus after milking the urethra will confirm urethritis. Absence of pus and clear urine passed subsequently will exclude urethritis.

Differential diagnosis

Differential diagnosis is from other causes of urethritis (Chapter 7.5) with which some patients may be concurrently infected, e.g. up to a third of the patients with gonorrhoea may also be infected with *C. trachomatis*. In general, the symptoms and signs in gonococcal urethritis are more severe, e.g. the discharge is more profuse and more purulent, than in non-gonococcal urethritis. However, there can be a considerable overlap, and without laboratory assistance it is not possible to confirm or exclude these infections.

Diagnosis

A presumptive diagnosis can be made immediately by examining a Gram-stained urethral smear which will detect the characteristic Gram-negative intracellular diplococci (Plate 85) accurately in over 95% of the symptomatic men with gonococcal urethritis. A urethral specimen should be obtained even if no discharge can be seen. If the patient has just urinated and the Gram stain is negative, but gonococcal infection is suspected, the patient should be advised to re-attend for a repeat smear after urine has been held for more than 4 h. Material for culture may be obtained from asymptomatic men for whom a Gram-stained smear may be less sensitive, and also for antimicrobial susceptibility tests as well as for medicolegal reasons. Other sites to be sampled include the pharynx in heterosexuals, and the pharynx and the rectum in homosexuals (see below).

Course of gonococcal urethritis

In most patients, the urethral discharge gradually becomes less purulent and scanty, may be present only in the mornings or may disappear altogether after 1–3 months. The majority become asymptomatic and non-infectious within 6 months, and hence cured. Others may develop complications and run the risk of metastatic spread. It is not clear whether the situation of the pre-sulphonamide era when almost one-fifth of the male cases developed complications still exists in tropical areas where patients remain untreated or are treated inadequately.

Local complications

Most of these complications are now extremely rare in developed countries.

INFECTION OF THE PARAURETHRAL DUCTS. If these minute channels are infected, a tiny bead of pus can be seen at their openings on the urinary meatus.

INFECTION OF TYSON'S GLANDS. Infection of the Tyson's glands may be diagnosed by the appearance of a bead of pus or a swelling on either side of the fraenum.

INFECTION OF THE MEDIAN RAPHE. The infection of the narrow blind tracts resulting from defects of the median raphe may give rise to small beads of pus on the ventral surface of the penile shaft in the midline.

PERIURETHRAL ABSCESS. This complication follows rupture of the infected Littre's glands, causing extension of the infection into the submucous tissue. This may result in a boggy, painful and tender local swelling. An abscess deep down may present in the perineum. Erection may be painful. The abscess may open into the urethra or point to the skin surface and burst open, the former resulting in urethral discharge and relief from pain and the latter resulting in the formation of a sinus or a fistula.

URETHRAL STRICTURE. It is a chronic sequel, the sequence of events being littritis, periurethral inflammation and fibrosis of the urethral mucosa. Predisposing factors include trauma and superimposed infection from inexpert bouginage, catheterization and irrigations. The symptoms which appear several months or years later include morning gleet, difficulty in passing urine, a narrow stream and eventually retention of urine. The bulbous urethra and urinary meatus are the sites commonly affected. Diagnosis is suspected from the history and by viewing the urine stream, and is confirmed by urethroscopy and urethrogram. Secondary bacterial infection with coliforms, etc., is common. Urine examination reveals heavy pyuria and bacteriuria.

INFECTION OF COWPER'S GLANDS. Posterior urethritis may extend to involve one or both Cowper's glands. If the ducts only are affected, there may be no symptoms. The infection of the gland(s) may result in painful and tender swelling(s) on either side of the perineal raphe, best felt between the thumb on the perineum and a forefinger in the rectum. The patient may be febrile and experience pain during defaecation and micturition. Rectal examination may be very painful. Rupture of abscess into the perineum may result in fistula formation.

ACUTE PROSTATITIS. Infection from the posterior urethra may spread to the prostate gland resulting in acute prostatitis. The patient is ill with general malaise, suprapubic pain, headache, fever, shivering and pain in the perineum. There may be urinary and rectal symptoms due to the proximity of the prostate to the trigone, urethra and rectum. The urinary symptoms include urgency, frequency, haematuria and retention due to spasm of the compressor urethrae muscle. The rectal symptoms include constipation and painful defaecation. Acute prostatitis may progress to abscess formation. The abscess may burst into the urethra or point to the perineum, the latter resulting in sinus formation. If it points to the rectum, secondary infection will follow. Prostatitis should be suspected if a patient with gonorrhoea develops symptoms mimicking flu or malaria. A gentle rectal examination will reveal an enlarged, warm and very tender prostate which may be fluctuant in the case of an abscess. The differential diagnosis is from acute prostatitis due to urinary pathogens. The two-glass urine test will show haziness in both glasses. A urine dip-stick will show proteinuria and haematuria. The diagnostic tests include urethral smear and culture for *N. gonorrhoeae*, a midstream urine culture for the urinary pathogens and transrectal ultrasound. (See Chapter 4 for contraindications of prostatic massage.)

CHRONIC PROSTATITIS. Chronic prostatitis is usually a sequel of non-gonococcal infection (Chapter 7.5) and often of unknown aetiology. Nevertheless, if a patient with a history of gonococcal urethritis does in due course develop symptoms and signs of chronic prostatitis (Chapter 7.5), gonococci are hard to find whether or not the patient had received an antibiotic.

SEMINAL VESICULITIS. Inflammation of seminal vesicles usually accompanies prostatitis. The symptoms and signs are largely similar to those of prostatitis. In addition, the ejaculate may be blood stained. The inflamed seminal vesicles may be felt rectally as tender sausage-like structures above the prostate.

VAS DEFERENTITIS. Inflammation of the intra-abdominal part of the vas deferens may cause lower abdominal pain on the same side.

Epididymitis

Pathogenesis

The infection may reach the epididymis as a result of retrograde passage of infected urine from the urethra or direct spread by surface continuity or by lymphatics. The inflammatory process begins in the tail and then extends to the rest of the epididymis and the testicle.

Clinical features

The condition is usually preceded by symptomatic urethritis. The onset of gonococcal epididymitis is usually acute and the patient presents with an acutely painful unilateral scrotal swelling. The other side may occasionally be affected later. There may be malaise, fever, and pain in the groin and lower abdomen. In addition, the testicle is often enlarged due to orchitis and hydrocoele. Clinical examination will reveal red and oedematous scrotum, a very tender epididymal swelling, and testicular swelling – the swellings being separated by the groove. Occasionally, the spermatic cord may also be swollen and tender (funiculitis) which may give rise to pain in the iliac fossa. Although with the development of epididymitis, urethral discharge becomes scanty, urethritis is easily evident in gonococcal epididymitis when the patient presents.

Differential diagnosis

The differential diagnosis is from other causes of epididymitis, torsion of the testicle and neoplasm. The other causes of epididymitis include: (i) *C. trachomatis* (Chapter 7.5) which may coexist; (ii) urinary tract pathogens such as *Escherichia coli*, and *Pseudomonas* spp., which may be associated with urinary tract abnormalities, or may occur in homosexuals who practise insertive rectal intercourse, or in men over 35 years of age with prostate disorders; (iii) systemic infections due to *Brucella* spp., *N. meningitidis, Streptococcus pneumoniae, T. pallidum, Mycobacterium tuberculosis*, mumps virus, and fungal infections in patients with HIV infection; and (iv) filariasis (Chapter 11.6). Tuberculous epididymitis, which is nearly always associated with tuberculosis of kidneys, prostate and seminal vescles, is usually bilateral; the epididymis is firm, swollen but not usually tender, the vas may be thickened or beaded. The investigations include a chest X-ray and the diagnosis is confirmed by the demonstration of tubercle bacilli in the smears and cultures of urine sediment, prostatic fluid and sputum.

Torsion of the testicle and neoplasm require urgent differentiation. There is no pyuria in either of these conditions, and ultrasound examination is useful. Torsion, which usually occurs under the age of 20, is associated with sudden intense scrotal pain, and an enlarged and tender testis which lies at higher level than its counterpart. Surgical opinion must be sought without delay.

Diagnosis

Laboratory tests include Gram-stained urethral smear, culture or antigen detection tests for *N. gonnorhoeae* and *C. trachomatis*, a two-glass urine test, microscopy and culture of a midstream specimen of urine for other bacteria. Five or more polymorphonuclear leukocytes (PMN) per high power field in the Gram-stained urethral smear will confirm urethritis, and the presence of Gram-negative diplococci indicates gonococcal infection. Mixed infection, for example with *C. trachomatis*, can only be confirmed by detecting its presence.

Epididymal aspiration, although occasionally helpful in the detection of causative agent, is not a routine investigation.

Sequelae and complications of acute epididymitis

In the absence of appropriate treatment, an abscess and infarction of the testicle may result, requiring surgical referral. With or without treatment, the inflammation subsides leaving a residual thickening of the lower pole of the epididymis (this may be confused with the lumpy lower pole of the epididymis following vasectomy). In some cases, the adjacent part of the body is also thickened. There may be azoospermia, but blockage of the lumen is certain. Some patients may experience a dull ache in the scrotum. If both epididymes are blocked, sterility will result.

Clinical features of urogenital gonococcal infections in females

Symptoms

The number of those with or without symptoms may vary with the setting/ clinic where the patient is seen. Over half of the infected women seen at STI clinics may be asymptomatic. The symptoms, when present, may be due to primary infection, secondary spread, complications or concurrent infection(s) with *C. trachomatis* (the most common), bacterial vaginosis organisms, *T. vaginalis*, *Candida albicans*, herpes simplex virus or warts, etc. One or more of these infections may coexist in over 80% of the cases of gonorrhoea in some settings.

The incubation period of primary infections is similar to that in men. Primary infection of the urethra may manifest as transient and mild dysuria. Frequency of micturition will indicate trigonitis or cystitis. Periurethral gland ducts may be affected. Bartholin's duct involvement is common and often asymptomatic. Involvement of the cervix may cause 'vaginal' discharge, occasionally low backache, menorrhagia and intermenstrual bleeding. The discharge is often minimal unless the cervicitis is severe or, as is often the case, other infections coexist (see above).

See below for symptoms of extragenital gonococcal infections of the rectum, throat and conjunctivae as primary sites or due to secondary spread. Complications and their symptoms are described later.

Signs

Many patients infected with *N. gonorrhoeae* only may not show any abnormal signs. Others may reveal some or all of the following features. The urethral meatus may be red and pouting, and mucopus may be expressed on massaging the urethra (Plate 86). Beads of pus may be seen at the paraurethral duct orifices if Skene's glands are affected. Likewise, if Bartholin's gland or duct is infected, a bead of pus may be seen at the Bartholin's duct orifice (Plate 87). In less than a quarter of the patients, there may be evidence of acute cervicitis, i.e.

the cervix is congested, enlarged and mucopurulent discharge may be seen exuding from the endocervix. A cervical ectopy may be reddened, oedematous and associated with bleeding when swabbed. Mucopus may be expressed from any of the above sites without any obvious signs of inflammation (see below for signs of extragenital gonococcal infections).

Differential diagnosis

None of the above symptoms and signs are specific to gonorrhoea. Urinary symptoms associated with cystitis may be due to urinary pathogens. Vaginal discharge may be physiological or due to gynaecological causes, or vaginal or cervical infections, described in the relevant chapters (see also Chapter 10.2). The macroscopic appearance of the cervix does not discriminate between gonococcal and chlamydial infections. Mixed infections are common (Plate 88).

Diagnosis

Regardless of symptoms, whether present or absent or their type, gonococcal infection can be confirmed or excluded only with the help of the laboratory. In view of the possibility of different sites being infected with varying sensitivity to the antibacterials and also the possibility of a single site being infected, swabs should be taken from all sites likely to be the routes of infection (see below for extragenital sites). The opposite sides of the same culture plate can be used for specimens from two sites. It should be noted that in about 5% of patients only the rectal swab, only the urethral swab or only the throat swab may yield gonococci. However, constraints may permit swabs from only one site, in which case the cervix is the preferred site to be sampled (or the urethra if the patient has had a hysterectomy). In addition, some may take a urethral swab if there was a history of dysuria or a demonstrable mucopurulent urethral discharge, and a swab from Bartholin's duct orifice if showing a bead of pus (occasionally even clear mucus at the orifice after massaging the Bartholin's duct may yield gonococci).

A presumptive diagnosis of gonorrhoea can be made immediately by examining the Gram-stained smears. However, due to the presence of other Gram-negative cocci, the sensitivity of Gram staining of material from the cervix, even in experienced hands, is less than 65%. Cultures are, therefore, essential to diagnose or exclude gonorrhoea in females. The sensitivity of only one culture of cervical specimens is about 90%.

Course of untreated urogenital gonococcal infection in females

In a proportion of patients, the infection may resolve spontaneously with time. In some, the infection may remain latent for several months, during which the patient is infectious. Others develop local and systemic complications.

Local complications

Salpingitis is the most common and most serious complication and is described in Chapter 10.3.

Abscess of Skene's glands or paraurethral cyst may occur as a result of blockage of their ducts. Extension of infection to periurethral tissues posteriorly may result in periurethral abscess. Urethral stricture is extremely rare in females.

Bartholin's gland abscess

Bartholin's gland abscess (Plate 89) is a common complication as is chronic infection (Bartholin's cyst). In the former, the swelling is painful and tender. Walking aggravates the pain. Clinical examination may reveal a fluctuant pointing abscess, and the insertion of a vaginal speculum is painful. Bartholin's cyst is a sequel of blockage of Bartholin's duct due to previous inflammation. Other causes of acute infection include *C. trachomatis*, *E. coli*, staphylococci, *Proteus mirabilis* and *T. vaginalis*. A specimen from the abscess cavity may be overgrown by other organisms and fail to show *N. gonorrhoeae*. However, gonococci may be isolated from the specimens of the other Bartholin's duct and the endocervix.

Extragenital gonococcal infections

These include gonococcal infections of the eyes, oropharynx and rectum, disseminated gonococcal infection and perihepatitis; the last is described in Chapter 10.3. They may occur in any combination and, with the exception of perihepatitis, with or without urogenital involvement.

Gonococcal infection of the eyes

Infection of the conjunctivae in adults and children may be acquired accidentally, the infection being carried to the eyes by contaminated fingers. The condition may be mild or severe. The symptoms and signs include pain in the eyes, discharge, photophobia, redness of the conjunctivae and oedema of the eyelids. If neglected, keratitis and eventually panophthalmitis may occur. Differential diagnosis is from other causes of conjunctivitis. The diagnosis is aided by Gram-stained smear of the conjunctival exudate and confirmed by culture. Gonococcal ophthalmia neonatorum is described below.

Gonococcal infection of the oropharynx

Mode of infection

The mode of infection is by orogenital or possibly oroanal intercourse with an infected person. With regard to the former, fellatio would appear to be a more effective mode of transmission than cunnilingus. Consequently, oropharyngeal gonorrhoea is more common in homosexuals, and more common in women than in heterosexual men. Gonococcal pharyngitis and tonsillitis are more common than gingivitis, stomatitis or laryngitis. Pharyngeal gonorrhoea seems to have become rather common in some areas because oral sex has been considered to be safer than other forms of penetrative sex in the context of prevention of HIV infection. In about 5% of patients, the oropharynx may be the only site yielding a positive culture.

Symptoms

Oropharyngeal gonorrhoea is often asymptomatic. Symptoms, when present, are no different from common throat infections. A person may have concurrent pharyngeal and rectal gonorrhoea and both may be asymptomatic.

Signs

Clinical examination of the oropharynx is often normal. In others, the appearance may be similar to that of other common throat infections, i.e. redness of the fauces, uvula and tonsillar area with or without visible pus.

Diagnosis

A high index of suspicion is essential. The patient should be questioned frankly about a history of orogenital contact. Often, this is denied at first interview and yet the throat swab is reported positive. The diagnosis is confirmed by culturing the material from the throat; the material is obtained by applying the swab vigorously on the posterior pharyngeal wall and the tonsillar crypts. Selective media are used and the organism differentiated from the other *Neisseria*. The ubiquitous presence of the latter organisms in the throat excludes the use of smear for the diagnosis.

Course of oropharyngeal gonorrhoea

Although the infection may resolve spontaneously, reportedly within 3 months, the patient will, in the meantime, continue to remain infectious, e.g. by receptive fellatio, as well as run the risk of developing gonococcal septicaemia.

Gonococcal infection of the rectum

Mode of infection

The principal mode of anorectal gonococcal infection in males is by receptive anal intercourse. It may also happen, albeit extremely rarely, following rupture of a gonococcal prostatic abscess. In females, the rectum may be the primary site of infection by anal coitus, or the rectum can be involved as a result of secondary spread, via menstrual flow or vaginal discharge, from the primary urogenital site in about 30–50% of such cases. In about 5% of women with gonorrhoea and 40% of homosexual men with gonorrhoea, the rectum may be the only infected site. In both sexes, accidental infection by contaminated fingers, gloves or instruments is extremely rare.

The pathology is in the anorectal crypts and the glands of Lieberkühn lined by columnar epithelium.

Symptoms

There are usually no symptoms. When present, they include a change in bowel habits, constipation, loose stools, tenesmus, anal irritation, moisture around the anus, a mucoid, purulent or blood-stained discharge per rectum, or a discharge visible on the stools.

Signs

On proctoscopy, the rectal mucosa may look normal or mildly congested, friable, or acutely inflamed and oedematous with mucopus on it (Plate 90).

Differential diagnosis

Differential diagnosis is from other causes of proctitis (*C. tractomatis*, herpes simplex viruses, *Treponema pallidum*, etc.), other causes of colitis and enteritis (*Campylobacter* spp., *Shigella* spp., *C. trachomatis* LGV strains, *Entamoeba histolytica*, *Giardia lamblia*, etc.), and HIV-related alimentary tract problems.

Diagnosis

The diagnosis is made by microscopic examination of a Gram-stained smear and culture on selective medium of the material obtained from the rectal mucosa. The interpretation of the smear is difficult because of the large number of bacteria, and hence its sensitivity is no more than 40%. The isolates, especially from homosexual men, will need to be differentiated from *N. meningitidis*.

Disseminated gonococcal infection

Epidemiology

The incidence of disseminated gonococcal infection in tropical countries is unknown. It is around 1% of the cases of gonorrhoea in industrialized countries. It is more common in females and relatively uncommon in homosexuals.

Pathogenesis

The pathogenesis is not entirely clear. There is a blood-borne dissemination of gonococci which are more resistant to complement-mediated killing by normal human serum, and more susceptible to antibiotics than the other strains. Additionally, a possible immune mechanism rather than direct gonococcal invasion of the tissues has been suggested.

Clinical features

The condition is often mild and hence termed 'benign gonococcaemia'. It may present as a pyrexia of unknown origin and/or few skin lesions and minimal arthralgia. This combination of symptoms should arouse suspicion. The other more serious but rare manifestations include endocarditis, myocarditis, pericarditis and meningitis. Perihepatitis may also occur. There may be concurrent urogenital or extragenital gonococcal infection in men and women. In women, gonococcaemia may occur in the first week of the menstrual cycle, or following abortion, confinement, dilatation and curettage.

SKIN LESIONS. The skin lesions may be due to gonococcal embolization and the release of endotoxins following phagocytosis. The lesions, which are difficult to see on dark skin, may be petechial, vesicular, pustular, necrotic or haemorrhagic (Plate 91). They are usually painless and not itchy. They are few to several in number, occurring anywhere on the body but usually have a distal distribution. They may resolve within a week and then reappear. The differential diagnosis is from meningococcal septicaemia, pyoderma, drug rashes, erythema nodosum, typhoid, etc.

TENOSYNOVITIS. This frequently encountered feature presents as reddened, tender, swelling of the tendon sheaths, usually of the hands and feet.

ARTHRITIS. The initial migratory polyarthralgia is often followed by the development of multiple non-suppurative arthritis or acute septic arthritis of one or two larger joints. The joints of the extremities are the ones most frequently involved. In septic arthritis, the joints are painful, swollen, hot and tender. The overlying skin is reddened. The patient may be febrile, the erythrocyte sedimentation rate elevated and the synovial fluid purulent. Gonococcal infection should be considered in any young sexually active adult presenting with arthritis. The differential diagnosis is commonly from rheumatic fever (high fever, signs of carditis, typical skin rash and joints not septic), Reiter's syndrome (Chapter 7.5), meningococcal septicaemia (patient very ill with symptoms and signs of meningitis), acute pyogenic arthritis (culture of blood and synovial fluid to find the cause), brucellosis (relevant history, intermittent pyrexia and a positive blood culture and agglutination test).

Diagnosis

The specimens should be obtained from the usual urogenital and extragenital sites for smear and cultures for gonorrhoea whether or not the patient has any symptoms relating to these sites. The additional samples include blood, joint aspirate, material from skin lesions and cerebrospinal fluid if indicated, to detect gonococci. As the gonococcal septicaemia is usually associated with very sensitive strains, non-selective media should be used for materials when contaminating organisms are not a problem. Despite this precaution, in many of these patients gonococci are hard to find in skin lesions, joint aspirates and blood.

Gonococcal infection in pregnancy

Pregnancy is not a special risk factor for gonococcal infection. However, disseminated gonococcal infection is thought to be more common than in non-pregnant women. Salpingitis can occur in early pregnancy, i.e. before the chorioamnion obliterates the uterine cavity at about the fourth month of pregnancy. Nevertheless, other events such as chorioamnionitis, spontaneous abortion, pre-term rupture of membranes and low birth weight have been attributed to gonococcal infection. Postpartum sepsis is a distinct possibility.

Gonococcal infections in infants and children

Ophthalmia neonatorum

N. gonorrhoeae is the most serious cause of conjunctivitis in the newborn in many tropical countries (see Chapters 1 and 12.1). The infection occurs by direct contact with infected cervical secretions during delivery, the transmission rate being 30%.

Clinical features

The incubation period is usually less than 5 days. The condition is often bilateral, starting with watery or slightly blood-stained discharge which soon becomes purulent. There is severe conjunctivitis and inflammation and swelling of the eyelids (Plate 92). The pus under the oedematous eyelids may be under tension and spurt out when the lids are separated. The clinical severity is variable. Nevertheless, if left untreated, corneal involvement and serious visual impairment may occur.

Differential diagnosis

Differential diagnosis is from other causes of conjunctivitis (see Chapter 7.5). Concurrent infection with *C. trachomatis* also occurs.

Diagnosis

A presumptive diagnosis of gonococcal infection can be made immediately by the presence of Gram-negative intracellular diplococci in a Gram-stained smear of the conjunctival exudate. For culture, a non-selective medium such as an enriched chocolate agar should be used.

Vulvovaginitis

The child's thin, immature vaginal epithelium and its alkaline pH are susceptible to the gonococcus. Gonococcal vulvovaginitis in pre-pubertal girls may be acquired accidentally by direct contact with infected towels or sharing a bed with infected parents or relatives in crowded bedrooms. Sexual abuse, and voluntary sexual activity in older children are other possibilities and call for care and tact in interviewing these children.

After the incubation period of a few days, the child may complain of vulvovaginal itching, dysuria and soreness aggravated when walking. The mother may notice stains on the underwear. The purulent discharge is often obvious as are also inflammation and swelling of the vulva and vaginitis. Differential diagnosis is from other causes of vulvovaginitis (see Chapter 7.5). Examination must be gentle and specimens for smears and cultures should be obtained from the vaginal orifice and, if necessary, from the urethra and rectum. The household contacts may need to be investigated.

Urethritis in male children

The infection may occur as a result of voluntary sexual activity, especially after the age of 10 years, or seduction by prostitutes or older women. The patient may experience urethral discharge and dysuria. The diagnosis is made by examining a smear, and is confirmed by culture.

Other manifestations

Gonococcal infection of the oropharynx and the rectum may follow sexual assault. Other manifestations such as salpingitis and disseminated infection may also occur rarely.

HIV infection and gonorrhoea

Many studies have failed to find any association between gonococcal infection and HIV seropositivity. Others have reported gonorrhoea to be a risk factor for HIV infection. HIV-positive men with gonococcal urethritis have been reported to have significantly higher concentrations of HIV-1 RNA in semen than HIV-positive controls. This may have implications in the sexual transmission of HIV-1 in view of the fact that treatment of gonorrhoea resulted in significant reduction in the concentration of HIV-1 RNA. HIV infection does not have any significant effect on the clinical manifestations of gonococcal infection in men, but has been suggested to promote development of pelvic infection in women. Response to therapy, however, is not affected. The treatment recommendations in the following pages apply to both HIV-positive and HIV-negative patients.

Management of gonorrhoea

General considerations

An ideal drug for the treatment of gonorrhoea should be 100% effective in a single oral dose, cheap, safe and completely abort or cure a simultaneously acquired or frequently concurrent chlamydial infection which is the case in up to a third of the men and well over half of the women with gonorrhoea. Such a drug is not yet available. However, single oral drug regimens are now available which will cure at least 98% of the cases of gonorrhoea. This could be followed by an antichlamydial treatment regimen in areas where concurrent chlamydial infection rates are known or suspected to be high. Azithromycin is highly or potentially effective against multiple sexually transmitted bacterial infections. However, it is not currently recommended to treat gonorrhoea, firstly because a single 2.0 g dose required to match the high cure rates with alternative regimens is comparatively more expensive and has significant gastrointestinal side effects, and secondly because of a recent report of emergence of azithromycin-resistant *N. gonorrhoeae* as a result of the increased selective pressure associated with the long half-life of the drug.

The choice of standard regimen should be made with the full knowledge of the antimicrobial susceptibility patterns of the circulating strains. The antimicrobial regimen selected should achieve serum levels equal to or greater than three times the minimum inhibitory concentration (MIC) of the local gonococcal strains and maintained for at least 8 h to cure uncomplicated infections. If this information is not available then, as a temporary measure, the one pertaining to the neighbouring area or country, if known, could be used and clinical efficacy monitored.

PPNG and TRNG are now widespread. Consequently penicillins and tetracyclines should no longer be used for the treatment of gonorrhoea.

The cost of the drugs in different countries is variable. Thus the correct choice of an affordable drug can only be made locally. If a patient is allergic to a drug or when a drug is contraindicated, as in pregnancy, then an alternative drug of a different group should be used. About 10% of penicillin-sensitive patients are also allergic to cephalosporins, which should certainly not be used if there is a history of penicillin anaphylaxis.

All patients should be assessed for concurrent STI (as outlined in Chapter 4) and managed accordingly.

Treatment of uncomplicated urogenital and extragenital gonococcal infections in adults

(see also Chapter 10 for problem-oriented approach at the PHC level)

The recommended regimens are given in Box 7.4.1, though the list is not comprehensive.

Need for the addition of antichlamydial treatment

A high proportion of the patients may contract gonococcal and non-gonococcal (including chlamydial) infections of the urethra, cervix, rectum or conjunctiva, at the same time. The figures may vary. In the author's experience, up to a third of the males with urethritis and up to half of the females with gonococcal infection of the cervix may also be infected with *C. trachomatis*. This concurrent chlamydial infection will not be affected by any of the above recommended regimens to treat gonorrhoea. About half of the males so treated will develop post-gonococcal urethritis (PGU) (see below), 70% being associated with *C. trachomatis* infection. Similar considerations apply to post-gonococcal cervicitis (see below), post-gonococcal proctitis (see below) and ophthalmia neonatorum. Therefore, in areas where concurrent chlamydial infection or PGU rates are high, it is recommended that treatment for presumed chlamydial infection (Chapter 7.5) should be added to the regimens listed in Box 7.4.1 for the treatment of gonorrhoea.

Surveillance

The patients who have been treated with any of the recommended regimens, including additional antichlamydial treatment, and feel well need not return for tests of cure, except for the final blood tests for syphilis, if considered necessary, at the end of 3 months. Others may be managed as follows.

The male patient may be advised to return on the fourth day and then 1 week and 2 weeks after treatment, each time after having held urine for over

Box 7.4.1. Treatment regimens for uncomplicated gonococcal infections in adults.

Single dose regimens

Ceftriaxone, 250 mg intramuscularly (may also abort incubating syphilis)

or

Cefixime, 400 mg orally

or

Cefotaxime, 1 g intramuscularly

or

Cefoxitin, 2 g intramuscularly plus probenecid, 1 g by mouth

or

Ciprofloxacin, 500 mg orally

or

Ofloxacin, 400 mg orally

or

Norfloxacin, 800 mg orally

Reports of resistant strains in Southeast Asia; 10% of PPNG strains reported to be resistant to ciprofloxacin; not recommended during pregnancy and lactation, not for children or adolescents.

or

Spectinomycin, 2 g intramuscularly

Geographical variation in efficacy; may not be effective for pharyngeal gonorrhoea.

or

Kanamycin, 2 g intramuscularly

Multiple dose regimen

Cotrimoxazole [trimethoprim (80 mg)/ sulphamethoxazole (400 mg)], four tablets twice daily for 2 days (extended to 4 days for pharyngeal gonorrhoea)

(Kanamycin and cotrimoxazole:) Geographical variation in efficacy; contraindicated in pregnancy; discontinue cotrimoxazole if skin rash appears.

The patients should be advised to abstain from sexual intercourse until they and their partners are cured and to avoid excessive alcohol for 2 weeks (see p. 229 for management of partners).

For gonococcal conjunctivitis, some specialists prefer a single session treatment comprising ceftriaxone, 1 g intramuscularly and irrigation of the eye with saline solution.

3 h. At each visit, the patient is interviewed briefly about any symptoms, treatment compliance, interim medication, time since last voided, further sexual intercourse and whether or not the partner has attended. The patient is then examined for urethral discharge and urethral swabs are taken for a smear for Gram staining (and culture if possible), regardless of symptoms and signs. Urine is examined by the two-glass test. In a successfully treated case, the urethral discharge disappears in 48 h and urine becomes clear within a week or a few flakes/threads may persist a little longer. If necessary, the threads may also be sampled for smear and if possible culture. Up to about half of the patients will develop PGU after gonococcal infection has resolved. The discharge may persist or reappear after having resolved. If initially copious and purulent, the discharge may now be scanty or demonstrable only on stripping the urethra after the patient has not voided urine for over 3 h. The symptoms are also much milder and often absent. The Gram-stained urethral smear will usually show more than ten PMN in several high power fields, but no

diplococci. Urine will show heavy flakes in the first glass. Most of these cases of PGU are associated with concurrently acquired chlamydial infection. If indicated, the pharyngeal, conjunctival and rectal swabs are also repeated.

Female patients are also asked to return 1 and 2 weeks after treatment for tests of cure. After taking an appropriate history as for male patients (see above), the patient is examined and specimens obtained from the same sites as before treatment. Macroscopic cervicitis (see above) and proctitis (in both sexes) may still be evident in those with concurrent chlamydial infection (post-gonococcal cervicitis and post-gonococcal proctitis).

If the follow-up tests for gonorrhoea are positive, it is often difficult to distinguish relapse from re-infection. However, in all treatment failures, sensitivity studies should be carried out. If that is not possible, the patient should be treated with an alternative regimen. PGU, post-gonococcal cervicitis and post-gonococcal proctitis should be managed as for non-gonococcal urethritis/chlamydial infection (Chapter 7.5).

Treatment of local complications in males

Infection of Tyson's glands

Most cases will respond to the standard treatment of gonorrhoea.

Infection of the paraurethral ducts

The standard treatment of gonorrhoea should be adequate.

Infection of the median raphe

Most cases will respond to the standard treatment; the rest may require surgical referral.

Periurethral abscess

Treat as for acute epididymitis (see below). Aspiration may help but incision should be avoided.

Urethral stricture

These cases should be referred to a urologist. Treatment is by dilatation. Some cases may benefit from urethroplasty. A neglected case of urethral stricture may present as an emergency with acute retention of urine requiring suprapubic cystostomy.

Infection of Cowper's glands

In addition to the standard treatment of gonorrhoea, an abscess may require aspiration. Referral to a surgeon may be necessary, especially in the presence of sinus formation.

Acute prostatitis

The patient should be admitted and treatment commenced with a cephalosporin such as cefoxitin, 2 g intravenously four times daily until symptoms subside. This is followed by ciprofloxacin, 500 mg orally twice daily to complete treatment for a total of 14 days. The patient is given a lot of fluids to drink. Laxatives may need to be prescribed. Hot sitz baths may be helpful in acute retention. If catheterization becomes necessary, gum elastic or a rubber catheter is used. Most cases will respond to these measures. Surgical intervention may be necessary in the case of abscess formation.

Chronic prostatitis

Chronic prostatitis is usually due to a non-gonococcal infection (see Chapter 7.5).

Vesiculitis

Vesiculitis often accompanies prostatitis and will be covered by the treatment of the latter complication.

Epididymitis

The patient should rest in bed with the scrotum elevated until there is no tenderness, and given analgesics. Because of the possibility of mixed infection the antibiotic regimen comprises standard treatment of uncomplicated gonorrhoea (see Box 7.4.1) followed by: doxycycline, 100 mg orally twice daily for at least 10 days, *or* tetracycline, 500 mg orally four times daily for at least 10 days, *or* erythromycin, 500 mg orally four times daily for at least 10 days, *or* ofloxacin, 300 mg orally twice daily for 10 days (ofloxacin should not be given to those under 18 years of age). The diagnosis and treatment should be reviewed after 3 days from the start of therapy. The subsequent follow-up is once weekly for 4 weeks, and tests for gonorrhoea are repeated on the first two follow-up visits. The persistence of scrotal swelling for longer than 1 month, despite treatment, should alert one to the possibilities of tuberculosis, neoplasm and fungal infection. See below for the management of sexual partners.

Treatment of local complications in females

Skenitis

Standard treatment of uncomplicated gonorrhoea will be adequate.

Bartholin's gland abscess

The patients in the early stages will usually respond to the standard dosage regimen extended to 3 or 4 days. Analgesics are given for pain. A fluctuant abscess may require repeated aspirations, using a wide bore needle under local anaesthesia by ethyl chloride spray. Those with a recurrent abscess or cyst formation will need gynaecological referral for marsupialization.

Salpingitis

See Chapter 10.3.

Treatment of disseminated gonococcal infection

Patients with septic joints or other serious complications will need to be hospitalized. The recommended regimens are as follows: ceftriaxone, 1 g intramuscularly or intravenously daily, *or* cefotaxime, 1 g intravenously every 8 h, *or* spectinomycin, 2 g intramuscularly every 12 h.

Any of the above treatment regimens should be continued until 24 h after the patient shows improvement, followed by either cefixime, 400 mg orally twice daily, *or* ciprofloxacin, 500 mg orally twice daily to a total of 7 days. Consideration should also be given to treat a presumed chlamydial infection.

Severely affected joints may need splinting for about 48 h and possibly also arthrocentesis. Analgesics are prescribed for pain. The skin and joint lesions usually improve within 3 days. Passive and later active movements are then commenced. Endocarditis and meningitis may be treated with ceftriaxone, 1–2 g intravenously every 12 h for 4 weeks in the former and for 10–14 days in the latter condition.

Education of the patient and management of partners

The patient is likely to be very receptive to education when an episode of STI has occurred. The education should include the cause and the mode of infection, the importance of treatment compliance and the treatment of partners, as well as disease prevention in the future. The patient may be given an information leaflet on gonorrhoea and other STI.

All partners (primary and secondary) within the last 2 weeks before symptoms developed and within 1 month for asymptomatic patients, or the most recent partner if the last sex was more than a month ago, will need to attend the clinic. Many of the partners, including those of patients with disseminated infection, may be asymptomatic. They should all be examined and specimens taken for smears and, if possible, culture. If laboratory facilities are not available locally, the specimens could be processed at the nearest facility even though at a later date (see Chapter 5 for storage and transport). The need for epidemiological treatment of the partners will be determined by the local availability of diagnostic facilities, ease of access to the clinic and the patient's willingness to attend again for the results. Most of the contacts of proven gonorrhoea will have the disease. The treatment regimen should be the same as for those known to have the infection.

Management of gonococcal infections in children

Ophthalmia neonatorum

TREATMENT. Recommended regimens are as follows: ceftriaxone, 25–50 mg kg^{-1} body weight (maximum 125 mg) intramuscularly or intravenously in a single dose, *or* spectinomycin, 25 mg kg^{-1} (maximum 75 mg) intramuscularly in a single dose, *or* kanamycin, 25 mg kg^{-1} (maximum 75 mg) intramuscularly in a single dose.

Topical treatment is with saline only.

FOLLOW-UP. The infant should be reviewed after 48 h and again 2 days later. The tests for gonorrhoea should be repeated. If a chlamydia swab was not taken at the initial visit and/or if the improvement is unsatisfactory, treatment for presumed chlamydial infection should be considered (Chapter 7.5).

PARENTS. In many instances, the genital infection in parents is asymptomatic. Both the parents will need to be examined, investigated and treated. The father may still have a demonstrable urethral discharge especially if examined after an overnight bladder. If left untreated, complications may occur.

For management of ophthalmia neonatorum in the absence of laboratory facilities see Chapter 10.1.

PREVENTION (see also Chapter 12.1). Detection and treatment of infection in the mother before she goes into labour (and examination and treatment of her partner) is the method of choice to prevent gonococcal ophthalmia neonatorum. Other methods immediately after birth include cleaning the infant's eyes and instilling into each conjunctival sac:

1% aqueous silver nitrate solution (one or two drops), i.e. Credé's method, *or* 1% tetracycline eye ointment, *or* 0.5% erythromycin eye ointment. The efficacy of the latter two treatments may vary because of resistant strains.

Silver nitrate should be freshly prepared since it might become concentrated through evaporation and, therefore, cause chemical conjunctivitis. Single dose containers are free from this risk. Chemical conjunctivitis should be treated with normal saline washes and usually clears in a couple of days.

The 2.5% povidone–iodine ophthalmic solution recently claimed to be effective needs further evaluation.

Vulvovaginitis

TREATMENT. This is based on CDC guidelines and is also applicable to cervicitis, urethritis, pharyngitis or proctitis. If the patient's weight is ≥ 45 kg, the treatment regimen is the same as for adults. For those weighing less than 45 kg, the treatment is ceftriaxone, 125 mg intramuscularly – single dose, *or* spectinomycin, 40 mg kg^{-1} (maximum 2 g) intramuscularly – single dose (efficacy poor in pharyngeal infection).

SURVEILLANCE AND MANAGEMENT OF CONTACTS. Surveillance should be continued for 2 weeks. The child's mother should be advised about not allowing children and others in the house to share towels and beds. Parents and household contacts should be examined and offered treatment where appropriate.

Disseminated gonococcal infection

Every child with suspected gonococcal infection should be examined for any evidence of disseminated infection such as skin lesions, arthritis and meningitis, and investigated appropriately.

TREATMENT. This is based on CDC guidelines. The recommended regimen for infants is ceftriaxone, 25–50 mg kg^{-1} intravenously or intramuscularly in a single dose daily for 7 days (10—14 days if meningitis present), *or* cefotaxime, 25 mg kg^{-1} intravenously or intramuscularly every 12 h daily for 7 days (10—14 days if meningitis present).

The recommended regimen for children who weigh less than 45 kg is ceftriaxone, 50 mg kg^{-1} (maximum 1 g) intravenously or intramuscularly in a single dose daily for 7 days.

Epidemiological treatment of infants

Infants born to mothers with untreated gonococcal infection are considered to be at high risk. They may be treated on an epidemiological basis with any of the following single dose regimens: ceftriaxone, 25—50 mg kg^{-1} (maximum 125 mg) intramuscularly, *or* spectinomycin, 25 mg kg^{-1} (maximum 75 mg) intramuscularly, *or* kanamycin, 25 mg kg^{-1} (maximum 75 mg) intramuscularly.

Further reading

Centers for Disease Control and Prevention (1998) Guidelines for treatment of sexually transmitted disease. *Morbidity and Mortality Weekly Report* 47 (No.RR-1): 65–68.

Grosskurth, H., Mayaud, P., Mosha, F., Todd, J., Senkoro, K., Newell, J., Gabone, R., Changalucha, J., West, B., Hayes, R. and Mabey, D. (1996) Asymptomatic gonorrhoea and chlamydial infection in rural Tanzanian men. *British Medical Journal* 312, 277–280.

Isenberg, S.J., Apt, L. and Wood, M. (1995) A controlled trial of povidone-iodine as prophylaxis against ophthalmia neonatorum. *The New England Journal of Medicine* 332, 562–566.

O'Rourke, M., Ison, C.A., Renton, A.M. and Spratt, B.G. (1995) Opa-typing: a high-resolution tool for studying the epidemiology of gonorrhoea. *Molecular Microbiology* 17, 865–875.

PHLS Communicable Disease Surveillance Centre, London (20 June 1997) Sexually Transmitted Disease quarterly report: gonorrhoea in England and Wales. *Communicable Disease Report Weekly* 7, 225–227.

World Health Organization (1991) Management of patients with sexually transmitted diseases. *WHO Technical Report Series* 810, Geneva.

World Health Organization (1994) Management of sexually transmitted diseases. WHO/GPA/TEM/94.1.

Young, H., Moyes, A. and McMillan, A. (1997) Azithromycin and erythromycin resistant *Neisseria gonorrhoeae* following treatment with azithromycin. *International Journal of STD and AIDS* 8, 299–302.

CHAPTER 7.5
Chlamydial, other non-gonococcal and non-specific infections, and Reiter's syndrome

O.P. Arya
Department of Medical Microbiology and Genitourinary Medicine, University of Liverpool, Liverpool, UK

The main conditions covered in this chapter include chlamydial infections in males and females, non-gonococcal and non-specific urethritis in males, chlamydial and other non-gonococcal infections in children, and Reiter's syndrome.

The diseases caused by *C. trachomatis* are largely similar to those due to *N. gonorrhoeae* and include conjunctivitis, urethritis, infection of Bartholin's gland, cervicitis, endometritis, pelvic infection, perihepatitis, epididymitis, proctitis, arthritis, rarely endocarditis and meningoencephalitis, and possibly also pharyngitis and prostatitis. Other conditions caused by *C. trachomatis* include lymphogranuloma venereum, neonatal infections and, rarely, pneumonia in immunocompromised adults.

Epidemiology

Chlamydial infection of the genitalia is common worldwide, mainly because most female and many male patients have no symptoms. Thus they do not attend any clinic and the infection may continue to spread. The majority of such patients would be detected only by screening high-risk groups which is not often possible because of inadequate resources. Application of newer tests, such as PCR and LCR, might reveal higher incidences and prevalences than with the currently available tests. See also Chapter 1 for epidemiology in the tropics.

The causative organism

The genus *Chlamydia* comprises obligate intracellular small Gram-negative bacteria which contain both DNA and RNA and have a cell wall. There are four species: *C. trachomatis* (see below), *C. pecorum* which causes pneumonia and diarrhoea in cattle and sheep, *C. pneumoniae* which causes human respiratory disease and possibly is connected with atherosclerosis, and *C.*

psittaci which causes disease in birds and animals and psittacosis in humans.

C. trachomatis has three biovars: the murine biovar which does not infect humans; the LGV biovar which infects macrophages, and includes serovars L1, L2 and L3 of lymphogranuloma venereum (Chapter 7.6); and the trachoma biovar which infects squamocolumnar cells and includes serovars A, B, Ba and C which are the causative agents of trachoma, and serovars D–K associated with urogenital infections, inclusion conjunctivitis and pneumonia of newborns. Monoclonal antibodies specific to these serovars are now available.

The chlamydiae have two developmental forms, the elementary body and the initial or reticulate body. The infectious elementary bodies (which are adapted to extracellular existence) enter the host cell, and within 6–8 h change to the metabolically active initial bodies. The latter divide by binary fission. After 48–72 h, the cell ruptures and infectious elementary bodies are released.

Laboratory aspects

For sampling swabs and collection of clinical specimens see Chapters 4 and 5.

Diagnostic tests

Tests for diagnosis of chlamydial infections include isolation by cell culture, antigen detection by direct immunofluorescence staining of smears, ELISA, nucleic acid amplification assays (LCR and PCR), and serological methods. See Chapter 5 for details.

Choice of test

LCR and PCR are the most sensitive and specific tests for *C. trachomatis*, but are expensive. Culture is 100% specific, accepted for medicolegal purposes, but sensitivity is no more than 75–80%, is labour-intensive and expensive. Enzyme immunoassay (EIA) is the most convenient and widely available antigen detection test but its sensitivity is less than 80%; it can show false positives and hence, ideally, needs confirmation by another method such as immunofluoresence, which requires considerable expertise. EIA is unsuitable for pharyngeal and rectal samples. As urethral swabbing is painful and other invasive procedures (e.g. endocervical and rectal sampling) are unpleasant and may deter patients from attending, a non-invasive test would be an obvious advantage. Recently, researchers have evaluated first-voided urine (FVU), and vulval and vaginal introitus swabs for chlamydia antigen detection. To achieve an acceptably high sensitivity (>90%) these specimens need to be tested by nucleic acid amplification (LCR or PCR). More affordable and easier to perform versions of these tests are urgently required. Multiplex PCR aimed at several infective agents is a distinct possibility and may be more cost effective.

Time of sampling and menstruation

The findings, in females, with regard to any relationship between the phase of the menstrual cycle and chlamydia detection from the cervix have been contradictory.

Antimicrobial susceptibility

C. trachomatis is susceptible to tetracycline, erythromycin, ofloxacin, rifampicin, to a lesser degree to sulphonamides and ciprofloxacin, and less still to penicillin, but is insensitive to spectinomycin and aminoglycosides.

Transmission and predisposing factors

The modes of transmission of *C. trachomatis* are similar to those of *N. gonorrhoeae* (Chapter 7.4). In addition, cervical ectopy (often associated with use of oral contraceptives) facilitates chlamydial infection of the cervix. Oral contraceptive use may be an independent risk factor.

Pathogenesis and immunity

Chlamydial replication may cause tissue damage and an inflammatory response and possibly a hypersensitivity reaction. Initially there is infiltration with neutrophils followed by a localized lymphoproliferative response resulting in follicular urethritis, follicular cervicitis and follicular conjunctivitis. Eventually the affected mucous membranes may undergo fibrosis and scarring.

Chlamydial infection does not seem to confer significant immunity. Repeated infections are common. Low-level immunity may, however, develop after repeated infections.

Non-gonococcal and non-specific urethritis in adult males

Non-gonococcal urethritis (NGU), commonly known as NSU, i.e. non-specific urethritis, is perhaps the most common sexually transmitted disease in men worldwide. The term NSU should only be used when all known causes of urethritis have been excluded. This is neither feasible nor necessary except in research settings. The term NGU is, therefore, to be preferred, and serves well for clinical as well as management purposes. The aetiology, clinical features and management aspects of PGU (Chapter 7.4) are similar to those of NGU.

Aetiology

Bacteria

C. trachomatis is the undisputed cause in up to 40% of the cases of NGU. The role of mycoplasmas is unclear. Colonization of the genitourinary tract by

Ureaplasma urealyticum is common, and it is not known how and when it adopts a pathogenic role. Nevertheless, *U. urealyticum* is thought to account for about 20% of cases. *Mycoplasma genitalium* is another contender. *Haemophilus ducreyi* and *Treponema pallidum*, as a result of rare intrameatal or intraurethral lesions, may present with symptoms and signs of urethritis. Non-sexually transmitted bacterial urethritis may occur in association with urinary tract infection (coliform infection, urogenital tuberculosis), residual urine due to prostatic enlargement in older men, urethral stricture and trauma due to instrumentation. Commensals, when present in large numbers, may assume a pathogenic role, e.g. mixed anaerobes, *Staphylococcus saprophyticus*.

Viruses

Herpes simplex virus and human papillomavirus may be the cause of urethritis in less than 1% of the cases.

Fungi

C. albicans may rarely cause urethritis, especially in the presence of diabetes mellitus.

Protozoa

Trichomonas vaginalis, although very difficult to find in cases of NGU in industrialized countries, may account for over 10% of the cases in some tropical areas.

Helminths

Although the cardinal symptom of *Schistosoma haematobium* infection, causing vesical schistosomiasis, is haematuria, a male patient may occasionally present with features of NGU (see also Chapter 11.6).

Other causes

NGU may also occur as a manifestation of Reiter's syndrome (see below), Stevens–Johnson syndrome and isotretinoin therapy.

After all the above known causes have been excluded, there still remain about 30% of cases of NGU where no cause can be found.

Incubation period

The incubation period is usually longer than that of gonorrhoea. The range is 5–30 days but may be much longer, e.g. chlamydial infection may remain latent for a long time.

Symptoms and signs

Up to 40% of cases may be asymptomatic. The diagnosis in these patients is made after careful examination when they present to the clinic. Some attend because their partners have been found to be infected.

The symptoms and signs are usually much milder than in gonorrhoea. The patient may complain of mild dysuria, irritation or pricking sensation in the urethra, or scanty urethral discharge. Very rarely, a patient may present with acute haemorrhagic cystitis when the posterior urethra is involved, and the symptoms include intense dysuria, urgency and frequency of micturition.

A careful clinical examination, aided if necessary by massaging the urethra from the root of the penis to the meatus, will show urethral discharge in most cases, especially if the patient has not voided urine for over 4 h. In some, the discharge may be demonstrated only in the mornings after the patient has not passed urine overnight. In the majority, the discharge is minimal, clear, grey, mucoid or mucopurulent (Plate 93). In a few cases, the discharge may be profuse and purulent, i.e. indistinguishable from a typical case of gonorrhoea.

The two-glass urine test shows threads or haziness in the first glass and clear urine in the second. Haziness in both glasses may be due to phosphaturia (Chapter 4), excessive pus or the presence of posterior urethritis/cystitis. The last may be associated with haematuria. Proteinuria is uncommon in uncomplicated anterior urethritis.

Differential diagnosis

Gonorrhoea is the main condition to be excluded. Other causes and conditions associated with urethritis are listed above. Accordingly, other investigations, e.g. urine examination, radiology, cystoscopy and intravenous urography and possibly referral to a urologist, may be necessary.

Diagnosis

NGU is diagnosed if a Gram-stained urethral smear shows five or more PMN per high power field (×1000) and Gram-negative diplococci are absent. An alternative criterion is 15 or more PMN per field (×400) in a smear of urine threads or of the sediment of the first-catch urine (first 15–20 ml). In the subclinical cases with no demonstrable discharge, and if the above tests are inconclusive, the patient may need to be re-examined and tests repeated after the patient has not passed urine overnight.

The leukocyte esterase (LE) urine dip-stick test to screen urine for the detection of urethritis has a variable sensitivity (50–70%) in asymptomatic patients. A positive test should be confirmed with a Gram-stained smear of a urethral swab specimen, which is also essential to detect the presence or absence of Gram-negative intracellular diplococci.

Tests for the detection of *Chlamydia*, although not essential in the male patients, are desirable. The demonstration of a specific cause will facilitate information, education, counselling, partner notification and treatment compliance, as well as enhance the learning experience and morale of the medical attendant. In addition, the patient should be screened for any other STI.

Course of non-gonococcal urethritis

The condition may resolve spontaneously. However, the patient, if harbouring *C. trachomatis*, may remain infectious for several months. Recurrences are not uncommon. A small proportion of patients develop complications.

Complications

Complications or sequelae of untreated or inadequately treated NGU are uncommon. Local complications are essentially similar to those in gonorrhoea, and include infection of Tyson's and Cowper's glands, periurethral abscess, urethral stricture, epididymitis and possibly chronic prostatitis. In almost a quarter of the NGU patients, urethritis may persist or recur despite 'adequate' treatment (see below). With regard to systemic complications, Reiter's syndrome may be triggered in about 1% of cases of NGU.

The diagnosis of urethral stricture may be aided by examining the urine stream and the passage of a sound. These patients should be referred to a urologist for further investigations and management.

Epididymitis (Plate 94)

The most important sexually acquired non-gonococcal causative agent is *C. trachomatis*.

PATHOGENESIS. This is assumed to be similar to that of gonococcal epididymitis (Chapter 7.4).

CLINICAL FEATURES. The condition is usually preceded by urethritis which may have been asymptomatic. As epididymitis develops, the urethral discharge becomes scanty. The onset of epididymitis and the clinical features are usually less severe than in gonococcal epididymitis, but severe forms do occur. Thus clinical differentiation is almost impossible. A careful examination including a two-glass urine test will reveal evidence of urethritis especially if the patient has not voided recently.

DIFFERENTIAL DIAGNOSIS. This is as for gonococcal epididymitis (Chapter 7.4).

DIAGNOSIS. A Gram-stained urethral smear will show five or more PMN per high power field and absence of Gram-negative intracellular diplococci. If facilities are available, tests described in the section on gonococcal epididymitis should be considered.

Chronic prostatitis

Although chronic prostatitis may appear to be a common sequel of NGU, there is no reliable information on this relationship. Nevertheless, the condition is encountered frequently at STI clinics. The potential, but not proven, sexually transmitted causes include *C. trachomatis*, *U. urealyticum*, *T. vaginalis* and herpes simplex virus. Whereas the known causes include

Escherichia coli, *Klebsiella* spp., *Proteus* spp., *Enterococcus faecalis*, etc., no infectious agent is isolated in the majority of cases.

CLINICAL FEATURES. Chronic prostatitis is often asymptomatic. The symptoms include perineal discomfort, pain in the groin and in the tip of the penis, suprapubic pain, intermittent early morning penile discharge, low backache, urinary frequency, dysuria, post-micturition dribbling, pain on ejaculation and haemospermia. Rectal examination may reveal a normal or slightly enlarged prostate with localized tenderness.

DIFFERENTIAL DIAGNOSIS. Among other conditions, differential diagnosis is from benign prostatic enlargement, bladder neck dyssynergia and prostatodynia.

DIAGNOSIS. Diagnosis is established by examination of fractionated urine samples and expressed prostatic secretions (Chapter 4). Seminal fluid examination for this purpose is said to be less reliable. Consideration should be given to the inclusion of tests for STI although they are likely to be negative partly because most patients have received antibiotic therapy before the possibility of chronic prostatitis becomes an issue. Transrectal ultrasound may help in the diagnosis and localization of prostate disease but will not point to the cause.

Reiter's syndrome

Reiter's syndrome is described below.

Urogenital chlamydial infections in females

Symptoms and signs

The majority of the patients (60% or more) are asymptomatic. Symptoms, when present, are not diagnostic and are more or less similar to those in gonococcal infection. The symptoms include vaginal discharge, dysuria and frequency (urethral syndrome). The symptoms and signs may be due to associated infection(s), such as candidiasis, trichomoniasis and gonococcal infection. In the author's experience, only 30% of those harbouring *C. trachomatis* do not have a concurrent infection.

In the absence of concurrent infection, clinical examination in the majority of patients is normal. About a third of the patients show macroscopic cervicitis, i.e. mucopurulent discharge, oedema and congestion of the cervix, or friable cervix with contact bleeding. Cervical ectopy, if present, may become oedematous and congested (Plate 95). Mucopurulent discharge (which may look yellow on a white swab) of the endocervix is not always easy to recognize. In a patient with concurrent gonococcal infection, the endocervicitis, if present, may remain unchanged after treatment with a drug regimen with no effect on *Chlamydia* (post-gonococcal cervicitis, see Chapter 7.4). A small proportion of patients may show evidence of urethritis (e.g. urethral discharge) and infection of Bartholin's glands and their ducts (e.g. a bead of mucopus at the duct orifices after massaging the ducts).

Differential diagnosis

Differential diagnosis, apart from providing a valuable learning experience, may be an issue only in symptomatic patients (problem-oriented approach) and if clinical examination confirms an abnormal vaginal discharge, urethritis, infection of Bartholin's glands or mucopurulent cervicitis. The common conditions to be considered include gonococcal infection, trichomoniasis, bacterial vaginosis and yeast infection. None of these conditions can be excluded with certainty without tests. A very small proportion of patients may indeed have mucopurulent cervicitis without any known cause (non-specific cervicitis).

Diagnosis

Whereas NGU in men can be diagnosed easily by the number of PMN in a Gram-stained smear, there is no similar diagnostic criterion in women. In the author's experience a cut off point of 30 or more PMN per high power field of a Gram-stained cervical smear, used by some, has unacceptably low sensitivity and specificity. In the absence of any pathognomonic symptoms or signs, the only way to confirm or exclude chlamydial infection in women is by taking swabs for the detection of *Chlamydia*. As chlamydial infection in females is potentially a very serious infection, all women at perceived risk should have the benefit of tests for this infection. Hence, provision of this facility should be a priority. Various constraints may limit the number of swabs, in which case the cervix must be the preferred site to be sampled. However, the urethra may be the only positive site in up to 15% of patients. In some cases, *C. trachomatis* may be isolated from Bartholin's ducts and rectal mucosa (see below). The patients should also be screened routinely for gonorrhoea and other STI.

In the absence of laboratory facilities, the diagnosis will have to be made on epidemiological and clinical grounds (Chapters 10.1 and 10.2). In the author's experience, mucopurulent cervicitis, if correctly recognized (i.e. mucopus in the cervix and ≥30 PMN per high power field in a Gram-stained cervical smear), is the most reliable sign, but will detect only a minority of infected patients.

Natural course of chlamydial infection in females

The infection may clear spontaneously or persist for several months without causing symptoms. Eventually some patients will develop complications, such as pelvic infection and perihepatitis (see Chapter 10.3) or Reiter's syndrome (see below).

Chlamydial infection in pregnancy

In pregnancy, cervical ectropion is common, and may increase susceptibility to *C. trachomatis* infection. Whereas cervical carriage of *C. trachomatis* is a risk factor for post-abortal and postpartum infection, any aetiological link with abortion, intrauterine growth retardation or prematurity is not established. Postpartum endometritis (early: within 48 h after birth, or late: 3 days to 6 weeks after birth) may be asymptomatic or the patient may present with vaginal bleeding, lower abdominal pain, vaginal discharge and fever.

Extragenital chlamydial infections

These include chlamydial infections of the eyes, pharynx, lungs and rectum, perihepatitis (see Chapter 10.3) and Reiter's syndrome.

Chlamydial infection of the eyes

Inclusion conjunctivitis in adults

Occasionally, an adult, as a result of accidental infection (hand to eye contact) or infection directly during sexual activity, may develop inclusion conjunctivitis (follicular conjunctivitis). A considerable proportion of these men and women and/or their partners have asymptomatic chlamydial infection of the urogenital tract. Consequently, these patients initially are seen at the eye out-patient department (Plate 96). The condition may be self-limiting or become chronic, resulting in conjunctival scarring and keratitis.

A careful examination may reveal evidence of urethritis in the male and macroscopic cervicitis in some of the female patients in either or both partners. *C. trachomatis* may be detected in the conjunctival, urethral and cervical specimens. Gonococcal infection must always be excluded.

Chlamydial ophthalmia in the neonate is discussed below.

Chlamydial infection of the pharynx

Chlamydial infection of the pharynx is uncommon in adults. The mode of transmission is similar to that in gonorrhoea (Chapter 7.4). There are no specific symptoms or signs. Pharyngeal swab for the detection of *C. trachomatis* (by culture) in adults may be taken only on a selective basis. In children, chlamydial infection of the nasopharynx may be due to aspiration of the infected cervical secretion at delivery or extension of chlamydial infection from the conjunctiva, and may spread to the lungs. In these children, nasopharyngeal swabs for the detection of *Chlamydia* need to be taken for diagnosis as well as tests of cure (see below).

Chlamydial infection of the lungs

Pneumonia due to *C. trachomatis* in adults is rare but has been documented in immunocompromised patients. Chlamydial pneumonia in children is discussed below.

Chlamydial infection of the rectum

The mode of infection is similar to that in gonorrhoea in males and females (Chapter 7.4). Although *C. trachomatis*-associated proctitis may occur in homosexual males, NGU, in general, is less common in homosexuals than in heterosexuals. The symptoms and signs of chlamydial proctitis in males and females are similar to those of gonococcal proctitis (Chapter 7.4). LGV immunotypes of *C. trachomatis* are more invasive (Chapter 7.6). For the diagnosis, chlamydia culture is required. A Gram-stained rectal smear will show a large number of PMN. An excessive number of PMN in a rectal smear necessitates a search for sexually transmitted and other causes before making a diagnosis of 'non-specific' proctitis. The differential diagnosis will include infections due to *N. gonorrhoeae*, herpes simplex virus, human papillomavirus, *T. pallidum*, non-syphilitic spirochaetes, *Entamoeba histolytica*, *Campylobacter* spp., and *Shigella* spp., trauma, ulcerative colitis and Crohn's disease (see also Chapter 11.2).

Link between HIV and chlamydial infections

Up to now, the results of studies to demonstrate any link between *Chlamydia* and HIV infection have been contradictory. Nevertheless, there is no evidence that HIV infection alters the natural history of chlamydial infection.

Chlamydial infections in infants and children

Inclusion conjunctivitis of the newborn

The incidence of chlamydial conjunctivitis of the newborn in the tropics is unknown, but is thought to be much greater than in most industrialized countries. The infection occurs by direct contact with infected cervical secretions during delivery. The risk of chlamydial ocular infection in infants born to infected mothers is about 50%.

Clinical features

The incubation period is 5–14 days. The condition may be unilateral or bilateral. Many cases with mild infection may not be brought to the clinic. The infant develops sticky eyes, the conjunctivae are inflamed and the lids oedematous. The discharge may be thin, watery or mucoid, sometimes becoming mucopurulent and frankly purulent with or without secondary bacterial infection (Plate 97). The condition may resolve spontaneously after several weeks or progress to conjunctival scarring or even trachoma-like changes, especially in the presence of secondary bacterial infection. In some, the infection may extend to the nasopharynx and thence to the lungs, resulting in pneumonia (see below). Extension of infection to the middle ear resulting in otitis media has also been suggested.

Differential diagnosis

The most important condition to be considered is gonococcal ophthalmia (Chapter 7.4). Both infections may coexist. Other bacterial causes include *Staphylococcus aureus*, *Streptococcus pneumoniae*, *E. coli*, *H. influenzae*, *N.*

meningitidis, *Klebsiella*, *Proteus* and *Pseudomonas* spp. Chemical conjunctivitis, which develops within 24 h following the application of silver nitrate and associated with swelling of the lids, resolves within 3 days.

Diagnosis

A Gram-stained smear of conjunctival exudate will show PMN but no Gram-negative diplococci. If the smear shows many other bacteria, the aetiology may be non-gonococcal non-chlamydial. If the smear shows PMN but no other bacteria, the cause may possibly be *C. trachomatis*. A more precise diagnosis of chlamydial infection can be made by demonstrating intracytoplasmic inclusions in a Giemsa-stained smear of conjunctival scrapings. The diagnosis may be confirmed by culture or antigen detection methods.

Pneumonia

Chlamydial infection from the conjunctiva (see above) may extend to the nasopharynx, trachea and bronchi, leading to diffuse lung involvement. Alternatively, pneumonitis may result from aspiration of infected cervical secretions at delivery.

Clinical features

The condition usually manifests at 3–12 weeks of age. The child is afebrile or has mild fever, and has a staccato cough (pertussis-like cough without a whoop) and tachypnoea (rapid breathing). Some will also have conjunctivitis. Inspiratory crepitations can be heard on auscultation. The illness is generally mild and may resolve within 2 months. However, in some, the condition may progress to chronic obstructive lung disease.

Differential diagnosis

The conditions that may need to be considered in infant pneumonitis include viral pneumonia (due to respiratory syncytial virus, adenovirus, cytomegalovirus, influenza virus), *Pneumocystis carinii* pneumonia, whooping cough, tuberculosis and other bacterial infections.

Diagnosis

X-ray of the chest in chlamydial pneumonia shows hyperinflation and diffuse symmetrical interstitial infiltration. There is eosinophilia in the peripheral blood film and a chlamydia microimmunofluorescence (MIF) test may show elevated IgM and IgG levels. *C. trachomatis* may be detected in conjunctival scrapings and nasopharyngeal and bronchial aspirates. Because of the possibility of false-positive results due to cross-reaction of test reagents with *C. pneumoniae*, the culture method (confirmed by fluorescent antibody staining) is to be preferred.

Vulvovaginitis and infection of other sites

As stated earlier (see gonococcal vulvovaginitis, Chapter 7.4), the immature vaginal epithelium in pre-pubescent girls is susceptible to infection. In the case of chlamydial infection, the vulva is often, and urethra and rectum occasionally, also affected. In some children, chlamydial vulvovaginitis may occur in those with inclusion conjunctivitis. In others it may be the result of sexual abuse.

Clinical features

The clinical features are similar to those in gonococcal vulvovaginitis.

Differential diagnosis

Gonococcal infection must be excluded. The other causes of vulvovaginitis include *Staphylococcus* spp., *Streptococcus* spp., *H. influenzae*, *Corynebacterium diphtheriae*, coliforms, *C. albicans* and *T. vaginalis*. Threadworms (*Enterobius vermicularis*) which infest the lower bowel may also be found on the vulva and in the vagina. Vulvovaginitis may occur in systemic diseases such as measles, pneumonia, etc. If the discharge is blood stained, foreign body should be suspected.

Diagnosis

The diagnosis is confirmed by the detection of *C. trachomatis* (in cell culture for medicolegal cases) in material from appropriate sites such as the vagina, urethra, rectum, nasopharynx and conjunctivae.

Management of NGU and chlamydial infections

Treatment of uncomplicated NGU and genital and extragenital chlamydial infections in adults

Although the aetiology of NGU is diverse, it is possible to obtain an overall cure rate of over 80% with drug regimens (Box 7.5.1) which cure over 95% of men and women infected with *C. trachomatis*. The treatment regimen is the same for HIV-negative and positive patients. An ideal regimen for any area must be one which is highly effective locally, cheap, safe and easy to administer. Tetracycline is probably the cheapest of the drugs in Box 7.5.1. However, its absorption is decreased by milk, antacids, calcium, iron and magnesium salts, and it should be taken on an empty stomach. Tetracyclines (including doxycycline) and ofloxacin are contraindicated in pregnancy and nursing mothers. Erythromycin in the dosage regimen shown in Box 7.5.1 is not infrequently associated with gastrointestinal side effects, especially in pregnancy. The dosage regimen can then be changed to 250 mg, four times daily for 14 days. Some suggest, amoxycillin, 500 mg orally three times daily for 7 days for erythromycin-intolerant pregnant patients. Azithromycin has the advantage of being effective in a single dose but the cure rates have been

Box 7.5.1. Drug regimens for the treatment of uncomplicated non-gonococcal urethritis and chlamydial infections in adults.

Tetracycline, 500 mg orally four times daily for 7 days
or
Doxycycline, 100 mg orally twice daily for 7 days
or
Erythromycin, 500 mg orally four times daily for 7 days
or
Ofloxacin, 300 mg orally twice daily for 7 days
or
Azithromycin, 1 g orally in a single dose

See text for contraindications and other details.

lower than the doxycycline regimen in some studies. Furthermore, it is expensive, and the manufacturers advise its use in pregnancy and lactation only if adequate alternatives are not available.

The patients should be advised to abstain from sexual intercourse and excessive alcohol intake until treatment has been completed and symptoms resolved.

For management in the absence of laboratory facilities (problem-oriented approach), see Chapter 10.1.

Surveillance

Traditionally, surveillance is at intervals of 1–2 weeks until two consecutive tests are normal. The male patient is advised not to pass urine for about 4 h before each visit. Many patients will have become asymptomatic a week after the start of treatment; however, a successful outcome implies absence of urethritis (i.e. number of PMN in the urethral smear to fall below five per high power field which may take much longer than 1 week), normal urine in males and the absence of cervicitis, etc., in females (Plate 98), as well as a microbiological cure when a specific cause, such as *C. trachomatis*, has been found. Tests of cure for such patients who have been treated with a regimen in Box 7.5.1 and who have become asymptomatic are not considered to be cost effective. If, however, a test of cure is desired, then a follow-up of at least 4 weeks is probably necessary for the antigen detection tests. The timing of these tests needs clarification due to the prolonged detection of antigen although the bacteria may be dead. If possible, a final blood test for syphilis should be carried out at the end of 3 months in all cases.

Partner notification

Partners of symptomatic men over the previous 4 weeks and of women and asymptomatic men over the previous 8 weeks, or the most recent partner if last sex was over 2 months ago, should be examined, investigated and treated with one of the regimens in Box 7.5.1 to prevent re-infection and also for their own sakes. As stated earlier, a specific diagnosis will facilitate this process.

Management of complications

Persistent and recurrent NGU in males

In about 20% of patients, a low-grade NGU may persist or recur a few days to several weeks after treatment. Some patients may experience an early morning discharge, and their urine may contain persistent heavy threads. Others are asymptomatic but the Gram-stained urethral smears continue to show evidence of urethritis, i.e. more than five PMN per high power field. If re-infection has been excluded and compliance with treatment instructions is good, then some of these cases may be due to ureaplasmas resistant to tetracyline, or due to *T. vaginalis*, herpes simplex virus, intraurethral warts, *Mycobacterium tuberculosis*, chronic prostatitis, urethral stricture or perhaps delayed hypersensitivity response to *C. trachomatis* or other infection. These cases will, therefore, need to be investigated. Examination of female sexual partners may help, e.g. *T. vaginalis* is easier to find in vaginal specimens. The male partner can then be treated accordingly.

The above condition is certainly more common in *Chlamydia*-negative/ *Ureaplasma*-negative patients. Indeed, in most cases, no known pathogen can be found. In some cases, recurrence may be associated with excessive consumption of alcohol. In others, the symptoms may be associated with defaecation on account of faecal pressure on the prostate resulting in prostatorrhoea. Some of the patients become anxious and depressed and may resort to repeated self-examination and 'milking' the urethra, resulting in traumatic urethritis. The management of these patients requires considerable skill and understanding, as well as an appropriate clinical and microbiological reappraisal. If there is no evidence of urethritis, the patient should be reassured. However, if persistent urethritis is confirmed, a further course of antibiotic such as erythromycin, 500 mg orally four times daily for 14 days (which should clear ureaplasmas resistant to tetracycline) or doxycycline, 100 mg orally twice daily for 14 days, and/or metronidazole, 400 mg orally twice daily for 7 days might help some patients. Others may need referral for urological investigations, which may also be normal, exposing our inadequacy in the management of such patients.

Epididymitis

The patient is advised bed rest and elevation of the scrotum until scrotal tenderness resolves, and is given analgesics for pain. Any of the antibiotic treatment regimens shown in Box 7.5.1 may be prescribed, but the treatment is extended to 10–14 days. The dosage regimen for azithromycin in this condition is unknown. Surveillance is basically similar to that for gonococcal epididymitis (Chapter 7.4). See above for the management of sexual partners.

Chronic prostatitis

Any of the following treatment regimens, which achieve reasonable levels in the prostate, may be used: ciprofloxacin, 500 mg orally twice daily, *or* norfloxacin, 400 mg orally twice daily, *or* ofloxacin, 200 mg orally twice daily, *or* suphamethoxazole 800 mg/trimethoprim 160 mg orally twice daily, *or* doxycycline, 100 mg orally twice daily, *or* erythromycin, 500 mg orally four times daily. Azithromycin has not yet been evaluated. Treatment should be continued for 3 weeks and then the patient should be assessed. Further treatment may be necessary in some patients. The response in bacterial prostatitis is better than when no cause is found. Sexual partners should be checked for any STI and both partners then treated appropriately as indicated.

For treatment of pelvic infection and perihepatitis, see Chapter 10.3.

Management of chlamydial infection in infants and children

Inclusion conjunctivitis

TREATMENT. The recommended regimen is erythromycin (syrup), 50 mg kg^{-1} in four divided doses daily for 14 days. Topical treatment is unnecessary.

SURVEILLANCE. The infant should be reviewed after 48 h and treatment compliance checked and then reviewed after completion of treatment. If the condition has resolved, the chlamydia detection test should be repeated, if possible, at the end of 5 weeks. A second course of erythromycin should be prescribed if the condition has not resolved.

INFANT'S MOTHER AND PARTNERS. The infant's mother and the mother's sexual partners will need to be evaluated and treated with an appropriate regimen (Box 7.5.1). Breast-feeding mothers should be treated with erythromycin.

PREVENTION. The best way to prevent chlamydial infection in the infant is to detect and treat the infection in the mother before she goes into labour. Applications of 1% tetracycline eye ointment or 0.5% erythromycin eye ointment to the infant's conjunctivae at birth may prevent chlamydial ophthalmia but not nasopharyngeal colonization of *C. trachomatis* nor respiratory infection.

Pneumonia

TREATMENT. The recommended treatment regimen is erythromycin, 50 mg kg^{-1} body weight in four divided doses daily for 14 days. Oxygen may be required if there is respiratory distress.

SURVEILLANCE. The child should be followed up to ensure pneumonia has resolved.

INFANT'S MOTHER AND PARTNERS. The management of infant's mother and the mother's sexual partners is the same as in the case of conjunctivitis of the newborn (see above).

Vulvovaginitis and infection of other sites

The recommended treatment regimen is erythromycin, 50 mg kg^{-1} body weight divided into four doses daily for 14 days for children weighing less than

45 kg, and an adult dose for those weighing more than 45 kg. Tetracyclines should not be given to children under 12 years of age.

SURVEILLANCE. The child should be followed up to ensure the infection has cleared.

Reiter's syndrome (and sexually acquired reactive arthritis)

Reactive arthritis is an aseptic arthritis which follows an infection elsewhere in the body. Reiter's syndrome – a seronegative arthropathy (absence of rheumatoid factor) – is a triad of reactive arthritis, genital tract inflammation and ocular inflammation. Many patients also develop mucocutaneous lesions. Incomplete forms of Reiter's syndrome frequently are encountered. The true incidence of the condition is unknown.

Aetiology

The condition occurs in about 1–2% of men with sexually acquired NGU and in women with cervicitis, or may develop after an enteric infection caused by *Shigella flexneri*, *Yersinia enterocolitica*, *Salmonella* spp. and *Campylobacter* spp. As urethritis may also occur in the enteric infection category of patients, it cannot always be assumed to have been sexually acquired.

The aetiology is more likely to be multifactorial, comprising infective, immunological and genetic factors. Among sexually transmitted agents, *C. trachomatis* has been isolated from the genital tract of almost half of the men presenting with reactive arthritis or Reiter's syndrome. Chlamydial antigen, but not the viable organism, has been detected in the synovial tissue of patients with Reiter's syndrome. Other STI which may possibly be associated with reactive arthritis include gonorrhoea, syphilis, LGV, hepatitis B and HIV. The role of *U. urealyticum* remains unresolved.

Almost 80% of Caucasian patients with reactive arthritis have the histocompatibility HLA-B27 antigen which determines susceptibility to the condition. However, the immunological mechanisms in the pathogenesis of the various manifestations are not clear.

When associated with NGU, the disease predominantly affects males, occurring usually between the ages of 20 and 40 years. In many females the condition probably remains unrecognized.

Clinical features

As Reiter's syndrome is a multisystem disease, the patient may present initially at ophthalmology, rheumatology and other departments.

Genitourinary tract

The syndrome in males usually begins with NGU or PGU. The urethritis may be asymptomatic, detected only on careful examination after the patient has not voided urine for several hours. Occasionally, the patient may have symptomatic or asymptomatic prostatitis. Female patients may have cervicitis, urethritis, cystitis, salpingitis, and may give a history of vaginal discharge and/or dysuria.

Joints and entheses

The onset of non-suppurative (reactive) arthritis is acute or subacute, with or without an effusion, and asymmetrical. In some, joint involvement is limited to arthralgia. Synovitis develops usually within 4 weeks after urethritis. Joint symptoms may, however, precede genitourinary symptoms. Initially, the joints commonly affected are knees, ankles or metatarsophalangeal (Plate 99). Others involved include sacroiliac joints, and small joints of the hands, wrists and temporomandibular joints. The joints are painful, swollen, tender and warm, but the overlying skin is not greatly reddened. The muscles around the affected joints may become wasted. Involvement of sacroiliac joint during the course of the illness is very common and may be asymptomatic or associated with low backache. An X-ray may show erosions of articular surfaces, sclerosis and obliteration of the joint space. Similar changes may be seen in the other joints in chronically affected cases. There may also be extra-articular musculoskeletal lesions including inflammation of the plantar fascia and of the Achilles tendon and intercostal muscles at the insertion sites, giving rise to pain in the heels and chest wall.

Eyes

Conjunctivitis occurs in over half of the cases. It is usually mild and transient. The conjunctival secretion may be mucoid or mucopurulent, but no organisms are found. Iritis, which is more serious, occurs usually later in the disease and may be an isolated phenomenon in some patients with a previous history of Reiter's syndrome.

Skin and mucous membranes

The skin and mucous membranes show characteristic changes, developing in over a quarter of the patients. They may begin as erythematous macules developing into pustules, and then become hyperkeratotic (keratodermia blenorrhagica). They may develop on the soles of the feet (Plate 100), on the circumcized glans penis and in more severe cases may spread to legs and, rarely, to other parts of the body. These changes, which are painless, may also affect the nails, and are indistinguishable from some types of psoriasis (Plate 101). In uncircumcized men, the glans penis and prepuce are moist, the lesions are shallow superficial erosions, initially circular, which then coalesce to form polycylic outline, i.e. balanitis circinata (Plate 102). In a few patients, erythema and shallow erosions may occur in the mouth and on the palate (Plate 103).

Constitutional symptoms and signs

Those mildly affected generally feel well. Others may experience malaise, pyrexia and weight loss. There may be a moderate polymorphonuclear leukocytosis, hypochromic or normochromic anaemia, elevated erythrocyte sedimentation rate as well as α2-globulins. All these changes are non-specific.

Course and late effects

After the initial attack, urethritis and conjunctivitis clear within a few weeks but the arthritis may take longer, i.e. 3–6 months. In HLA-B27-negative individuals, the disease, in general, seems to run a milder and shorter course. Overall, about half of the patients experience one or more relapses. The remissions may last for months or years. The relapse may be associated with re-infection or some unknown factor. In some HLA-B27-positive individuals, the relapse of reactive arthritis may be triggered by an infection different from that in the initial episode.

Late effects include calcanean spur as a result of plantar fasciitis and periosteal reaction, progressive involvement of the spine indistinguishable from ankylosing spondylitis, subluxation and destruction of the metatarsophalangeal joints, impairment of vision as a result of uveitis, and, more rarely, aortic incompetence, pericarditis, myocarditis, encephalitis, peripheral neuritis, pleurisy and pneumonitis.

Differential diagnosis

The differential diagnosis will include disseminated gonococcal infection, other forms of septic arthritis, rheumatoid arthritis, gout, rheumatic fever, tuberculosis, brucellosis, other reactive arthritides, other seronegative arthropathies (idiopathic ankylosing spondylitis, Bechçet's disease, Crohn's disease, psoriatic arthritis, ulcerative colitis and Whipple's disease), serum sickness, systemic lupus erythematosus, Stevens–Johnson syndrome and iritis due to other causes.

Diagnosis

There is no specific test for the diagnosis of Reiter's syndrome. Nevertheless, there is not much difficulty in the presence of a full-blown syndrome. A systematic approach will include a detailed history, a thorough physical examination including that of the urogenital tract, appropriate specimens for Gram-staining and detection of *C. trachomatis* and *N. gonorrhoeae*, and tests for other STI as indicated.

Other investigations include X-ray of the sacroiliac joints and examination of the synovial fluid which in Reiter's syndrome is turbid and sterile on culture but shows an elevated PMN count initally. Other tests on synovial fluid include examination for crystals and bacteria, and detection of chlamydial antigen.

Some non-specific laboratory tests have already been mentioned above. Depending upon the indications and the facilities available, other investigations include: MIF test for chlamydia antibody, HLA typing, rheumatoid factor, antinuclear antibodies, antistreptolysin O titre, serum uric acid levels, circulatory immune complexes and synovial biopsy.

Prognosis

The majority of the patients recover completely. The prognosis is less favourable in those with severe initial illness and who are HLA-B27-positive. These individuals, albeit a small proportion, will be left with residual disability.

Treatment

Triggering infection

Any sexually transmitted triggering infection, such as due to *C. trachomatis*, presumed or confirmed, including urethritis and prostatitis, should be treated appropriately. The sexual partners should also be checked and offered treatment. Whether or not this influences the course of illness remains to be resolved.

Arthritis

It is preferable to manage these patients jointly with a rheumatologist. The mild cases may respond to simple analgesics such as soluble aspirin (600–900 mg) or paracetamol (1 g), orally three times daily. Alternatively, and in more severe cases, a non-steroidal anti-inflammatory drug such as indomethacin is usually very effective. The dose is 25 mg (may be increased to 50 mg) orally three times daily.

Swollen and painful joints may require aspiration, rest (a short stay in hospital) and support with a firm bandage, followed by passive and active movements as soon as possible. For more severe symptoms limited to one or two sites, a local steroid injection may help. For patients with persistent aggressive arthropathy, the options include: methotrexate, 5–15 mg orally weekly, *or* azathioprine, 1–2 mg kg^{-1} orally daily, *or* sulphasalazine, 500 mg (initially), orally daily.

Conjunctivitis and iritis

Conjunctivitis usually clears spontaneously. If secondary infection is suspected, tetracycline eye ointment may be used after obtaining appropriate specimens to identify the cause. Iritis is more serious, and an ophthalmologist's assistance should be sought. It usually subsides with topical hydrocortisone and atropine eye drops.

Keratodermia

Most mildly affected patients do not require any treatment. Others, including those with balanitis, will respond to topical hydrocortisone.

Surveillance

Because of tendency to relapse, these patients need to be kept under surveillance. Their morale needs to be kept high because patients with a positive attitude seem to do better. They should be advised to use a condom for sexual intercourse, and to return should any symptoms recur or if new symptoms appear.

Further reading

Berger, R.N. (1990) Acute epididymitis. In: Holmes, K.K., Mardh, P.A., Sparling, P.F., Wiesner, P.J., Cates, W., Lemon, S.A. and Stamm, W.E. (eds) *Sexually Transmitted Diseases*, 2nd edn. McGraw-Hill, New York, pp. 641–651.

Keat, A. and Rowe, I. (1990) Reiter's syndrome and reactive arthritis. In: Csonka, G.W. and Oates, J.K. (eds) *Sexually Transmitted Diseases – a Textbook of Genitourinary Medicine.* Bailliere Tindall, London, pp. 66–82.

Luzzi, G. (1996) The prostatitis syndromes. *International Journal of STD and AIDS* 7, 471–478.

Thin, R.N. (1997) Diagnosis of chronic prostatitis; overview and update. *International Journal of STD and AIDS* 8, 475–481.

CHAPTER 7.6
Lymphogranuloma venereum

A.O. Osoba
Division of Microbiology, King Khalid National Guard Hospital, Jeddah, Saudi Arabia

Lymphogranuloma venereum (LGV) is a sexually transmitted infection caused by *Chlamydia trachomatis* serotypes, L1, L2 and L3. It is characterized by a transient and often unrecognized by the patient or undiagnosed primary cutaneous or mucosal lesion, with a later development of lymphadenitis of the regional lymph glands. It is manifested by other generalized constitutional symptoms and a wide spectrum of genital lesions, which may be acute or chronic with gross devastation of genital and perineal tissues. LGV is so protean in its manifestations, especially in females, that it can mimic any of the venereal diseases and genital carcinoma.

Aetiology

LGV is caused by *C. trachomatis* serovars L1, L2 and L3. They are biologically and serologically distinct from *C. trachomatis* strains which cause trachoma (types A–C) or the more common sexually transmitted chlamydial diseases (types D–K) such as cervicitis and urethritis and their complications. They are more invasive *in vivo* and *in vitro* than the related trachoma-inclusion conjunctivitis agents.

Epidemiology

LGV is distributed worldwide, but accurate data are not available. It is prevalent in many tropical countries, such as those of South America, the West Indies, West Africa, East Africa, India and Southeast Asia. It may account for about 10% of cases of STI seen in some parts of Africa where, due to lack of diagnostic facilities, LGV frequently is under-reported and inaccurately diagnosed. In the developing countries, LGV is more common in urban than in rural areas, particularly among the sexually promiscuous, and among the lower socioeconomic classes. However, in developed non-tropical countries such as the USA, the UK and France, sporadic cases of LGV have been reported in travellers from endemic areas or in patients with sexual contacts in endemically infected populations. In addition, rectal LGV is being encountered among male homosexuals.

The age distribution of LGV matches that of all other sexually transmitted diseases, with most of the infections occurring in patients aged between 15 and 40 years.

Acute LGV is seen more commonly in men than in women, with a ratio of 5:1 or more. However, the late manifestations of the disease are more common in women, suggesting the greater incidence of minimal symptoms and asymptomatic carriage of the LGV agent in women. Active LGV is rarely documented in sex partners of infected patients, suggesting that asymptomatic carriage is common.

Several studies have shown that genital ulceration, including that caused by LGV, increases the risk of transmission of HIV infection.

Pathogenesis

LGV is primarily a systemic infection involving lymphoid tissues, the main features being thrombolymphangitis and perilymphangitis, with spread of the inflammatory process from the infected lymph nodes into the surrounding tissue. LGV bacteria predominantly infect mononuclear cells, specifically macrophages, with predilection towards lymph node involvement as opposed to the other *C. trachomatis* strains which infect squamocolumnar cells. Since they are obligate intracellular parasites, and kill host cells at the end stages of their growth cycle, they usually cause cell damage where they persist. The disease process and clinical manifestations of LGV infections probably represent the combined effects of tissue damage resulting from chlamydial replication as well as the inflammatory responses caused by the presence of *Chlamydia* and necrotic material from the destroyed host cells.

On entering the body through microscopic abrasions or lacerations of the skin of the external genitalia, the tissue response to invasion tends to follow a definite pattern, resulting in the characteristic appearance of stellate abscess and suppurative granuloma of the lymph nodes. The organism can spread systemically in the bloodstream and enter the central nervous system. Dissemination and local extension of the disease is limited by the host immunity. The microscopic picture is the same in the primary lesion and in the lymph nodes. In the primary lesion, the base of the ulcer is made of granulation tissue with a narrow border zone of necrosis with undermined margins, while in the corium there is a dense infiltration of plasmacytes and lymphocytes, with occasional areas of necrosis with a marginal fibroblastic palisade.

Occasionally, the corium exhibits tiny tuberculous lesions without necrosis, i.e. epithelioid cells and a few giant cells. The lymph nodes draining the site of the initial lesion undergo characteristic changes, whether located in the inguinal region as is usually the case in men, or in the deep pelvic nodes which drain the areas which are most apt to be the seat of the primary infection in women. The characteristic changes found in the lymph nodes are the focal accumulation of the neutrophils in the tiny necrotic foci and, later, rapid hyperplasia of lymphocytes associated with a striking influx of plasmacytes. The small suppurative foci enlarge and coalesce to form a classical 'stellate abscess' typical of LGV. Later, a marginal zone of epithelioid cells and fibroblasts develops to form the so-called suppurative granuloma. The matting of lymph nodes is due to involvement of the capsules and perinodal tissue by acute abscess and extensive scarring. The contraction of the scar tissue produces chronic lymphoedema of the drainage areas.

Antibodies to *C. trachomatis* may be detected in the blood of patients with LGV by various immunological techniques (see below). As indicated by the Frei skin test (see below) and by *C. trachomatis* lymphocyte transformation *in vitro*, cell-mediated immunity also develops. However, these responses do not seem to protect against reinfection.

Clinical manifestations

The incubation period is usually 4–21 days. The clinical course of the disease may be divided into three stages: the primary stage includes the initial infection and early lesions; the secondary stage involves the regional lymph nodes; and the tertiary stage includes the late sequelae with the destruction of the perineum.

Primary stage

The earliest manifestation of the disease, which occurs probably in about a third of patients, is the production of a localized genital lesion. This primary lesion, which is often transient and unnoticed by some patients, is usually an ulcer, vesicle, papule or pustule, not more than 5–6 mm in diameter. In the male, the primary lesion usually appears on the glans penis and is painless, and heals spontaneously within a few days without scar formation. In the female, the site is usually the posterior aspect of the vulva, the inside of the labia minora, or on the cervix, producing a moderate cervicitis that may mimic cervical cancer. The infection of the cervix may ascend to cause salpingitis. Primary LGV lesions of the mouth and pharynx and tonsil may occur as a result of oral sex with an infected partner.

Secondary stage ('inguinal syndrome' and extra inguinal lymphadenitis)

The lymph gland involvement depends on the site of infection and the lymphatic drainage (see Chapter 2).

Acute inguinal lymphadenitis is the most frequent and principal manifestation of LGV, developing 4 days to 4 months after the primary lesion. It is the commonest manifestation in men, but comparatively rare in women. The male/female ratio is greater than 10 : 1. It is more often unilateral than bilateral. It is frequently the cause of medical consultation in most patients because of the painful nature of the lesion. The affected lymph nodes are usually inguinal, although both inguinal and femoral nodes may be involved. When the swellings are separated by the inguinal ligament, the so-called 'groove sign', which is considered pathognomonic of LGV, may become apparent (Fig. 7.6.1). The glandular mass becomes attached to the skin and subcutaneous tissue and fluctuation can be noted. Subsequently, the mass (bubo) may rupture through the skin and discharge purulent material (Fig. 7.6.2). Some buboes, however, never reach this stage, and involution of the firm masses without suppuration may occur – the so-called 'abortive form' of LGV. A small percentage of patients may develop chronic lymphadenopathy which may persist for years.

About 20–30% of women present with 'inguinal syndrome'. Simultaneous involvement of the deep iliac lymph nodes occurs in about 75% of cases, and may cause the formation of a large pelvic mass, which seldom suppurates. These patients may complain of lower abdominal pain, especially when supine (this symptom may be mistaken for appendicitis). Numerous adhesions may form, fixing the pelvic organs together.

Perforation of the bubo through the skin results in the formation of numerous sinuses, giving the inguinal region the appearance of a 'watering can' and the condition the name poradenitis. The abscess may contain thin, sticky yellowish fluid, blood-stained pus or thick caseous material. Healing of such a fistulous mass is usually slow, and the sinuses continue to drain pus for months, or even years. The scars which form later in the inguinal region are callous and contracted and should suggest the diagnosis when encountered.

If the infection is in an extragenital site, lymphadenopathy may occur

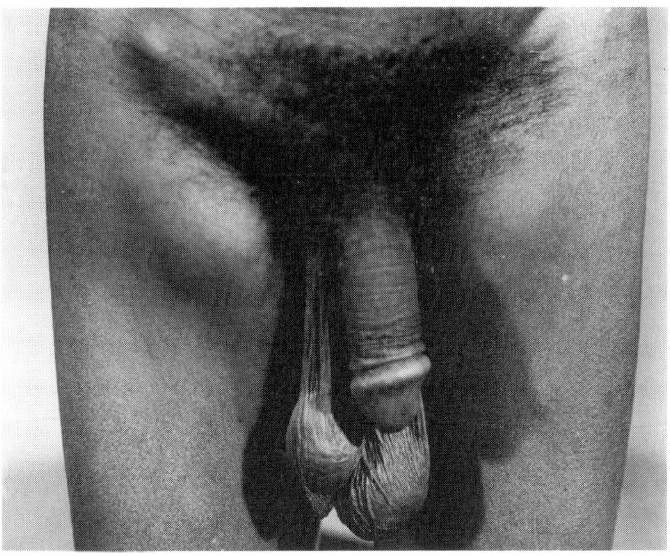

Fig. 7.6.1. Lymphogranuloma venereum: inguinal and femoral lymphadenopathy showing the 'sign of the groove'.

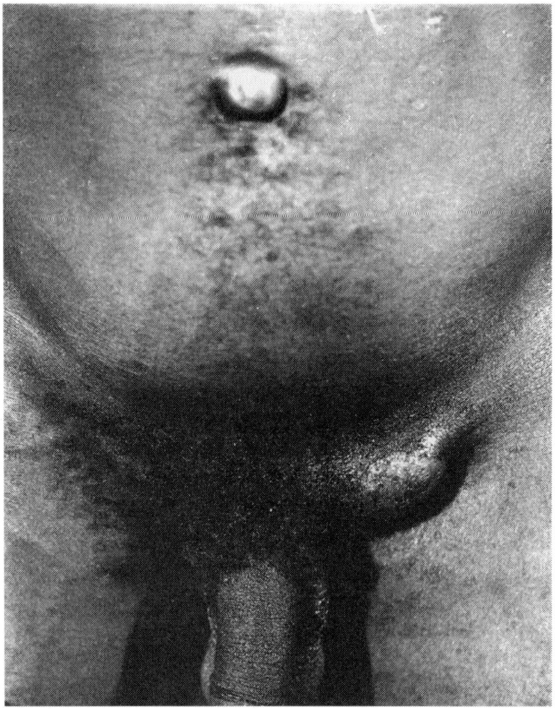

Fig. 7.6.2. Lymphogranuloma venereum: bubo at the point of rupture.

correspondingly at other sites such as axilla, submaxillary or cervical regions. Systemic spread of the bacterium to various organs, such as the liver, lungs, central nervous system and joints, can occur. The patient may experience fever, chills, sweating, headache, loss of appetite, nausea and vomiting.

Tertiary stage: genito-anorectal syndrome

The tertiary stage, i.e. genito-anorectal syndrome, is a late manifestation of the disease. The progressing infection results in obstruction of lymphatics, oedema and hypertrophic and necrotic lesions. The symptoms and clinical and/or radiological features may be indistinguishable from rectal and genital neoplasia. The early lesions are proctocolitis and hyperplasia of the intestinal and perirectal lymphatic tissue. The late manifestations are perirectal and ischiorectal abscesses, rectovaginal and anal fistulae, and rectal strictures. The vast majority of patients with genito-anorectal syndrome are women or homosexual men, but increasingly cases are being described in heterosexual males.

In women, the organisms reach the rectal mucosa either directly during anal intercourse or by contamination with infected vaginal secretion or by lymphatic spread from the cervix and the posterior vaginal wall. The early symptoms of rectal infection are anal pruritus and mucous rectal discharge associated with oedema of the anorectal mucosa. The mucosa becomes hyperaemic and friable, and after a period of several weeks bleeds easily when traumatized. If left untreated, the granulomatous process progressively involves all layers of the bowel. The muscle layers are replaced by fibrous tissue and in some women the rectovaginal septum may be eroded, giving rise to a rectovaginal fistula. Contraction of the fibrous component of the granulation tissue over a period of months or years results in rectal stricture. The development of rectal stricture is usually accompanied by constipation and passage of 'pencil stools', with colic, abdominal distention and weight loss. Characteristically, rectal stricture in LGV develops 3–10 cm above the anocutaneous margin where the perirectal lymphatic tissue is the richest. It is usually annular or tubular in shape and its proximal margins are granular. The mucous membrane below the stricture generally shows ulcerative and granulomatous proctitis. Although the rectal stricture is often very narrow, complete bowel obstruction is rare, but may be associated with bowel perforation and peritonitis, which is the usual cause of death in LGV.

The rectal mucosa below the stricture and the skin around the anus are frequent sites of formation of perirectal abscesses and anal fissures. This may be the only manifestation of chronic genito-anorectal LGV. Obstruction of the lymphatic and venous drainage of the lower rectum produces perianal outgrowths of the lymphatic tissue, which grossly resemble haemorrhoids but are called 'lymphorrhoids' (Fig. 7.6.3).

A causal relationship between rectal stricture and malignant transformation has been suggested. Hence it is necessary to exclude rectal malignancy in patients with LGV-associated stricture.

Another relatively early presentation called 'esthiomene' (Greek meaning eating away) begins as a primary infection of the lymphatics of the scrotum, penis or vulva, and eventually results in oedema, sclerosing fibrosis of the subcutaneous tissues and ulceration. In women, papillated lobular growths of the labia, clitoris and vulvoanal region may be associated with induration of the perivaginal tissues and marked vulval elephantiasis (Fig. 7.6.4). If left untreated, the lesion may destroy the genitalia, and coitus becomes impossible. In the males, penile and scrotal enlargement due to lymphatic obstruction may result in distortion of the penis (Fig. 7.6.5).

Urethral and/or vaginal stenosis as well as fistula formation may sometimes occur. Destruction of the urethra, especially in women, may lead to incontinence of urine. Fenestration of the labia may also occur. The anorectal and colonic syndromes are the more serious of the late manifestations of LGV. They are very distressing for the patient and an exercise in futility for the attending physician. Destructive lesions of the external genitalia, such as urethral loss, fenestration of the labia as well as palpable discrete inguinal glands, inguinal scars and patulous anus should be regarded as 'tell-tale' lesions of LGV infection (Fig. 7.6.6).

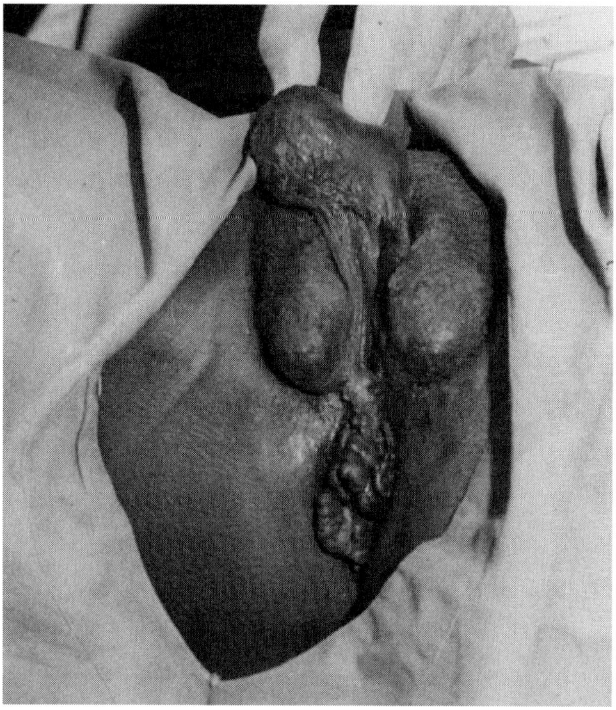

Fig. 7.6.3. Lymphogranuloma venereum: elephantiasis of the labia and clitoris in late LGV. Note the perianal outgrowths called 'lymphorrhoids'.

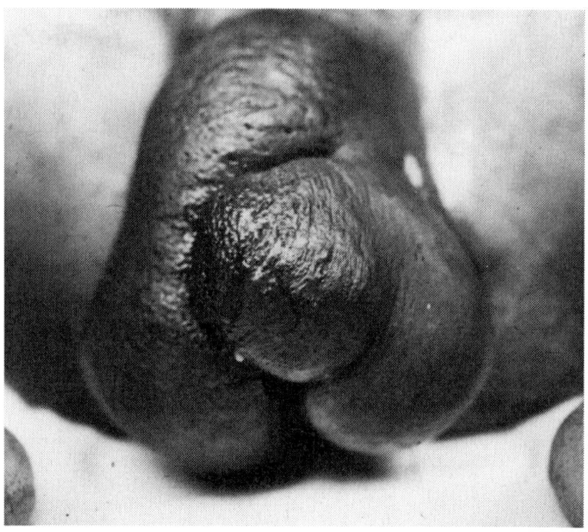

Fig. 7.6.4. Lymphogranuloma venereum: genital syndrome in a female with massive elephantiasis of the labia.

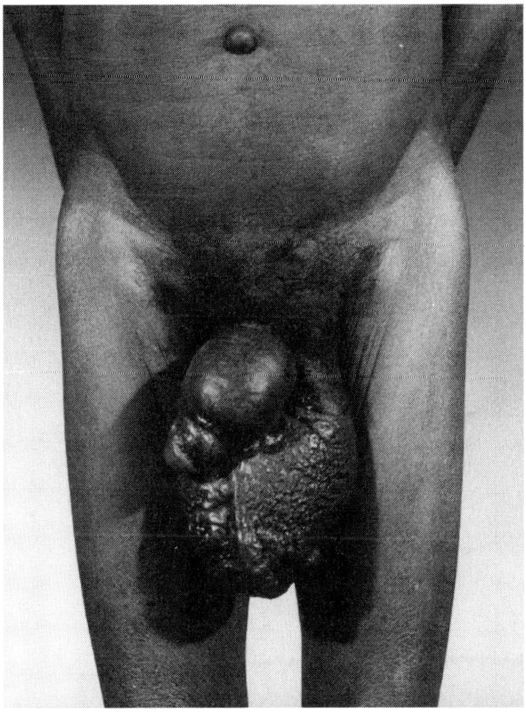

Fig. 7.6.5. Lymphogranuloma venereum: late stage showing elephantiasis of the penis and scrotum.

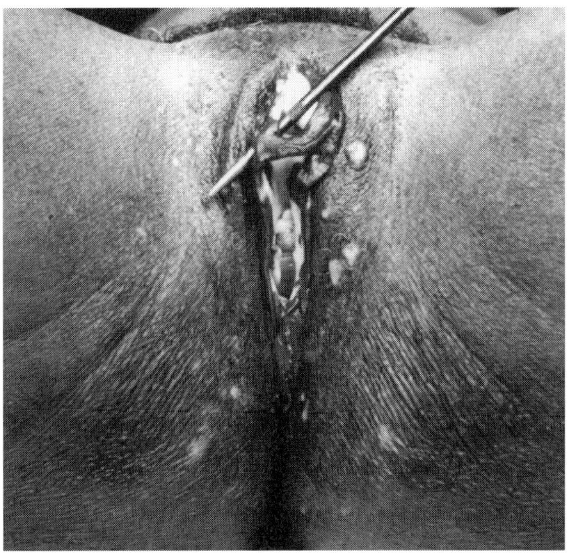

Fig. 7.6.6. Lymphogranuloma venereum: late stage showing fenestration of the labia and destruction of the urethra.

Differential diagnosis

The differential diagnosis should include all common causes of genital ulceration and inguinal lymphadenopathy such as syphilis, chancroid, granuloma inguinale, genital herpes, tuberculosis and filariasis. Anorectal LGV should be distinguished by appropriate tests from ulcerative colitis, Crohn's disease, amoebiasis and other causes of proctocolitis and perineal abscesses. Most especially, in cases of chronic LGV, neoplasm must be excluded in all instances.

Diagnosis

The diagnosis of LGV commonly is based on clinical features of the lesion and serological evaluation of the patient's serum. The diagnosis is confirmed by isolation of the LGV agent and histological identification of the chlamydia in infected tissues, where appropriate facilities are available.

Frei's test

This is a delayed hypersensitivity reaction using intradermal inoculation of material obtained from the growth of LGV agent in chick embryo yolk sac. It is genus-specific and will react in the presence of other chlamydia infections. Because of its low specificity and sensitivity, it is not now commercially available.

Serological tests

Complement fixation test (CFT)

This tests employs a heat-stable antigen common to all chlamydiae. Over 80% of LGV patients will give a titre of 1:64. Demonstration of a fourfold rise in titre of paired sera is diagnostic but uncommon. It is a more sensitive and specific indication of LGV than the Frei's test, but it is also limited by cross-reactivity in other chlamydial infections. Once positive, it may remain so for several years.

Single L-type Chlamydia *immunofluorescence test*

This test appears to be more sensitive than the LGV CFT, but also broadly cross-reacts with serovars of *C. trachomatis* and possibly *C. pneumoniae*, and thus suffers the same drawbacks as the LGV CFT.

Microimmunofluorescence (MIF) test

This is a highly sensitive and specific test for the detection of different immunoglobulin classes of type-specific antibody, and hence will differentiate LGV serologically from other chlamydial infections. During the active phase of LGV, patients usually demonstrate high levels of IgM titre greater than 1:32 and IgG greater than 1:512 with the antigen type of the infecting strain and much lower cross-reactivity with other *C. trachomatis* strains. The major disadvantage of the MIF test is that the reagents are not yet commercially available and the test is confined to a few specialized centres.

Culture of LGV agent

The definitive diagnostic test is the isolation of the causative agent. *C. trachomatis* can be isolated from bubo pus, genital ulcer and rectal tissue on inoculation into tissue culture. A recovery rate of about 50% can be achieved using cycloheximide-treated McCoy cells or DEAE-treated HeLa 229 cells. Material aspirated from the fluctuating bubo is most likely to give the best results.

Antigen detection

Cytological procedures have been used to diagnose LGV infections by demonstrating inclusion bodies in patient's cells, and include the direct immunoperoxidase assay, the MicroTrak direct smear immunofluorescence test and the monoclonal antibody indirect immunofluorescence test. Smears taken from bubo pus, genital and rectal lesions are more likely to be positive, but the sensitivity of these procedures is reported to be about 50% that of culture.

Histopathology

Biopsy is rarely used in the diagnosis of early stages of LGV. However, it may prove useful in the genito-anorectal syndrome and proctocolitis. It is especially indicated when neoplastic change is suspected. Although biopsies of colonic lesions may show histological findings similar to those found in ulcerative colitis, some workers believe that features of LGV are sufficiently distinct to permit a reasonably accurate diagnosis. In biopsy materials, the elementary bodies of *Chlamydia* can be identified both intra- and extracellularly by using Giemsa, iodine and fluorescent antibody staining methods.

Radiology

Radiological examination is of little use in the early stages of LGV. Lymphography can be used to demonstrate the retroperitoneal involvement in the late stages of LGV and to monitor the therapeutic response in cases of rectal stricture, rectovaginal fistulae and esthiomene. Buboes are not usually outlined by lymphography. Barium enema findings in LGV rectal strictures are said to be characteristic and quite different from cancer. In contrast to strictures due to carcinoma, the strictures in LGV are usually elongated and produce little alteration in the mucosal pattern of the bowel.

Treatment

Response to therapy in the early stages of the disease is usually satisfactory, while in the late stages could be an exercise in futility. The treatment of choice is doxycycline, 100 mg orally twice daily for 2–3 weeks. Alternative regimens include: oxytetracycline, 500 mg orally four times daily for 21 days, *or* erythromycin, 500 mg orally four times daily for 21 days. Sulphonamides such as sulphadimidine, using a dose of 1.0 g four times daily for 14–21 days, have been reported to give a satisfactory result, especially in the early stages of the disease. The advantage of the sulphonamides is that they are cheap and would not mask concurrent syphilitic infection. Pregnant women should be treated with erythromycin.

Azithromycin is a new macrolide antibiotic that has substantial activity against *C. trachomatis*, is concentrated intracellularly and has a long half-life in serum and tissues. This new agent has been shown to be effective in a single dose therapy of 1 g for chlamydial urethritis and endocervicitis. So far, no clinical studies have been carried out to demonstrate its effectiveness in LGV.

The bubo seldom suppurates after therapy begins, but fluctuant buboes may require aspiration to prevent rupture. Generally, fluctuant lymph nodes should be aspirated through normal skin using a wide bore needle; incision and drainage are best avoided.

Antibiotic therapy of proctocolitis gives a dramatic response, with early relief of symptoms and healing of lesions. However, anal and rectovaginal fistulae are not usually cured by antibiotic therapy. Surgical management of some late cases may be required to relieve the misery of the patient, but the results frequently are disappointing due to the impairment of blood supply and extensive fibrosis. In cases of genital elephantiasis, reconstructive surgery may be attempted following antibiotic therapy for several weeks.

Prevention and control

The control of LGV is similar to that of other STI causing genital ulceration. Early diagnosis and treatment of the patients and their sexual contacts, whether symptomatic or not, with antibiotics is the main method of control. In endemic areas and in particular among the lower socioeconomic classes, health education must be intensified to encourage infected patients to present early for treatment. Genital hygiene after sexual exposure is of limited value.

Further reading

Osoba, A.O. (1983) Lymphogranuloma venereum. In: Holmes, K.K. and Mardh, P.A. (eds) *International Perspectives on Neglected Sexually Transmitted Diseases*. Hemisphere, Washington, DC, pp. 193–204.

Osoba, A.O. (1987) Lymphogranuloma venereum. In: Osoba, A.O. (ed.) *Clinical Tropical Medicine and Communicable Diseases*. Balliere Tindall, London, pp. 143–152.

Osoba, A.O. (1993) Lymphogranuloma venereum in Western Nigerian. In: Carenza, L., Atlante, G., Pozzi, V. and Luciani, S. (eds) *Recent Advances in Cervical Pathology and Colposcopy*, Advances in Gynecological and Obstetrics Research Series, No. 3, Proceedings of the 7th World Congress of Cervical Pathology and Colposcopy, May 1990. Pathenon, Carnforth, pp. 115–121.

Perine, P.L. and Osoba, A.O. (1984) Lymphogranuloma venereum. In: Holmes, K.K., Mardh, P.A., Sparling, P.F. and Wiesner, P.J. (eds) *Sexually Transmitted Diseases*. McGraw-Hill, New York, pp. 281–291.

Schachter, J. and Osoba, A.O. (1983) Lymphogranuloma venereum. *British Medical Bulletin* 39, 151–154.

Van Dyck, E. and Piot, P. (1992) Laboratory techniques in the investigation of chancroid, lymphogranuloma venereum and donovanosis. *Genitourinary Medicine* 68, 130–133.

CHAPTER 7.7
Donovanosis (granuloma inguinale)

J. Richens
Department of Sexually Transmitted Disease, University College London Medical School, London, UK

Donovanosis is a tropical STI characterized by genital ulcers in which distinctive intracellular Gram-negative bacteria (*Calymmatobacterium granulomatis*) are found.

Early descriptions refer to the disease as an ulcerating, often 'lupoid', granuloma of the pudenda and groins. The term granuloma inguinale is used by *Index Medicus*, but the disease is also known as donovanosis, after Donovan who first noted the presence of intracellular inclusion bodies (Donovan bodies). Confusion with leishmaniasis sometimes occurs because it was the same Donovan who described the protozoal inclusions, sometimes referred to as Leishman–Donovan bodies, in that infection.

Aetiology

The infection is caused by the Gram-negative bacterium, *Calymmatobacterium granulomatis* which forms the characteristic inclusions known as Donovan bodies. They have been grown in the chick embryo yolk sac but will not grow on any conventional solid media. However, recent work in South Africa and Australia has shown that it is possible to grow *C. granulomatis* in tissue culture. Koch's postulates have not been fulfiled for this infection, but there is strong circumstantial evidence that the organisms visualized within lesions as Donovan bodies are the agent of the disease. Immunofluorescence studies have shown high levels of antibody to Donovan bodies confined to affected patients, and successful antibiotic treatment correlates well with healing and disappearance of Donovan bodies from lesions.

Epidemiology (Fig. 7.7.1)

Donovanosis remains common in many parts of India, where it was first described. It is an important infection of Melanesian communities in Papua New Guinea and Australia. In Africa, the condition seems to occur in Zimbabwe, Zambia and South Africa, and an important epidemic has been reported lately affecting Natal, Eastern Transvaal and Swaziland. The infection

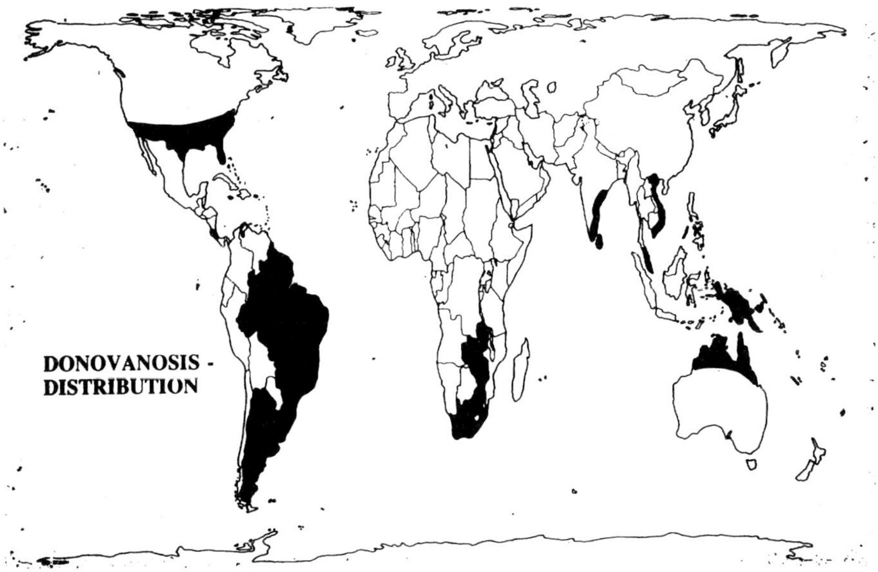

Fig. 7.7.1. Donovanosis: map showing principal known endemic areas.

is prevalent in many parts of South America, especially Brazil. The incidence in the Caribbean and southern USA has declined markedly in recent years.

Transmission

There is strong evidence that transmission is usually sexual. Lesions occur mostly in the genital area. A history of unsafe sexual exposure can usually be elicited, and coexisting STI, especially syphilis, are commonly found. Reported rates of infection in sexual partners tend to be lower than for other STI (rarely over 50%), and this has been cited as evidence for an alternative hypothesis of transmission, that *C. granulomatis* resides in the bowel and is an opportunistic invader of anogenital skin. This hypothesis rests on extremely slender evidence (a single case report). Rare cases of perinatal transmission have been documented when an infected child has been born to a mother with an untreated lesion of the cervix uteri. Infection can be auto-inoculated by patients to extragenital sites, and occasional cases of accidental (non-sexual) or experimental transmission have been described.

Pathogenesis and immune response

C. granulomatis shows a clear predilection for skin, but is capable of infecting deeper tissues occasionally. Organisms multiply at the site of inoculation and are then conveyed through lymphatics to regional lymph nodes. An unusual feature of this infection is a tendency for the bacteria to cause relatively little pathology within the lymph node itself and to migrate into overlying subcutaneous tissue to produce an abscess (pseudobubo) or, more commonly, to produce further cutaneous ulceration in the overlying skin. Untreated infection is characterized by a slow process of ulceration gradually extending along skin folds of the anogenital area. There is a vigorous humoral immune response with high levels of antibody produced. The infiltration within the lesions consists largely of plasma cells and histiocytes, a small number of neutrophils and rarely lymphocytes. Spontaneous resolution can occur, and in chronic cases healing in some areas and extension of lesions in others may be observed. Some patients display a cicatrizing variant of the infection where Donovan bodies are hard to demonstrate and large amounts of dense scar tissue form.

Clinical features

The incubation period in the majority of patients is in the range of 1–6 weeks.

A small nodule develops at the site of inoculation, usually the distal penis or vulva, which soon ulcerates. Primary lesions of the mouth and anus may develop following orogenital and anogenital sex. The early lesion generally is painless and difficult to distinguish from other types of genital ulcer. More established lesions take a variety of forms. The most distinctive is the hypertrophic type, where elevated exuberant granulomatous tissue, deep red in colour, bulges out above the level of surrounding skin (Plates 104 and 105). Flatter lesions with just the edge raised also occur. Dry, warty-looking lesions are less common. Primary lesions of the cervix are notorious for mimicking cervical carcinoma or cervical tuberculosis. Occasionally, an inguinal lesion may commence as a firm lymphadenopathy. As the infection moves towards the overlying skin, a subcutaneous abscess (pseudobubo) may develop transiently before a new ulcerative lesion appears in the groin (Plate 106). Similar lesions may develop on the neck when primary oral inoculation occurs. Established ulcers show a tendency to extend slowly along moist skin folds, especially along the inguinal creases and back towards the anus.

Complications

Lymphoedema frequently accompanies donovanosis, especially in women, and may lead to genital elephantiasis. Extensive, long-standing ulceration may cause genital mutilation, e.g. auto-amputation of the penis, and may be associated with development of squamous carcinoma. Some patients develop extensive tracts of scar tissue which can cause contractures and stenoses. Donovanosis in women occasionally involves the uterus, tubes and ovaries. Such patients may present with haemorrhage, hard pelvic masses and ureteric obstruction. Haematogenous dissemination of donovanosis to bone, liver, spleen and lung is a rare event, most commonly reported in women sustaining trauma to an untreated cervical lesion during labour. Secondary infection with fuso-spirochaetal organisms occasionally can transform a chronic ulcer into a rapidly advancing destructive lesion. Fatalities were not uncommon before the introduction of antibiotics, and still occur occasionally in women with extensive disease.

Differential diagnosis

The lesions that show the closest clinical similarity to donovanosis are: (i) condylomata lata of secondary syphilis; (ii) squamous carcinoma of the penis, vulva, anus or cervix; (iii) (for early lesions) other STI causing genital ulcers, e.g. chancroid; (iv) (for complicated cases) other conditions causing genital lymphoedema, e.g. filariasis, lymphogranuloma venereum; and (v) occasionally rarer infections of the genitalia such as tuberculosis and amoebiasis.

Diagnosis

Until the recently described culture methods are confirmed and perfected, the definitive diagnosis requires the demonstration of Donovan bodies in material from lesions, which may be collected in the form of biopsy material or scrapes, smears or crush preparations. The author's preference is to pinch off a small piece of tissue from the edge or base of a lesion and to crush this between two slides for staining with Giemsa or Leishman's stain. This can provide rapid, on-the-spot diagnosis, and can be supplemented by taking a punch biopsy for additional histopathological examination. Reliance on haematoxylin and eosin staining of pathological specimens can result in misdiagnosis, as Donovan bodies do not show up well with this stain and require silver stains or Giemsa to stand out clearly. The cardinal histological features are the presence of encapsulated Donovan bodies showing the classical 'closed safety pin' appearance within large histiocytes (Plate 107), a dense plasma cell infiltrate and epithelial hyperplasia at ulcer margins. A comprehensive screen for other STI is desirable, including, if possible, microscopy for syphilis and amoebiasis, cultures for *Haemophilus ducreyi* and *Chlamydia trachomatis*, and serological tests for syphilis, amoebiasis and LGV.

Treatment

Donovanosis responds to a wide variety of broad-spectrum antibiotics which need to be administered in standard doses until lesions have healed, and possibly longer to lower the incidence of relapse. Antibiotics used for donovanosis have been studied mostly in small open trials. Lack of *in vitro* data on sensitivities and the absence of any randomized trials precludes any objective recommendations about treatment of choice. Local experience is often of value in selecting antibiotics in endemic areas. The most widely used drug regimens include: tetracycline, 500 mg, four times daily, *or* erythromycin 500 mg, four times daily, *or* doxycycline, 100 mg twice daily, *or* co-trimoxazole, two tablets twice daily.

Treatment should be given for at least 1 week and, if re-epithelialization is not then complete, treatment should be extended until this occurs. Treatment response is assessed by examination of lesions for signs of healing and repeat smears for Donovan bodies if re-epithelialization fails to occur. Signs of healing should be apparent within 1 week of starting treatment. Otherwise, a change to an alternative antibiotic or combination should be considered.

Recent publications have demonstrated the usefulness of norfloxacin, 400 mg twice daily, *or* azithromycin, 500 mg daily or 1 g weekly, *or* ceftriaxone, 1 g intramuscularly daily, the last proving useful in the management of chronic, resistant cases. In addition to the above drugs, the following second line drugs have been reported to be useful in some cases: ampicillin, chloramphenicol, thiamphenicol, lincomycin, streptomycin and gentamicin. Treatment failure is more likely to occur in pregnancy and in patients coinfected with HIV. Such patients may respond better to combination therapies. Secondary infection can be treated either topically using dilute potassium permanganate or by the addition of penicillin or metronidazole to antibiotic regimens. Plastic surgical procedures may be required to correct genital deformity.

Prevention

Attempts should be made to trace and treat the source of a patient's infection. Secondary contacts should be offered examination and epidemiological treatment if considered appropriate. It seems reasonable to assume that condoms could prevent transmission, but this has not yet been documented for donovanosis specifically. Health education, as for other STI, is appropriate. Major epidemics of donovanosis in New Guinea have been brought under control by regular surveys of affected populations and administration of treatment to cases detected. Donovanosis is very much associated with poverty, and its disappearance from former endemic areas such as the southern USA has been attributed to a general improvement in living standards.

Further reading

Bowden, F.J., Mein, J., Plunkett, C. and Bastian, I. (1996) Pilot study of azithromycin in the treatment of genital donovanosis. *Genitourinary Medicine* 72, 17–19.

Kharsany, A.B.M., Hoosen, A.A., Kiepiela, P., Naicker, T. and Strum, A.W. (1997) Growth and cultural characteristics of *Calymmatobacterium granulomatis* – the aetiological agent of granuloma inguinale (Donovanosis). *Journal of Medical Microbiology* 46, 579–585.

Merianos, A., Gilles, M. and Chuah J. (1994) Ceftriaxone in the treatment of chronic donovanosis in central Australia. *Genitourinary Medicine* 70, 84–89.

Rajam, R.V. and Rangiah, P.N. (1954) *Donovanosis (Granuloma Inguinale, Granuloma Venereum)*. WHO Monograph Series 24, World Health Organization, Geneva.

Richens J. (1991) The diagnosis and treatment of donovanosis (granuloma inguinale). *Genitourinary Medicine* 67, 441–452.

Richens, J. (1998) *Calymmatobacterium granulomatis*. In: Yu, V.L., Merigan, T.C., White, N.J. and Barriere, S. (eds) *Antimicrobial Chemotherapy*. Williams and Wilkins, Philadelphia, in press.

CHAPTER 7.8
Bacterial vaginosis

O.P. Arya
Department of Medical Microbiology and Genitourinary Medicine, University of Liverpool, Liverpool, UK

Bacterial vaginosis (BV) is a very common cause of vaginal discharge. The condition is encountered frequently in STI clinics and commonly is concurrent with chlamydial, gonococcal and trichomonal infections. Although sexually active women are predominantly affected, there is no evidence that BV is sexually acquired. An association between BV and NGU in male sexual partners has been observed, but needs further study.

Aetiology and pathogenesis

The mixture of organisms associated with BV includes strict and facultative anaerobic bacteria, such as *Bacteroides*, *Prevotella*, *Porphyromonas*, *Peptostreptococcus* and *Mobiluncus* spp., *Gardnerella vaginalis* and *Mycoplasma hominis*. Many of these bacteria are found in the normal vagina of asymptomatic women, but in BV their numbers increase by 1000-fold. What triggers this change remains a mystery. The events include a marked reduction in the number of the normally predominant hydrogen peroxide-producing lactobacilli, and production of amines and ammonia by other organisms resulting in a higher pH of the vagina (normal 3.5–4.5). This in turn allows the anaerobes and other organisms to increase by 1000-fold. The numbers of these organisms may decrease or increase intermittently in some individuals, perhaps due to hormonal changes. Some of these organisms may produce cytotoxins which may damage vaginal epithelium, resulting in vaginal discharge. The precise mechanism of the formation of clue cells (which provide a clue to the diagnosis) is not known. The exact role of *M. hominis*, apart from that of a colonizer in a favourable environment, is also unclear.

The cofactors include use of an intrauterine contraceptive device (IUCD), low socioeconomic status and smoking.

Clinical features

Symptoms

The main symptom is malodorous vaginal discharge, often worse after unprotected vaginal intercourse. Many women are asymptomatic but some will admit to smelly discharge if specifically asked. Vulval irritation and soreness may be mentioned, but very rarely.

Signs

In the absence of a concomitant infection, the vaginal discharge is greyish white, thin, homogeneous and adherent to the vaginal walls (Plate 108). There is no obvious inflammation – hence the term vaginosis rather than vaginitis. Occasionally, however, the discharge may be bubbly and there may be minimal vaginitis or vulvitis, or even cervicitis.

The pH of vaginal fluid is >4.5 (see Chapter 4 for the pH measurement methods). One should be aware that the pH may be elevated by the presence of semen for up to 48 h and by blood of menses or if the vaginal material is mixed with cervical mucus.

The amine test is always positive (one or two drops of vaginal discharge are mixed with one or two drops of 10% potassium hydroxide on a glass slide; alkali releases volatile amines, giving rise to a fishy odour).

Differential diagnosis

See Chapter 10.2 for the other causes of vaginal discharge and Table 7.8.1 for the common vaginal conditions.

Diagnosis

Appropriate specimens should be taken to exclude any STI. The diagnosis of bacterial vaginosis can be made in the presence of the following criteria:

- Thin greyish white homogeneous discharge adherent to the vaginal walls. (This can be unreliable. The following three criteria when present together, are adequate to diagnose BV.)
- Vaginal pH >4.5.
- Positive amine test.
- Presence of clue cells on microscopy of a wet mount of a sample of vaginal discharge from the posterior fornix. (Clue cells are vaginal epithelial cells covered by coccobacilli obscuring the cell outline and producing a rather granular cytoplasmic appearance.)

A wet film will also show masses of small bacilli and actively motile *Mobiluncus* spp. However, clue cells are best seen on a Gram-stained smear of

Table 7.8.1. Comparison of vaginal infections.

Feature	Normal	Yeast vaginitis	Trichomoniasis	Bacterial vaginosis
Symptoms when present				
Vaginal discharge smell	–	Yeasty	'Bad' smell	Fishy
Vulvar irritation	–	+	+	Rare
Vulval soreness	–	+	+	Rare
Dysuria	–	External	Internal/external	–
Dyspareunia	–	+	+	–
Signs when present				
Vulvitis/vaginitis	–	+	+	Rare (minimal)
Discharge				
Amount	Scanty	Varies	Profuse	Slightly increased
Colour	Clear or greyish	Watery or white	Lime green	Greyish white
Consistency	Floccular	Thin, watery, or curdy or cheesy plaques	Watery, frothy, or purulent	Thin, homogeneous, occasionally frothy
Diagnosis				
Vaginal pH	3.5–4.5	≤4.5	>4.5	>4.5
Amine test	–	–	+ (often)	+
Microscopy (wet mount/Gram stain)	Epithelial cells, lactobacilli (Gram-positive rods) abundant, pus cells scanty	Pseudohyphae and yeast spores (Gram-positive)	Motile trichomonads, pus cells abundant	Clue cells, BV morphotypes, lactobacilli scanty or absent, pus cells scanty in most cases

the vaginal specimen, and a Gram-stained smear is considered to be the definitive diagnostic method. It confirms paucity or absence of lactobacilli and paucity of pus cells (in most cases), and facilitates identification of various morphotypes, i.e. *Lactobacillus* morphotypes (large Gram-positive rods), *G. vaginalis* morphotypes (small Gram-variable rods), *Prevotella/Porphyromonas* morphotypes (small Gram-negative rods) and *Mobiluncus* morphotypes (curved Gram-variable rods) (Plate 109). It also allows a scoring system mainly for research purposes (each morphotype is assigned a score; a total score of 7 or more equates to bacterial vaginosis, a score of 4–6 suggests 'intermediate' category, and 0–3 is normal).

HIV infection and bacterial vaginosis

HIV-1 infection has been shown to be more frequent among younger women with abnormal vaginal flora and BV. It has been speculated that reduction in hydrogen peroxide-producing lactobacilli may enhance HIV-1 survival in the genital tract and that a high pH in BV may facilitate an increase in activated HIV-1 target cells in the vagina. Whether or not BV does facilitate HIV-1 acquisition is not proven.

Management

All symptomatic patients should be treated. Metronidazole is highly effective, with short-term cure rates (clinical and microbiological) of around 85%. The dose is 400 mg orally twice daily for 5–7 days, or 2 g orally in a single dose. The cure rate with the latter regimen is believed to be lower than with the longer regimen. The patient should be advised to abstain from alcohol during treatment. Clindamycin cream 2%, 5 g intravaginally at night for 3–7 nights is as effective as the metronidazole regimens. A small proportion of patients may develop *Candida* vaginitis after either of the above treatment regimens. Metronidazole gel 0.75%, 5 g intravaginally once daily for 5 days has also been reported to be effective, but experience with it is limited. Topical treatment, however, may not eliminate the potential for upper genital tract complications (see below).

Sex partners

Although BV-associated bacteria have been isolated from subpreputial swabs and some males may develop balanitis/balanoposthitis, their treatment has not proved to be of any benefit with regard to recurrences in the female partners.

Recurrences

The condition usually resolves within 1 week after treatment. However, recurrences are common; almost 50% relapse within 6 months. The reasons are not clear. One possibility is that the rectum, where these bacteria reside, may serve as a reservoir of infection. Some patients continue to experience frequent recurrences. There is no effective treatment regimen available to prevent these recurrences. The options include the use of an alternative treatment regimen to the one initially used, intravaginal treatment with clindamycin cream for longer than 1 week, use of vaginal preparations (such as acetic acid vaginal jelly) to restore normal acidity, 3% hydrogen peroxide used as a single wash, treatment of sex partners, removal of IUCDs and use of condoms.

Treatment in pregnancy

Recently, a meta-analysis confirmed the safety of metronidazole in pregnancy, including in the first trimester. However, manufacturers advise avoidance of high-dose regimens in pregnancy, and some specialists avoid the oral regimens in the first trimester. A low-dose regimen is metronidazole, 200 mg orally three times daily for 7 days. Clindamycin (rather expensive) is not known to be harmful in pregnancy and the dose is 300 mg orally twice daily for 7 days. Intravaginal preparations may not reduce perinatal morbidity (see below).

Complications and their prevention

BV may be a risk factor for chorioamnionitis, premature rupture of membranes, pre-term labour, late miscarriage, postpartum endometritis, pelvic infection and infective complications following gynaecological surgery.

Randomized controlled trials are needed to prove that treatment of BV during pregnancy will prevent the related complications. A definitive outcome will also resolve the uncertainty about the treatment of asymptomatic patients. In addition, to be cost effective, the preventive measures (detection of BV and treatment) will probably need to be applied on a selective basis (e.g. those at high risk with a history of pre-term birth), bearing in mind that the majority of the patients will deliver at term even without treatment, and that there are several other causes of pre-term birth which will need to be sorted out. Then there will be the question of timing, i.e. when best to treat such patients in view of the fact that in many treated patients the condition will relapse within 1–3 months. In addition, logistic problems will also need to be addressed. Nevertheless, some experts now recommend that pregnant women, with a history of second trimester fetal loss, if found to have BV, should be treated with oral metronidazole early in the second trimester. It is certainly prudent to screen for BV and treat those testing positive prior to termination of pregnancy and before gynaecological surgery.

Further reading

Burtin, P., Taddio, A., Ariburnu, O., Einarson, T.R. and Koren, G. (1995) Safety of metronidazole in pregnancy: a meta-analysis. *American Journal of Obstetrics and Gynecology* 172, 525–529.

Hay, P.E., Lamont, R.F., Taylor-Robinson, D., Morgan, J.D., Ison, C. and Pearson, J. (1994) Abnormal bacterial colonisation of the genital tract and subsequent preterm delivery and late miscarriage. *British Medical Journal* 308, 295–298.

Hillier, S.L., Nugent, R.P., Eschenbach, D.A., Krohn, M.A., Gibbs, R.S., Martin, D.H., Cotch, M.F., Edelman, R., Pastorek, J.G., Rao, A.V., McNellis, D., Regan, J.A., Carey, J.C. and Klebanoff, M.A. (1995) Association between bacterial vaginosis and preterm delivery of a low birth-weight infant. *The New England Journal of Medicine* 333, 1737–1742.

Keane, F.E.A., Thomas, B.J., Whitaker, L., Renton, A. and Taylor-Robinson, D. (1997) An association between nongonococcal urethritis and bacterial vaginosis and the implications for patients and their sexual partners. *Genitourinary Medicine* 73, 373–377.

Nugent, R.P., Krohn, M.A. and Hillier, S.L. (1991) Reliability of diagnosing bacterial vaginosis is improved by a standardized method of Gram stain interpretation. *Journal of Clinical Microbiology* 29, 297–301.

Priestley, C.J.F., Jones, B.M., Dhar, J. and Goodwin, L. (1997) What is normal vaginal flora? *Genitourinary Medicine* 73, 23–28.

Schwebke, J.R. (1997) Bacterial vaginosis – more questions than answers. *Genitourinary Medicine* 73, 333–334.

Sewankambo, N., Gray, R.H., Wawer, M.J., Paxton, L., McNairn, D., Wabwire-Mangen, F., Serwadda, D., Li, C., Kiwanuka, N., Hillier, S.L., Rabe, L., Gaydos, C.A. and Quinn,T.C. (1997) HIV-infection associated with abnormal vaginal flora morphology and bacterial vaginosis. *The Lancet* 350, 546–550.

Taylor-Robinson, D. and Hay, P.E. (1997) The pathogenesis of the clinical signs of bacterial vaginosis and possible reasons for its occurrence. *International Journal of STD and AIDS* 8 (Suppl.1), 13–16.

CHAPTER 8
Fungal infections

CHAPTER 8.1
Candidiasis

O.P. Arya
Department of Medical Microbiology and Genitourinary Medicine, University of Liverpool, Liverpool, UK

Genital candidiasis (or 'thrush') is a common condition. It is estimated that 50% of the female population will experience at least two episodes in their lifetime.

Aetiology

The aetiology in 80–90% of cases is *Candida albicans*. The rest may harbour *C. glabrata*, *C. tropicalis* or other species.

Transmission and predisposing factors

Candida spp. inhabit the mouth and gastrointestinal tract of the normal population, and may be commensal organisms of the human genitalia in about 20% of individuals of both sexes. *Candida* spp. may gain entry into the vagina from the adjacent perianal area during intercourse, when inserting a tampon or through migration. Sexual transmission or acquisition, although possible, is thought to be unimportant. Vaginal infection may not be associated with overt candidiasis in the partner.

The predisposing factors include uncontrolled diabetes mellitus, use of broad-spectrum antibiotics and antitrichomonal therapy, pregnancy, immunosuppressive therapy, HIV infection, depressed T-cell function, tight and synthetic underwear, bubble baths, scented soaps, vaginal deodorants, disinfectants and douches, poor anal hygiene and a tight foreskin in men. In the author's experience, oral contraception was not a predisposing factor. Besides, very few women now take high-strength oral contraceptives.

Pathogenesis

Candida organisms adhere to the epithelial cells. In general, the blastospore form is associated with asymptomatic vaginal colonization, and the germinating form with active symptomatic disease. The latter form penetrates deeper into the mucous membrane, and this tissue invasion is associated with inflammation and erythema. Certain factors such as oestrogens and pregnancy promote germination. Lactobacilli may be suppressed in some patients.

Clinical features

Females

Many individuals harbouring yeasts are asymptomatic. The most common symptoms are vulval irritation and/or soreness with or without vaginal discharge. Other symptoms include external dysuria (burning when urine touches the sore vulva), superficial dyspareunia, pruritus ani and a yeast-like smell. The symptoms are often worse in the days preceding menses and relieved with the onset of menstrual flow.

On examination, there may be dry congestion of the vulva (Plate 110), and excoriation of the affected skin. Speculum examination may show a watery or thick white curdy discharge in the vagina. In more severe cases, speculum examination is painful, there is vaginal mucosal erythema and cheesy-white plaques, which if removed may result in bleeding (Plate 111). The cervix may be reddened. Occasionally a patient with undiagnosed diabetes may present to the clinic with severe vulvovaginitis due to *Candida*.

Males

Overt candidiasis of the genitalia is less common in males than in females. Some may develop a transient rash, erythema and itching of the glans penis within a few hours after sexual intercourse with an infected female with or without symptoms. This is self-limiting and disappears after washing, and is thought to be a hypersensitivity reaction to *Candida*. Others may develop micropapular lesions with diffuse erythema of the glans penis and mucosal surface of the prepuce, or severe balanoposthitis with a cheesy exudate, fissuring, oedema and phimosis, especially in patients with uncontrolled diabetes. There may be inflammation of the groin and scrotum and, very rarely, the urethra may be involved (Plate 112).

Differential diagnosis

The conditions for the differential diagnosis include allergic and chemical reactions, other vaginal infections (Chapter 7.8, Table 7.8.1) and genital herpes, which usually can be excluded by careful clinical examination. See also Chapter 11.5 for other causes of balanitis.

Diagnosis

Tests should include those for other STI. The urine should be checked for sugar in all cases of vulvovaginitis and balanoposthitis due to *Candida* infection. A history of any other predisposing factor should be obtained (see above).

Microscopy of a wet mount of the vaginal secretions may show pseudohyphae. A Gram-stained smear of the material from the vagina in females, and from the glans penis and coronal sulcus in males, may show Gram-positive pseudohyphae and large Gram-positive yeasts (Plate 113). Culture should be considered if the condition is suspected and microscopy negative; otherwise almost half of the cases may be missed. The swab for culture may be sent to the laboratory in Feinberg–Whittington medium which will also do for *Trichomonas vaginalis* culture (see also Chapter 5).

Management

Personal hygiene

The female patients, especially those experiencing frequent recurrences, should be advised to avoid tight clothing, synthetic underwear, scented soaps, deodorants, bubble baths, douches, and to wipe from front to back and wash after defaecation. The male patients should retract the prepuce and wash the glans penis with water at least every other day and after intercourse.

Antifungal treatment

In general, only the symptomatic patients need to be treated. The imidazoles (e.g. clotrimazole, econazole and miconazole) are more popular than the polyenes (e.g. nystatin) because the shorter courses needed of the former category ensure better compliance. The clinical and mycological response is about 80–90%, the patients becoming asymptomatic within 3 days.

Females

The recommended dosage regimens for clotrimazole which is the commonly used drug are as follows: a 100 mg vaginal pessary, insert one each night for 6 nights, *or* a 200 mg vaginal pessary, insert one each night for 3 nights, *or* a 500 mg vaginal pessary, insert one at night as a single dose, *or* 10% vaginal cream, insert 5 g at night as a single dose.

If vulvitis is also present, clotrimazole 1% cream may be applied locally twice daily for 1 week. Vaginal pessaries containing econazole and miconazole formulated for single dose therapy are also available.

ORAL ANTIMYCOTIC REGIMENS. Oral treatment with itraconazole (200 mg twice daily for 1 day) *or* fluconazole (150 mg single dose) is becoming increasingly popular in industrialized countries because of its convenience, but it is expensive. The efficacy is comparable with that of topical therapy.

FOLLOW-UP. Follow-up after treatment is not necessary unless symptoms recur.

TREATMENT IN PREGNANCY. Topical treatment with azoles as recommenced above is usually adequate. Oral antimycotic agents are contraindicated in pregnancy.

Management of recurrent attacks

A small proportion of women, probably as a result of antigen-specific immunological deficiency, experience recurrent attacks (more than three in a year) which may cause personal misery and marital discord. Although it is not possible to rid the patient of yeasts, all patients can be helped to become asymptomatic. The patient must, therefore be reassured.

ANTIFUNGAL THERAPY. After the usual initial treatment, antifungal therapy may need to be prolonged. One option is clotrimazole, 500 mg vaginal pessary on day 7 and day 21 of the menstrual cycle for a couple of months and then once a month on day 21 for a few months.

OTHER MEASURES. Although the majority of patients with recurrent episodes do not have any predisposing factors, the latter should be checked for. The personal hygiene measures should be emphasized. A broad-spectrum antibiotic, when necesssary, may be combined with topical antifungal therapy. Other measures, such as change of oral contraceptive or of diaphragm (for patients using these), avoidance of receptive orogenital sex, application of yoghurt to the vagina, use of systemic antifungal treatment (itraconazole is more potent against *C. glabrata*), treatment of sex partners, may be tried but none has been proven to prevent recurrent attacks.

Males

Mild cases of balanitis with a transient rash and erythema often clear up by washing. More severe cases are usually associated with glycosuria or uncontrolled diabetes mellitus and should be managed with an antifungal cream (such as clotrimazole cream applied to the glans penis twice daily for at least 1 week) and control of diabetes. Others may require a mixed topical preparation of antifungal agent and hydrocortisone. *Candida* urethritis may resolve spontaneously. Alternatively, a systemic antifungal might be appropriate (needs evaluation).

Candidiasis in infants and children

Intrapartum infection of the neonate may result in primary mucocutaneous candidiasis involving the mouth, umbilicus and napkin areas. After that age, *Candida* spp. may become part of the normal flora. Transmission as a result of sexual abuse has been reported.

Vulvovaginitis may be mild to severe; see Chapter 7.5 for the differential diagnosis. The diagnosis is confirmed by the demonstration of spores and pseudohyphae in a Gram-stained smear of vulval and/or vaginal swab which may also be sent for culture, if possible. Any predisposing factors should be excluded. The treatment includes attention to hygiene and toileting and use of an antifungal cream and oral suspension.

Candidiasis and HIV infection

The genital candidiasis in patients with HIV infection may be severe, with frequent relapses. The patients should be managed as described above but the treatment may need to be prolonged. Sooner or later extragenital sites are also involved, requiring topical, systemic and intermittent suppressive therapy (see also Chapters 10.4 and 11.5).

CHAPTER 8.2
Other fungal infections

C.A. Hart
Department of Medical Microbiology and Genitourinary Medicine, University of Liverpool, Liverpool, UK

Fungi, like human cells, are eukaryotic. They have a nucleus and possess intracellular organelles which differentiates them from the more primitive prokaryotic bacteria. The fungus kingdom contains thousands of genera and species but most are not pathogenic for man. They may grow in a unicellular mode (i.e. yeasts) or in a more complex multicellular mode with filaments called hyphae which intermesh to form a mycelium. The latter may also reproduce sexually, but most of the fungi pathogenic for man do not. The most useful classification of pathogenic fungi is based on disease associations, namely superficial, subcutaneous and disseminated mycoses (Table 8.2.1). Some mycoses can be transmitted sexually (e.g. candidiasis) and, since some of the superficial mycoses are transmitted by contact, they may also be transmitted by sexual contact. Some mycoses have an altered clinical presentation and course in patients with AIDS.

Dermatophytoses

Dermatophytes are subdivided into anthropophilic (transmitted between humans), zoophilic (transmitted from animals) and geophilic (transmitted from the inanimate environment). Only the anthropophilic dermatophytes are likely to be transmitted by sexual contact, but they are just as, or more, likely to be transmitted by non-venereal routes. The diseases they cause are named tineas followed by the body site. Thus tinea unguium is infection of the nails, tinea cruris of the groin, tinea pedis of the foot and tinea corporis (also called ringworm) of the body. Causes of tinea corporis include *Trichophyton rubrum, T. mentagrophytes, Epidermophyton floccosum* and *Microsporum canis.* If infection occurs in patients with AIDS, the lesions tend to be more widespread, more persistent and difficult to treat.

Diagnosis is by taking skin, hair or nail samples, treating them with KOH (30%) and examining them microscopically for fungal hyphae. The precise diagnosis depends upon culturing the fungus on Sabouraud's agar at 37°C or at room temperature for up to 2 weeks. Treatment is with oral griseofulvin

Table 8.2.1. Fungal infections.

Disease	Fungi	Sexually transmissible	Altered disease in AIDS
Superficial mycoses			
Dermatophytosis (tinea)	*Trichophyton* spp.	?	Yes
	Microsporum spp.	?	(more
	Epidermophyton floccosum	?	widespread)
Pityriasis	*Malessezia furfur*	?	Seborrhoeic dermatitis (unproven)
Subcutaneous mycoses			
Sporotrichosis	*Sporothrix schenckii*	No	Yes (more widespread)
Chromomycosis	*Phialophora verrucosum*		
	Phialophera piedrosis	No	Not known
	Cladosporium carrionii		
Mycetoma	*Actinomadura madurae*		
	Nocardia asteroides, N. brasiliensis	No	Not known
	Streptomyces somaliensis		
Rhinosporidiosis	*Rhinosporidium seeberi*	No	Not known
Zygomycosis	*Basidiobolus heptosporus*	No	Not known
	Conidiobolus coronatus		
Systemic mycoses			
Primary pathogens			
Histoplasmosis	*Histoplasma capsulatum*	No	Yes
Coccidioidomycosis	*Coccidioides immitis*	No	Yes
Blastomycosis	*Blastomyces dermatitidis*	No	Yes
Paracoccidioidomycosis	*Paracoccidioides brasiliensis*	No	Not known
Cryptococcosis	*Cryptococcus neoformans*	No	Yes
Penicilliosis	*Penicillium marneffei*	No	Yes
Opportunistic pathogens			
Aspergillosis	*Aspergillus fumigatus*	No	Yes
Candidosis	*Candida albicans*	Yes	Yes
	C. krusei, C. parapsilosis, C. tropicalis	Yes	Yes
Pneumocystosis	*Pneumocystis carinii*	No	Yes
Mucormycosis	*Mucor pusillus*	No	Yes

(10 mg kg^{-1} day^{-1}) for 6 weeks, which for some infections (e.g. tinea corporis) can be combined with topical clotrimazole, ketoconazole or miconazole for 2 weeks longer. Topical treatment will be needed in AIDS patients (see also Chapter 11.5).

Seborrhoeic dermatitis

Seborrhoeic dermatitis may manifest in a severe form of AIDS. *Malassezia furfur* and other species are found in large quantities on the desquamated skin in seborrhoeic dermatitis, and patients with the condition have raised antibody levels to *Malassezia*. However, these yeasts are also part of the normal skin flora so the association remains unproved (see also Chapter 11.5).

Sporotrichosis

Of the subcutaneous mycoses, only *Sporothrix schenckii* is reported to have altered expression in AIDS. This dimorphic fungus exists as a mould in the environment but as a yeast in patients. Infection occurs following introduction of the fungus through the skin into the dermis or subcutaneous tissues. It presents either as a small ulcer at the site of inoculation which may enlarge slowly and produce satellite lesions, or in a lymphangitic form. In the latter there is spread from the initial ulcer to form secondary lesions along the lymphatics draining the area. In patients with AIDS, many foci of infection develop throughout the body which can be ulcers, nodules or both. It must be differentiated from cutaneous leishmaniasis and atypical mycobacteriosis, in particular due to *Mycobacterium marinum*. Culture from swabs or curettings on Sabouraud's agar is the most reliable diagnostic test. Treatment is with potassium iodide (saturated solution) 1–2 ml orally three times per day, increasing slowly to a maximum of 4–6 ml thrice daily. Treatment is continued for 2–4 months. Alternatives include itraconazole (100–200 mg daily) or terbinafine (250 mg daily) but there are no controlled trials of therapy.

Histoplasmosis

Histoplasma capsulatum var. *capsulatum* is another dimorphic fungus (a mould in the environment and a yeast in patients) that is found in soil or areas where bats and birds have defaecated (although it is not part of their faecal flora). Infection by *H. capsulatum* var. *capsulatum* (~ 5 μm) is endemic in the USA, Central and South America, the Caribbean, Africa, India and the far East, but is most prevalent in the Americas. In Africa, histoplasmosis is due to the larger (~ 12-20 μm) *H. capsulatum* var. *duboisii*. Infection is probably acquired by inhalation into the lungs and, in AIDS patients, disseminates rapidly throughout the body. The presentation is usually non-specific, with weight loss, fever and hepatosplenomegaly, but multiple skin lesions (papules, nodules and ulcers) can occur. It may also progress to meningitis and endocarditis. The differential diagnosis in AIDS includes cutaneous cryptococcosis, coccidioidomycosis, blastomycosis, penicilliosis and molluscum contagiosum. Diagnosis is by demonstration of the yeasts by culture of blood, bone marrow, sputum or material from skin lesions. On Giemsa-stained bone marrow they can be seen as multiple yeasts within macrophages. Serology and antigen detection are also possible. Treatment is with itraconazole (200–400 mg per day) or amphotericin B (0.6–1.0 mg kg^{-1} day^{-1}), but long-term, suppressive therapy with itraconazole continuously or amphotericin B intermittently is needed in AIDS patients to prevent relapses (see also Chapter 11.5).

Coccidioidomycosis

Coccidioides immitis is found in the soil in arid parts of the Americas. It is inhaled as a small arthrospore (2.5 × 6 μm) which in the tissues grows to a large (50–80 μm) spore containing numerous endospores (2–5 μm). The endospores then disseminate throughout the body. Reactivation of latent infection can also occur in AIDS patients. In Tucson, Arizona, USA, coccidioidomycosis is the third most frequent opportunist infection in AIDS patients. Common complaints include fatigue, fever, weight loss, night sweats and dyspnoea. Disseminated disease occurs in 15–20% of cases, with skin lesions (papules, pustules, plaques, nodules, ulcers and abscesses), osteomyelitis, arthritis and meningitis being more common manifestations. In the lungs, there may be reticular nodules, focal or diffuse nodular infiltrates, and the latter has the worst prognosis. Pleural effusions may also occur. Diagnosis is by demonstration of *C. immitis* in sputum, CSF, tissue and, rarely, blood by stained smear or culture. Tests for detection of specific IgM by immunodiffusion or agglutination are positive in 80% of cases. Treatment is as for histoplasmosis, but fluconazole (400–800 mg daily) is an alternative. Again suppression therapy is needed to prevent relapse.

Blastomycosis

Blastomyces dermatitidis is a dimorphic fungus which is found in soil enriched with animal faeces. Its geographic distribution is limited to the east and mid-west USA. It is acquired by inhalation of conidia and presents either as pulmonary or disseminated disease. Dissemination is common to the meninges, spleen, liver, kidney and thyroid. Cutaneous lesions are more common in non-AIDS patients. Diagnosis is by demonstration of the fungus by culture or stained smear of lung biopsy, bronchoalveolar lavage, CSF or, less, commonly, blood. Treatment is with amphotericin B (0.6–1.0 mg kg^{-1} day^{-1}) with itraconazole maintenance to prevent relapse.

Cryptococcosis

There are two variants of *Cryptococcus neoformans*, var. *neoformans* which causes infection in the immunocompromised host including in AIDS, and var. *gattii* which is a rare cause of disease in immunocompetent patients in Australia and the Far East. It is a dimorphic yeast which in clinical samples has a thick polysaccharide capsule (Fig. 8.2.1). *C. neoformans* var. *neoformans*

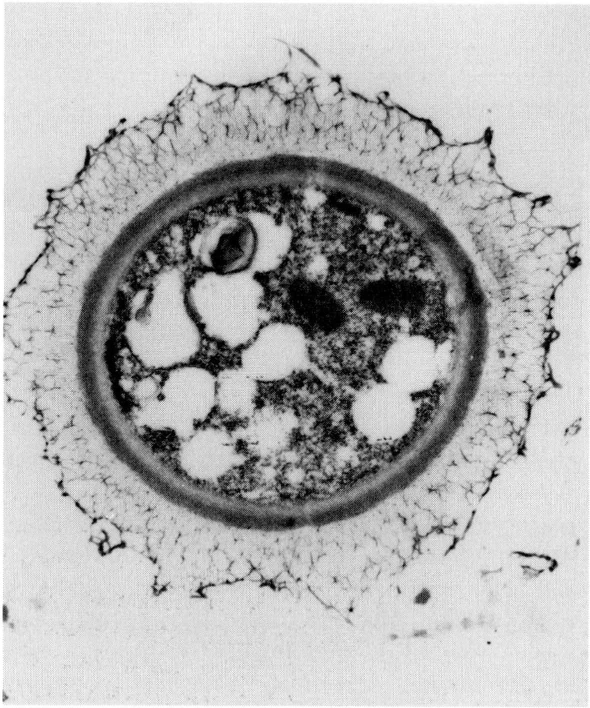

Fig. 8.2.1. *Cryptococcus neoformans*: thin section electron micrograph showing its thick polysaccharide capsule.

appears to be present in soil contaminated with bird and particularly pigeon excreta, whereas *C. neoformans* var. *gattii* is present in the environs of certain eucalyptus trees. Infection is thought to be acquired by inhalation, but in immune-deficient patients disseminates to other parts of the body. In the USA and Europe, about 6–10% of AIDS patients will develop cryptococcosis, but in sub-Saharan Africa it is encountered more frequently (15–20% of AIDS patients). Meningitis and meningoencephalitis are the most frequent presentation. In African AIDS patients, cryptococcal pneumonia is not an uncommon presentation, which contrasts with the picture in the USA and Europe. However, cryptococcal antigen can be detected in serum from 30% of African patients with pulmonary cryptococcosis and in the CSF of 25%.

Cryptococcal meningitis presents as a subacute meningitis and meningoencephalitis, with fever, malaise and headache for up to 4 weeks prior to presentation. Cryptococcal pneumonia presents with cough, weight loss, fever, dyspnoea, thoracic pain and, rarely, haemoptysis. Cutaneous lesions resembling molluscum contagiosum are a relatively common presentation. Because cryptococcosis can disseminate, focal infections such as mycocarditis, arthritis and gastroenteritis have been reported. The cryptococcal pneumonia must be differentiated from that due to HHV-5, *Pneumocystis carinii, Mycobacterium tuberculosis* and atypical mycobacteria. The differential diagnosis of cryptococcal meningitis includes *M. tuberculosis,* and that of cutaneous cryptococcosis includes molluscum contagiosum and the fungal infections described earlier.

Laboratory diagnosis is by demonstration of capsulate yeasts in CSF or sputum using the India ink stain, or by detection of capsular antigen in serum or CSF. Culture on Sabouraud's agar can take up to 2 weeks. In cryptococcal meningitis, the CSF white cell response is low in AIDS patients (<20 cells mm^{-3}).

The definitive treatment of cryptococcosis is an intravenous combination of amphotericin B (0.4–0.8 mg kg^{-1} day^{-1}) and 5-flucytosine (120–150 mg kg^{-1} day^{-1} in four doses) for 4–6 weeks. Even with therapy, 8–15% of patients die within 2 weeks. Even when CSF and blood are sterilized, relapse is common and suppressive therapy with fluconazole (200 mg orally daily) is necessary.

Penicilliosis (see also Chapters 6.1 and 11.5)

Penicillium marneffei is the only dimorphic *Penicillium* species, growing as a mould at 25°C and a yeast at 37°C. Although the bamboo rat is naturally and asymptomatically infected (90% of rats in one survey), it is thought that man and rat are infected from the environment. It has been isolated from bamboo from Southeast Asia. Human infections are particularly associated with living in or visiting Vietnam, Laos, Singapore, Malaysia, Thailand, Indonesia and Hong Kong. Infection can occur in apparently immunocompetent patients but, numerically, infections in AIDS patients are much more important. The yeast form enters and multiplies within macrophages. The most frequent clinical features in AIDS are fever (90% of cases), weight loss (72%), cutaneous eruptions (70%), lymphadenopathy (52%), cough (50%), hepatomegaly (44%) and diarrhoea (23%). The skin lesions consist of necrotic papules, nodules and pustules, and must be distinguished from molluscum contagiosum and the other fungal infections described previously.

Diagnosis is based on determining whether the patient has been to an endemic area and by staining of smears of bone marrow, skin scrapings or lymph node biopsy by Giemsa or silver stains. Over 50% of the patients are fungaemic, and fungi can be cultured (2 days at 37°C on Sabouraud's agar) from blood, bone marrow, skin, abscesses, lymph nodes, sputum or urine with varying degrees of success. Early institution of therapy (for 2 weeks) with intravenous amphotericin B and 5-flucytosine or ketoconazole followed by oral itraconazole suppressive therapy for 6 weeks has a high (70–90%) success rate.

Aspergillosis

Aspergillus fumigatus has been reported to cause pneumonic infiltration in AIDS patients. Treatment can be difficult, but itraconazole and a new imidazole, voriconazole, might be effective.

Candidiasis

Infection with *C. albicans* has been described in Chapter 8.1. Infections with other *Candida* are increasingly encountered in AIDS patients with clinical pictures similar to *C. albicans*. These (especially *C. krusei*) are more likely to be resistant to fluconazole. All can be distinguished from *C. albicans* in not producing a germ tube (pseudohypha) on incubation in serum.

Pneumocystosis

Pneumocystis carinii has, until recently, been classified as a protozoan, but genomic evidence now places it in the fungus kingdom. The infective form is a cyst which can survive in the environment. Infection occurs following inhalation of cysts which mature to grape-like clusters of trophozoites. Since *P. carinii* is found in some animals, questions have been raised over its zoonotic potential. However, little cross-species transmission has been described. Subclinical and asymptomatic infection is common in immunocompetent children. It is only when immunity is compromised (in particular children given chemotherapy for leukaemia, those on corticosteroids, and AIDS patients) that infection becomes manifest. It was commonly assumed that infection in adult AIDS was a reactivation of latent infection acquired in childhood. However, it is now clear that a proportion of cases result from exogenously acquired *P. carinii*. There is evidence that elderly apparently immunocompetent patients can develop *P. carinii* pneumonia (PCP).

PCP is the commonest opportunist infection in AIDS, with 80–90% of patients developing PCP in their lifetime. It was thought that PCP was rare in Africa, but recent data indicate that this is not the case.

In AIDS patients, PCP has a subtle and slow onset, with increasing dyspnoea, fever and cough over a period of weeks to months. On examination, there will be tachypnoea, tachycardia and cyanosis but surprisingly few signs on auscultation. The chest X-ray will reveal diffuse bilateral infiltrates initially in the perihilar regions and, eventually, with air bronchograms. Nodules and unilateral infiltrates can be seen occasionally. Dissemination of *P. carinii* to skin, liver, kidney and eyes has been described on occasions. Specific diagnosis is by demonstration of *P. carinii*. Samples for detection, in decreasing order of sensitivity, are lung biopsy, bronchoalveolar lavage, induced sputum and nasopharyngeal aspirate. Methods for detection again in decreasing order of sensitivity are PCR, immunofluorescence, immunoperoxidase and methenamine silver staining.

Although cotrimoxazole orally or intravenously (trimethoprim 20 mg kg^{-1} day^{-1}, sulphamethoxazole 100 mg kg^{-1} day^{-1} in four divided doses) is an effective treatment for PCP, up to 50% of AIDS patients experience serious side effects including fever, rash, neutropenia, thrombocytopenia and hepatitis. Rashes can progress to Stevens–Johnson syndrome. Pentamidine is an alternative given intramuscularly or by slow intravenous infusion (4 mg kg^{-1} day^{-1}). Toxicity does occur and includes cardiovascular instability, neutropenia and sterile injection abscesses. Both therapies should continue for 3 weeks. Once an AIDS patient has developed PCP and recovered, there is a 50% chance of recurrence within a year. Thus chemoprophylaxis is advised. Cotrimoxazole (trimethoprim 5 mg kg^{-1} day^{-1}, sulphamethoxazole 25 mg kg^{-1} day^{-1}) given orally daily or three times per week is effective and relatively non-toxic. If PCP occurs whilst on cotrimoxazole prophylaxis, treatment should be given with pentamidine and, if possible, secondary prophylaxis with aerosolized pentamidine.

CHAPTER 9
Protozoal and arthropod infections

CHAPTER 9.1
Trichomoniasis

O.P. Arya
Department of Medical Microbiology and Genitourinary Medicine, University of Liverpool, Liverpool, UK

Trichomoniasis is a common cause of vaginal discharge. Although often asymptomatic in men, it is the most common curable STI worldwide. It is encountered in sexually active women of all age groups, but is less common after the age of 40. See Chapter 1 for the epidemiology in the tropics.

Aetiology

The causative organism, *Trichomonas vaginalis*, is a protozoan with four free anterior flagella and a fifth directed posteriorly along the free edge of an undulating membrane (Fig. 9.1.1). It is larger than a pus cell, being 10–12 μm in length and 7–10 μm in width. Its shape in the vagina varies, and may be circular, oval, pyriform or amoeboid. It has a nucleus and an axostyle. It reproduces by binary fission. In a wet preparation, it can be recognized easily by the lashing movements of the flagella. A variety of media has been used for its culture, and the one commonly used is Feinberg–Whittington medium (see also Chapter 5).

Transmission, pathogenesis and immunity

Sexual contact is the usual mode of infection in adults. Accidental infection from inadequately sterilized instruments, gloves, toilet seats, moist contaminated towels and communal baths is possible but difficult to prove.

The infection is confined to the urogenital tract. The pathogenic mechanisms are uncertain. The organisms have an affinity for squamous epithelium. The vaginal infection is associated with elevation of vaginal pH, suppression of lactobacilli and an increase in the anaerobic flora and *Mycoplasma hominis* in many cases. The inflammatory response includes infiltration with polymorphonuclear leukocytes (PMN).

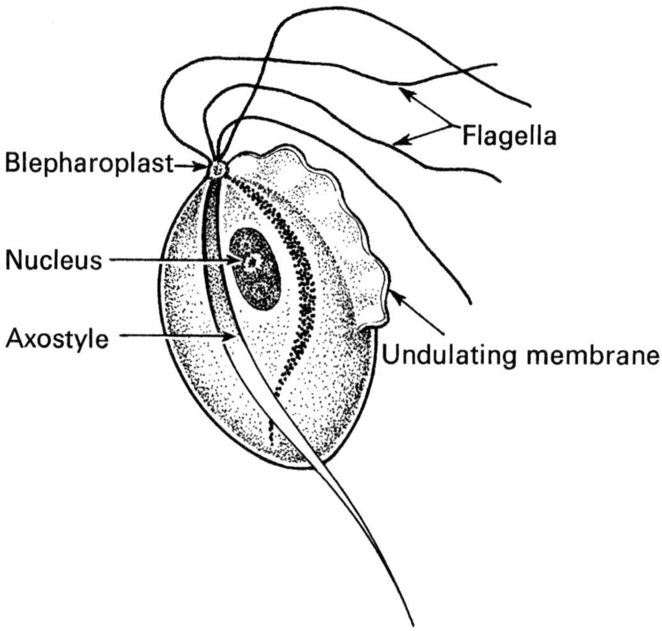

Fig. 9.1.1. *Trichomonas vaginalis.*

The infection does not confer significant protective immunity. Repeated infections are common.

Clinical features

Females

Symptoms

In the author's experience at a Genitourinary Medicine Clinic (with comprehensive screening for STI and bacterial vaginosis), around 10% of the patients with *T. vaginalis* infection are asymptomatic. In other settings, this proportion may be higher. About half of the patients have one or more other conditions concurrently, including chlamydial and gonococcal infections, genital warts, bacterial vaginosis and, occasionally, candidiasis. The incubation period, as far as can be assessed, is between 5 and 28 days. The majority of patients (infected only with *T. vaginalis*) present with vaginal discharge, usually offensive, and vulvovaginal irritation. Other symptoms with or without vaginal discharge and irritation, include dysuria, frequency of micturition, soreness of the vulva and of the skin of adjoining thighs, superficial dyspareunia and, rarely, lower abdominal discomfort. The symptoms may begin or worsen during or soon after menstruation, probably because the elevated pH is favourable to the organisms.

Signs

About 75% of patients have abnormal signs of the vulva or vagina or both. The vulval signs include discharge (which may be smelly) at the introitus, redness and oedema of the vulva, mucopurulent urethral discharge, discharge from Skene's ducts, and excoriation of the vulva extending to the inner thighs (Plate 114). The speculum examination may be painful. The vaginal walls may be reddened. The characteristics of the vaginal discharge vary; the discharge may be grey or lime green in colour, frothy or purulent, usually copious and offensive (Plate 115). Rarely, the ectocervix may have a 'strawberry' appearance as a result of areas of increased vascularity and punctate haemorrhages.

Males

Symptoms and signs

Males are often asymptomatic. Some may experience penile irritation, mild dysuria, early morning penile discharge, i.e. symptoms of NGU. Clinical findings are also similar to those in NGU (Chapter 7.5). Occasionally, a milky white bead may be expressed from the urethra after the patient has not passed urine overnight. A Gram-stained urethral smear often shows five or more PMN per high power field. A few patients may develop balanoposthitis.

Differential diagnosis

Differential diagnosis in females is from other causes of vaginal discharge (see Chapter 10.2 and Table 8.1.1), and in males from other causes of NGU (Chapter 7.5) and balanoposthitis (Chapter 11.5).

Diagnosis

Tests for other STI should be carried out in all cases, and those for trichomoniasis include wet smears and cultures. The wet smear is made by mixing the vaginal material with a drop of normal saline on a glass slide, a coverslip is placed on it and then examined immediately by direct illumination or darkfield examination or by phase contrast microscopy. The trichomonads are easily recognized by their shape, size and rotatory flagellar movements. Smears alone or cultures alone may miss 7–12% of the cases. *T. vaginalis* can also be identified on Papanicolaou-stained smears for cervical cytology. The organisms are difficult to demonstrate in male patients, probably because they are washed out with each act of micturition. Attempts should, therefore, be made to obtain specimens for wet smears and cultures from the early morning discharge and urethral scrape before passing urine, the centrifuged specimen of urine, and possibly also the prostatic secretion. Subpreputial smears and cultures should be made in the case of balanoposthitis.

Complications

Trichomoniasis does not usually produce any complications. Nevertheless, spread of the organisms to the fallopian tubes has been reported. There is no proof that trichomoniasis affects the outcome of pregnancy. In males, the possibilities, not proven, include epididymitis and chronic prostatitis.

Trichomoniasis in infants and children

Transmission

The female infant may acquire the infection from its untreated mother during birth (the risk being ~5%) or during routine child care with contaminated hands. In older children, the possibility of sexual abuse should be considered. However, trichomoniasis is uncommon in older children because the vaginal environment is unfavourable to the organisms until about adulthood. Nevertheless, the urinary tract as well as the vagina may be involved.

Clinical features

The child may remain asymptomatic and continue to harbour the organisms for several months. Some children may develop symptoms and signs of vulvovaginitis.

Differential diagnosis

See Chapter 7.5 (section on vulvovaginitis)

Diagnosis

The diagnosis is confirmed by microscopy and culture of material obtained from the vaginal introitus (with a swab or plastic loop), as well as microscopy and culture of the urine sediment. Tests for other STI, if appropriate, should be considered.

Trichomoniasis and HIV infection

There is, up to now, no proof of any interaction between trichomoniasis and HIV infection. The treatment of trichomoniasis, whether or not the patient has HIV infection, is the same as described below.

Management of trichomoniasis

Adults

Metronidazole, with up to 95% cure rates, is the drug of choice. The recommended regimens are: 200 mg orally, three times a day for 1 week, *or* 400 mg orally, twice daily for 5–7 days, *or* 2 g orally, as a single dose. The tablets should be taken with or following a meal to reduce the possibility of gastric side effects. Alcohol should also be avoided to prevent disulfiram-like reaction.

As metronidazole may give a bitter taste to the milk, large single doses should be avoided for lactating women.

Contact tracing

The infection may resolve spontaneously in some male patients. However, all sex partners, including those who are asymptomatic, should be examined and treated.

Follow-up

The patient should be advised to abstain from sexual intercourse until the patient and the sex partner(s) have completed treatment and the symptoms have resolved. If the symptoms persist, the patient should return and the swabs be repeated.

Treatment failure

Apart from re-infection, the causes of treatment failure include poor compliance, lack of absorption or inactivation of the drug by the vaginal flora such as haemolytic streptococci, and metronidazole resistance. Most refractory cases will respond to a double dose of metronidazole, i.e. 400 mg, orally three times daily for 7 days *plus* metronidazole, 500 mg intravaginally each night for 7 days. If possible, a high vaginal swab for culture may be taken to identify other bacteria which should then be treated appropriately (or treat with erythromycin or amoxycillin) before re-treating with a course of metronidazole. The other option is to try tinidazole, 2 g orally daily for 2 days. There is an urgent need for an alternative regimen which should be effective, safe and easy to administer, especially for those who persistently fail to respond to the above regimens, if the strains are resistant to metronidazole or for those allergic to metronidazole. In general, strains with MIC >8 $\mu g\ ml^{-1}$ will be resistant to oral therapy and those with MIC of more than 200 $\mu g\ ml^{-1}$ to topical therapy. For the present, if the above regimens fail, the patient may be treated with acetarsol, 250 mg suppository, two to be inserted intravaginally for 2–3 weeks, but to be avoided during menstruation; the side effects include gastrointestinal irritation, cutaneous irritation, anaphylaxis, etc.

Side effects of metronidazole

The side effects of metronidazole are uncommon, and include metallic taste, dizziness, headache, nausea, gastrointestinal disturbances, skin eruptions and superinfection with *Candida*. Prolonged intensive therapy may result in peripheral neuropathy and leukopenia.

Treatment in pregnancy

Although metronidazole appears to be safe in pregnancy (see Chapter 7.8), the manufacturers advise caution, and some specialists avoid it altogether in the first trimester. Instead, clotrimazole, 100 mg intravaginally each night for 6 days, may be used. It will provide symptomatic relief and may even cure some patients. If the infection persists, the patient can be treated with metronidazole, using the low-dose regimen, after the first trimester.

Infants and children

Symptomatic infection persisting after the age of 3 months may be treated with metronidazole, 5 mg kg^{-1} orally three times daily for 5 days. For older children, the dose may be increased to 7.5 mg kg^{-1} orally three times daily for 7 days.

CHAPTER 9.2
Scabies and pediculosis

A. Sivayathorn
Department of Dermatology, Siriraj Hospital, Bangkok, Thailand

Scabies

Scabies is caused by the mite, *Sarcoptes scabiei*. Mites are transferred between humans by close physical contact; therefore, the infestation is often sexually acquired. Itching, which is part of an allergic reaction to the mite faeces/saliva, etc., is the main symptom, often worse in a warm environment, for example when the patient is in bed. Characteristic lesions are the burrows which contain mites and their eggs. They are small tunneling lesions on the skin but are difficult to find because most of them are scratched away by the patients. The scabies mite prefers protected areas of the body. Patients, therefore, present with widespread excoriated papules most often found between the fingers, on the wrists, around the waist and on the legs. The penis and scrotum are frequently involved (Plate 116). In women, the bra line and the nipples are common sites of affliction. Sebum may have some inhibitory effect on the mites; so the face and scalp are usually spared, except in infants and immuno-compromised adults. Secondary bacterial infection is a common complication and, if streptococcal, may result in glomerulonephritis.

In HIV infection, deficiency in cell-mediated immunity allows unchecked proliferation of mites, resulting in hyperkeratotic lesions containing numerous mites. The intertriginous areas are more heavily involved than other areas of the skin. This highly infectious condition is known as 'crusted' or 'Norwegian' scabies. A uniform diffuse papular eruption has also been reported in HIV-associated scabies.

The diagnosis of scabies is usually made on clinical grounds. Patients presenting with an itchy papular eruption and burrows are readily recognized. Microscopic visualization of a mite or its eggs or faeces in a scraping taken from a papule or burrow verifies the diagnosis.

Treatment

Application of 1% lindane (γ-benzene hexachloride) cream from the neck to the toes for 12 h is effective, providing all areas including under the fingernails, between the toes, the pubic area and the umbilicus are treated. Help may be needed to reach the back and between the shoulders. Lindane, which is to be avoided in pregnant and lactating women and children under the age of 10 years, is no longer the preferred treatment in the UK. Aqueous malathion (0.5%) or permethrin cream are effective and safer if the recommended dose is not exceeded. The lotion is removed by washing after 24 h and the cream after 8–12 h. Less effective alternative treatments include 25% benzyl benzoate emulsion (daily for 2 or 3 days), crotamiton and 10% sulphur ointment.

In crusted and diffuse scabies (as in those with HIV infection), the medication should be applied from head to toes (avoiding the eye and mouth areas) daily for 2 or 3 days. Keratolytic ointment such as 10% salicylic acid may be applied to keratotic areas twice a day for removal of thick scales. There have been reports of lindane-resistant scabies especially in HIV-infected patients. Recently, ivermectin given orally has been shown to be highly promising.

The itching may persist for several days after treatment after the infestation has been eliminated. In such cases, application of calamine or crotamiton cream and an oral antihistamine at night may be helpful.

Clothes and bedding are laundered in the normal way and dried well. It is important that the sex partners and family contacts are examined and treated for their own sake and also to avoid re-infection.

Pediculosis pubis

The crab louse, *Phthirus pubis*, is the cause of pubic lice. This small wingless insect is about 1–2 mm in length and can be seen with the naked eye. It lives primarily in the pubic hair but occasionally infests other hairy parts of the body, with the exception of scalp hair and eye brows, although the eyelashes may be rarely infested. The transmission is by intimate body contact. Crab lice use their mouth parts to penetrate the skin, and they produce an anticoagulant to facilitate blood sucking. The eggs (nits) of pubic lice are cemented firmly to hair shafts and are seen as black dots attached to the hairs (Plate 117). Clinically, patients present with pruritus of the pubic area or complain of spots or observation of the louse itself.

The diagnosis is made by carefully examining the patient for lice and nits. The use of a hand lens and good light will facilitate the examination.

Treatment

Treatment is with an effective pediculocide that kills both the adult and nit stages of the infestation. Lindane (see also above) is applied to the infested and neighbouring hairy areas for 12 h and then washed off. Dead lice and nits are removed with a fine-tooth comb after 24 h. Treatment should be repeated in 1 week to kill any emerging young lice from nits which survive the first treatment. Aqueous malathion is equally effective, and is the preferred treatment in some countries. The infestation of eyelashes may be treated with vaseline applied to the eyelid margins daily for 7 days to smother lice and nits, which may be removed with fine tweezers.

Sex partners are examined and treated appropriately.

PART III
Problem-oriented approach, special topics and control aspects

Chapter 10 Problem-oriented approach

Chapter 10.1 Management of STI at the primary health care level

A.S. Latif
Departent of Medicine, University of Zimbabwe, Harare, Zimbabwe

General considerations

An important aspect in the control of STI is the rapid and effective treatment of persons who are infected. This requires almost universal access to high-quality care for persons with STI. In most developing countries, persons seeking care for STI attend primary health care (PHC) facilities in the first instance, where aetiological diagnosis of STI (essential for appropriate treatment) is often not possible. In addition, the clinicians working at the PHC level are already overworked and need to see a large number of patients, some of whom might have STI. Time constraints and pressure of work often lead to poor health care delivery. However, by integrating STI care within PHC centres (including PHC clinics, antenatal clinics and clinics for maternal and child health and family planning), effective and acceptable care could be made available at such facilities. This may be achieved by training PHC providers in delivering comprehensive case management using the problem oriented or the so-called 'syndromic approach'.

As the problem-oriented approach will usually result in treatment for more than one aetiological agent, the drawbacks of this approach include overdiagnosis and hence overtreatment. A serious limitation is exclusion of asymptomatic patients who do not attend and whose infections will remain undetected, and who may thus continue to spread the infection(s) and also be liable to suffer complications. It is desirable, therefore, to assess the cost-effectiveness of this approach.

Nevertheless, in order for specific treatment recommendation to be made, information on the prevalence of the various different pathogens in the given area, region or country, is required. If this type of information is not available for a given country, aetiologic studies may be necessary. In addition, periodic studies are needed in order to determine a change in the prevalence of the aetiologic agents and to determine whether a change in the pattern of antimicrobial susceptibility has occurred. If information on aetiology and antimicrobial susceptibility is not available in a country, then the recommendations may be based on the results of studies carried out in neighbouring countries.

STI-associated problems

The common clinical presentations of STI are urethral discharge, vaginal discharge and genital ulceration. Other clinical presentations include inguinal swelling, scrotal swelling, balanitis, lower abdominal pain in women, conjunctivitis with discharging eyes in neonates, a variety of skin lesions and rashes, generalized lymphadenopathy and genital warts. These symptoms and signs are easily recognizable provided the health worker is able to take a history and carry out an examination.

The above section heading has, until now, been universally presented as 'STI-associated syndromes'. However, the word 'syndrome', in this context, is inappropriate because a 'syndrome' is a concurrence of several symptoms or signs in a disease. On the other hand, urethral discharge, vaginal discharge, genital ulceration, scrotal swelling, etc. (Table 10.1.1) are symptoms or signs which may be due to more than one disease. These topics are dealt with individually in this chapter as a presenting problem.

A list of STI-associated problems and their common causes, for management at the PHC level, is shown in Table 10.1.1.

Case management of persons with STI

As a minimum, all patients seeking care for STI should be given the following:

- Appropriate antimicrobial and other therapy.
- Education on the nature of the infection, mode of transmission, treatment compliance and ways to prevent infection.
- A supply and use of condoms.
- Information on how sexual partners may also be treated.
- A date for a follow-up examination.

The delivery of this management 'package' is known as case management. The above components of case management are now briefly described.

Antimicrobial therapy

In general, it is preferable to recommend single dose, orally administered treatment regimens. Such treatments may be supervised at the clinic. Drugs should obviously be highly effective, free of side effects and available at the clinic. Unfortunately drugs that fall into all these categories may be too

Table 10.1.1. STI-associated problems and their causes. (For management at the PHC level.)

STI-associated presenting problems	Causes/conditions to be considered for management at the PHC level
Urethral discharge	Gonococcal and non-gonococcal urethritis
Genital ulcer	Syphilis, chancroid, genital herpes, granuloma inguinale, lymphogranuloma venereum
Inguinal swelling	Chancroid, syphilis, lymphogranuloma venereum, pyoderma
Scrotal swelling	Epididymitis (gonococcal/chlamydial infection, mumps)
	Surgical conditions (torsion, hydrocoele, haematocoele, varicocoele, hernia, tumour)
Balanitis/balanoposthitis	Poor genital hygiene, candidiasis, trichomoniasis, fusospirochaetosis
Vaginal discharge	Vaginal infections (candidiasis, trichomoniasis, bacterial vaginosis) cervical infections (gonococcal/chlamydial infection)
Lower abdominal pain in women	Pelvic inflammatory disease, ectopic pregnancy, appendicitis
Neonatal conjunctivitis	Gonococcal/chlamydial and other bacterial infections
Generalized lymphadenopathy	Syphilis, tuberculosis, HIV, CMV, infectious mononucleosis, lymphoma, Kaposi's sarcoma, toxoplasmosis, cryptococcosis, hepatitis B
Genital warts	Human papillomavirus

expensive to use on a nationwide scale. However, it should be borne in mind that the only weapon that is available to break the cycle of transmission is rapid treatment with a highly effective agent. The choice of the drug may vary from place to place depending on the common cause(s) of the STI-associated problem and on the pattern of antimicrobial sensitivity of pathogens.

Provision of health education (Box 10.1.1)

Patients with STI form an ideal target audience for health education as, apart from putting at risk the innocent partners (usually the wife or girlfriend), they have engaged in risky sexual behaviour and have placed themselves at risk for HIV infection.

The following aspects should be covered during the education exercise:

1. All patients should be educated regarding STI in general. The patient should understand how STI are acquired and transmitted and how he/she can prevent themselves becoming infected. Patients should be made to understand the possible risks of becoming infected, i.e. risks to oneself, risks of passing on the infection to the partner, and risk of infecting the newborn baby. Emphasis

Box 10.1.1. The health education component of STI case management.

The following information should be given to all patients
1. Mode of transmission of STI and possible complications of infection.
2. Safer sexual behaviour, i.e.
   delay sexual debut
   abstain from sexual activity
   engage only in a mutually faithful sexual relationship.
3. Engage only in safer sex acts, i.e.
   non-penetrative sex
   correct use of condoms with a demonstration of condom use.
4. The importance of treatment compliance.
5. The importance of having partner(s) treated.

should also be placed on the fact the HIV infection is acquired in exactly the same way as any other STI and that there is no cure for HIV infection.

2. Patients should be advised to complete the full course of treatment, even though symptoms improve or even disappear. The reasons for this advice are: (i) even though the patient feels much improved the infection may not have cleared and symptoms may return, and, complications of infection may occur; (ii) though the symptoms have improved the patient may still be infectious to his/her partner(s); and (iii) the chances of becoming infected with HIV are greater if the patient has sex with someone with HIV while he/she still has an STI. The patient should be advised to refrain from sexual activity while he/she is being treated for STI, and of the importance of having partners checked and treated.

3. The patient should be advised how to avoid becoming infected with any STI. The patient should be advised **to change his/her sexual behaviour**, and if he/she finds himself/herself in a risky situation then **he/she should engage only in safer sexual activity** as follows:

Safer sexual behaviour means:

- to abstain from sexual activity altogether; or
- to engage in a mutually faithful monogamous sexual relationship.

To engage only in safer sex acts means:

- to engage in sexual activity which does not involve penetration of the penis into the vagina, anus or mouth, i.e. non-penetrative sex, which in effect implies manual masturbation or rubbing of body parts; or to engage in penetrative sex acts provided the penis is covered with a condom.

It is important for the health care provider to take time to explain all these alternatives.

Provision and use of condoms

All patients with STI should be educated on proper condom use together with a demonstration of condom use on a penis model, and should be given a supply of condoms. It is important for the patient to understand that the condom should be on the penis during the entire period of penetration. The patient should also be told to keep condoms away from heat and direct sunlight and that as the condom is already lubricated no additional lubrication is necessary.

Finally, the patient should be advised on the safe disposal of the used condom, i.e. wrap the condom in paper and bury it or burn it, and if a flush toilet is available to wrap it in toilet paper and flush it down the pan.

The patient should be informed as to where further supplies of condoms may be obtained.

Treatment of sexual partners

The patient with STI should be informed as to how he/she became infected and should be advised that since he/she is the only one who knows the whereabouts of the source of the infection that he/she should have that person treated. If sexual intercourse has taken place with anyone subsequent to having sex with the source, then all such secondary contacts should also be treated. It is important for the patient to understand that if the source contact and all secondary contacts are not treated, then there is a risk of becoming infected again. Depending on the health care facility, the contact tracing exercise may be passive one whereby the index patient is counselled and given contact slips to pass on to his/her contacts, or the exercise may be an active one when a health worker visits the addresses given by the index patient in order to seek out the contacts. A combination of the two methods is often used. The patient should be assured that confidentiality will be maintained and that no information regarding himself/herself will be disclosed.

Follow-up examination

All patients should be advised not to engage in sexual activity until they are completely cured. Arrangements may be made for a follow-up examination if this is likely to be convenient for the patient. However, as it is recommended that only highly effective drugs be used in treating patients, a follow-up examination may not be necessary at all. Patients could be told to return if symptoms persist or if symptoms return after initial improvement.

If, however, patients do attend for follow-up examination, the opportunity should be used to reinforce health education.

Problem-oriented clinical management and flowcharts

As mentioned above, time constraints and often minimal or non-existent laboratory facilities may lead to health care of poor quality at the PHC level. One way to improve the outcomes in this setting is by the provision of clinical management flowcharts and standardized treatment protocols.

Clinical management flowcharts should be easy to read and simplify the decision-making process. The steps that need to be followed and the actions that the clinician needs to take should be clearly stated. Clinicians should be trained in using the flowcharts and in understanding the logic of the sequence of steps. Clinicians should be taught that all clinical management flowcharts should be read from top to bottom and from left to right. The clinicians should read the flowchart in order to understand the flow before actually using it.

Urethral discharge in men

The flowchart for the management of urethral discharge in men (Fig. 10.1.1) requires that the clinician takes a history and examines the patient. Once the presence of urethral discharge is confirmed, the patient is provided with the complete problem-oriented case management package (see above) The aetiology of urethral discharge may be gonococcal or non-gonococcal, such as chlamydial. It is not possible to differentiate between the two by clinical examination. If left untreated, the patient may develop serious complications such as epididymo-orchitis, infertility and urethral stricture. In over a third of the patients with urethral discharge, both gonococcal and non-gonococcal infections may occur at the same time. Therefore, it may be cost effective to treat all men with urethral discharge for both gonococcal and non-gonococcal infections.

Microscopic examination of Gram-stained urethral smears may assist in managing patients in that if after careful microscopic examination no intracellular Gram-negative diplococci are found then it is likely that the patient has NGU and may be treated as such in the first instance. If, however, Gram-negative intracellular diplococci suggestive of gonococci are found, then the patient is treated for both gonococcal and non-gonococcal infection as the test cannot rule out non-gonococcal/chlamydial infection, etc. This approach may be used where laboratory facilities are available. Box 10.1.2 lists the drugs that may be used in the treatment of gonococcal and non-gonococcal infection.

Genital ulcer disease in men and women

The common sexually acquired causes of genital ulcers include *Treponema pallidum* (syphilis), *Haemophilus ducreyi* (chancroid) and herpes simplex virus (HSV; genital herpes). Other causes are *Calymmatobacterium granulomatis* (granuloma inguinale or Donovanosis) and *Chlamydia trachomatis,* serovars L1, L2 and L3 (lymphogranuloma venereum).

There are also many other sexually and non-sexually acquired causes of genital ulceration such as gonococcal, *Candida, Trichomonas* and anaerobic infections, scabies, genital trauma, pyoderma, fixed drug eruption, Behçet's disease and neoplasm, etc. The sensitivity and specificity of the clinical diagnosis will, therefore, be determined by the locally prevalent clinical and aetiological patterns.

Figure 10.1.2 is an example of a clinical management flowchart that could

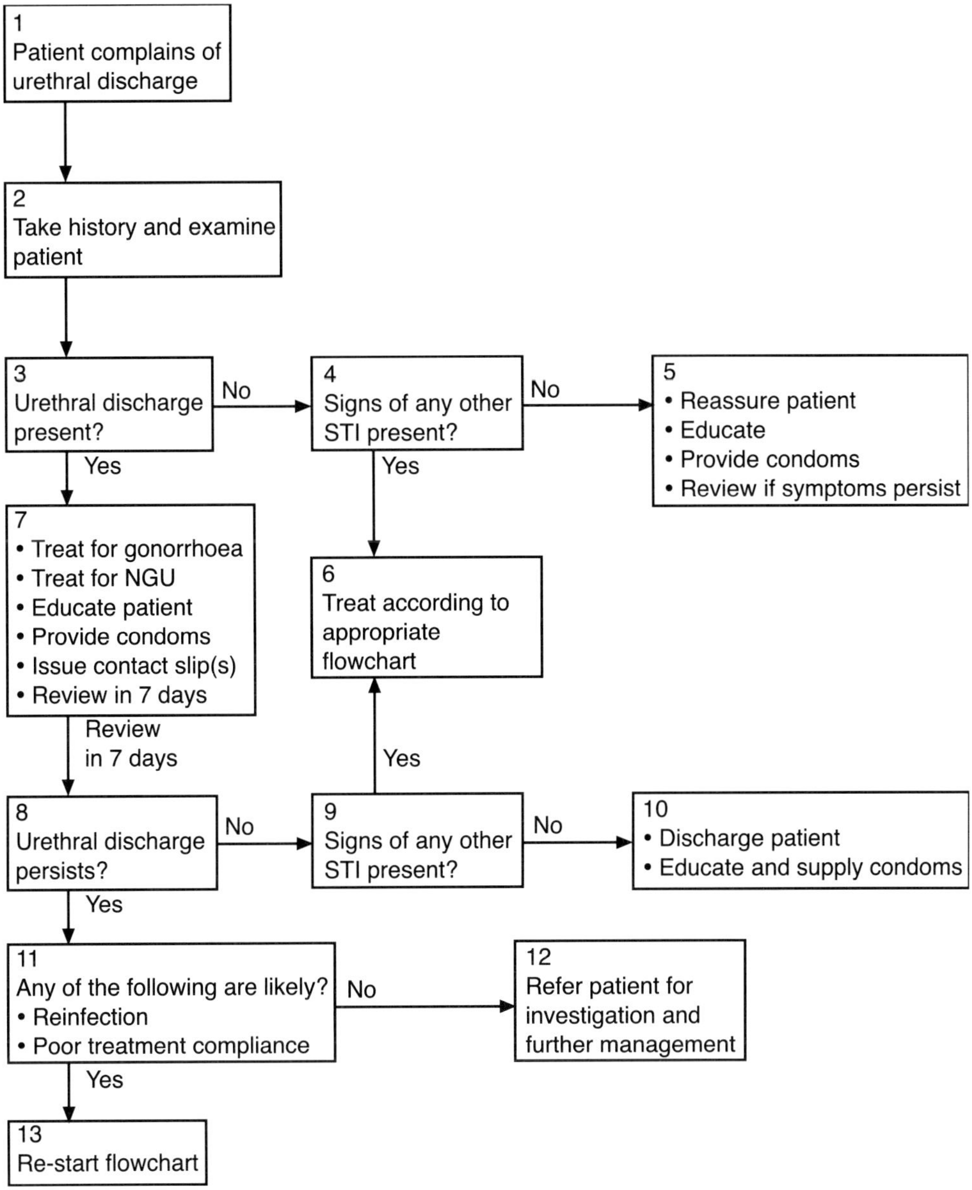

Fig. 10.1.1. Flowchart for the management of urethral discharge in men.

be used in providing comprehensive case management for persons with genital ulcers. Clinicians using the flowcharts are instructed to take a history and examine the patient. If the patient has an ulcer, and if syphilis and chancroid commonly occur, then he/she should be treated for both syphilis and chancroid for the following reasons:

Box 10.1.2. Antimicrobial therapy of STI-associated problems.

1. Urethral discharge
Treat for gonococcal and non-gonococcal infection:
For gonococcal infection use any ONE of the following:
Ceftriaxone, 250 mg i.m., *or*, spectinomycin, 2 g i.m., *or*, ciprofloxacin, 500 mg single oral dose, *or*, cefixime, 400 mg in a single oral dose, or kanamycin, 2 g i.m. in areas where susceptibility of gonococci to kanamycin has been demonstrated.
plus
For non-gonococcal infection: doxycycline, 100 mg orally twice daily for 7 days,*or*, tetracycline, 500 mg orally four times a day for 7 days. In persons who are unable to take doxycycline and tetracycline, give erythromycin, 500 mg orally four times a day for 7 days.

2. Genital ulcer disease
Treat for syphilis and chancroid:
For syphilis: benzathine penicillin, 2.4 million units i.m., *or*, if the patient is allergic to penicillin then doxycycline, 100 mg orally twice daily for 15 days, *or*, tetracycline, 500 mg orally four times a day for 15 days. Tetracycline should not be given to pregnant women. Hence pregnant women who are allergic to penicillin are given erythromycin, 500 mg orally four times a day for 15 days.
plus
for chancroid: erythromycin, 500 mg given orally four times a day for 7 days, *or*, ceftriaxone, 250 mg i.m., *or*, ciprofloxacin, 500 mg given in a single oral dose, *or*, spectinomycin, 2 g i.m., *or*, cotrimoxazole, two tablets (each containing trimethoprim 80 mg and sulphamethoxazole 400 mg) orally twice daily for 7 days. Over recent years, cotrimoxazole has become less effective in treating persons with chancroid.
Treatment of granuloma inguinale: cotrimoxazole, two tablets (each containing trimethoprim 80 mg and sulphamethoxazole 400 mg) orally twice daily for 14 days, *or*, doxycycline, 100 mg orally twice daily for 14 days, *or* tetracycline, 500 mg four times daily for 14 days, *or*, erythromycin, 500 mg four times daily for 14 days.

3. Bubo
In the presence of genital ulcers, treat the patient as for genital ulcer disease.
Patients with a bubo in whom no genital ulcers are found are treated for lymphogranuloma venereum as follows:
doxycycline, 100 mg orally twice daily for 14 days, *or*, tetracycline, 500 mg orally four times a day for 14 days, *or*, erythromycin, 500 mg orally four times a day for 14 days. Tetracycline and the tetracycline analogues should not be used in pregnant women, instead erythromycin should be used.

4. Acute scrotal swelling
Treat for both gonococcal and chlamydial infection as described above.

5. Ophthalmia neonatorum
The treatment of gonococcal ophthalmia neonatorum is with ceftriaxone 50 mg kg^{-1} body weight given as a single i.m. injection once. The maximum dose of ceftriaxone is 125 mg. Alternatively, a single i.m. dose of kanamycin, 25 mg kg^{-1} body weight is given (maximum dose 75 mg).
The treatment of chlamydial ophthalmia neonatorum is erythromycin in a dose of 50 mg kg^{-1} body weight daily orally in three divided doses for 14 days.

- From the clinical examination, it is often difficult to tell whether the patient has syphilis or chancroid; the presence or absence of pain or induration or the presence or absence of a bubo are not reliable discriminators.

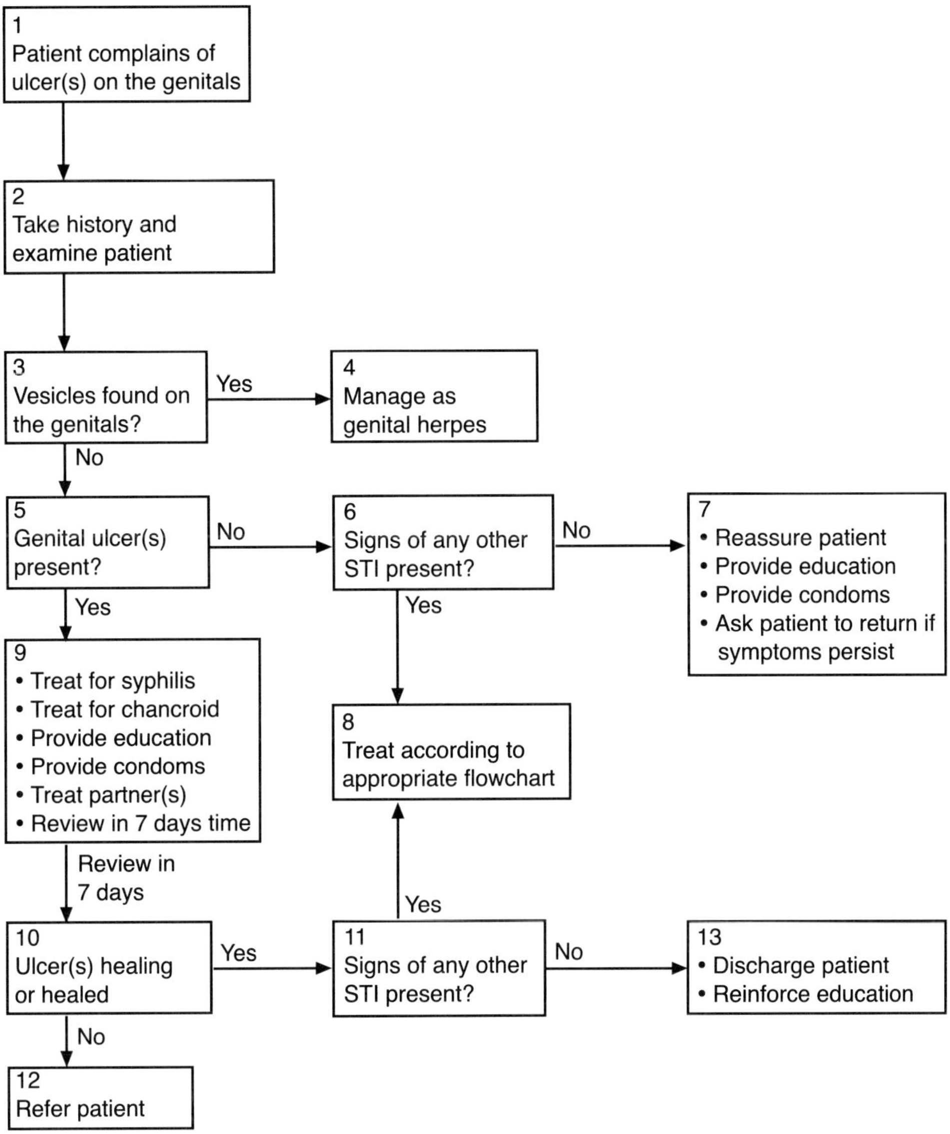

Fig. 10.1.2. Flowchart for the management of genital ulcers in men and women.

- Mixed infections are not uncommon.
- Both chancroid and syphilis are known to facilitate the acquisition and transmission of HIV.
- Only sophisticated laboratory tests can help in making an accurate aetiologic diagnosis.

Specific treatment recommendations for syphilis, chancroid and granuloma inguinale are listed in Box 10.1.2.

Herpetic ulceration usually cannot be distinguished from chancroid on a clinical basis. Nevertheless, if genital herpes is diagnosed, the patient should be informed of the natural history of genital herpes. The patient should understand that although there is no cure for this condition, there are usually no serious consequences. The patient should be advised to avoid sex during an attack of genital herpes and to use condoms at other times. (A supply of condoms should be issued.) Locally, no medication need be applied. The patient should be told to keep lesions clean and dry, to wash with soap and water if darkfield examination for *T. pallidum* is not envisaged but to use only saline baths if the darkfield examination is to be carried out or repeated.

For further details on various aspects of genital ulcer disease, the reader is referred to the chapters on individual diseases.

Inguinal bubo in men and women

A bubo is a painful swelling of the lymph nodes in the inguinal region. It occurs as a result of acute suppurative inguinal lymphadenitis. A bubo can result from any kind of acute infection of the skin on the pubic area, genitals, buttocks, anus, thighs, legs, feet and toes. A bubo may occur in STI such as chancroid and lymphogranuloma venereum (LGV). However, swollen and palpable lymph nodes may also occur in syphilis and in HIV infection, but as these are not painful or tender, they cannot really be considered as buboes.

If patients with enlarged non-painful inguinal lymph nodes also have generalized lymphadenopathy they should be referred for further investigations.

The flowchart in Fig. 10.1.3. describes the management of bubo in men and women. A history should be taken and an examination carried out in all patients who present with the complaint of having a swelling in the groin. From the examination, it should be determined whether the swelling is really a bubo or simply enlarged lymph nodes or any other pathology. A bubo is usually painful, warm and tender to palpation. The bubo may be one large mass (unilocular bubo) or a collection of smaller painful swellings (multilocular bubo). At times there may be abscess formation and fluctuation in the bubo.

Once it is confirmed that a bubo is present, the patient should be examined for ulcers on the external genitals, anus, perineum, labia minora, vagina, buttocks and lower limbs. The finding of any infected focus should be noted. If in a person with a bubo a genital ulcer is found, the patient should be treated for genital ulcer disease (Fig 10.1.2, Box 10.1.2). If the patient has only a bubo and no genital lesions, then he/she should be treated for LGV (Box 10.1.2).

The flowchart (Fig. 10.1.3) also instructs clinicians to aspirate fluctuant buboes. Fluctuant buboes may be aspirated as follows:

- If at the time of the first visit, or at any following visit, the bubo has become fluctuant and an abscess has formed, the abscess should be

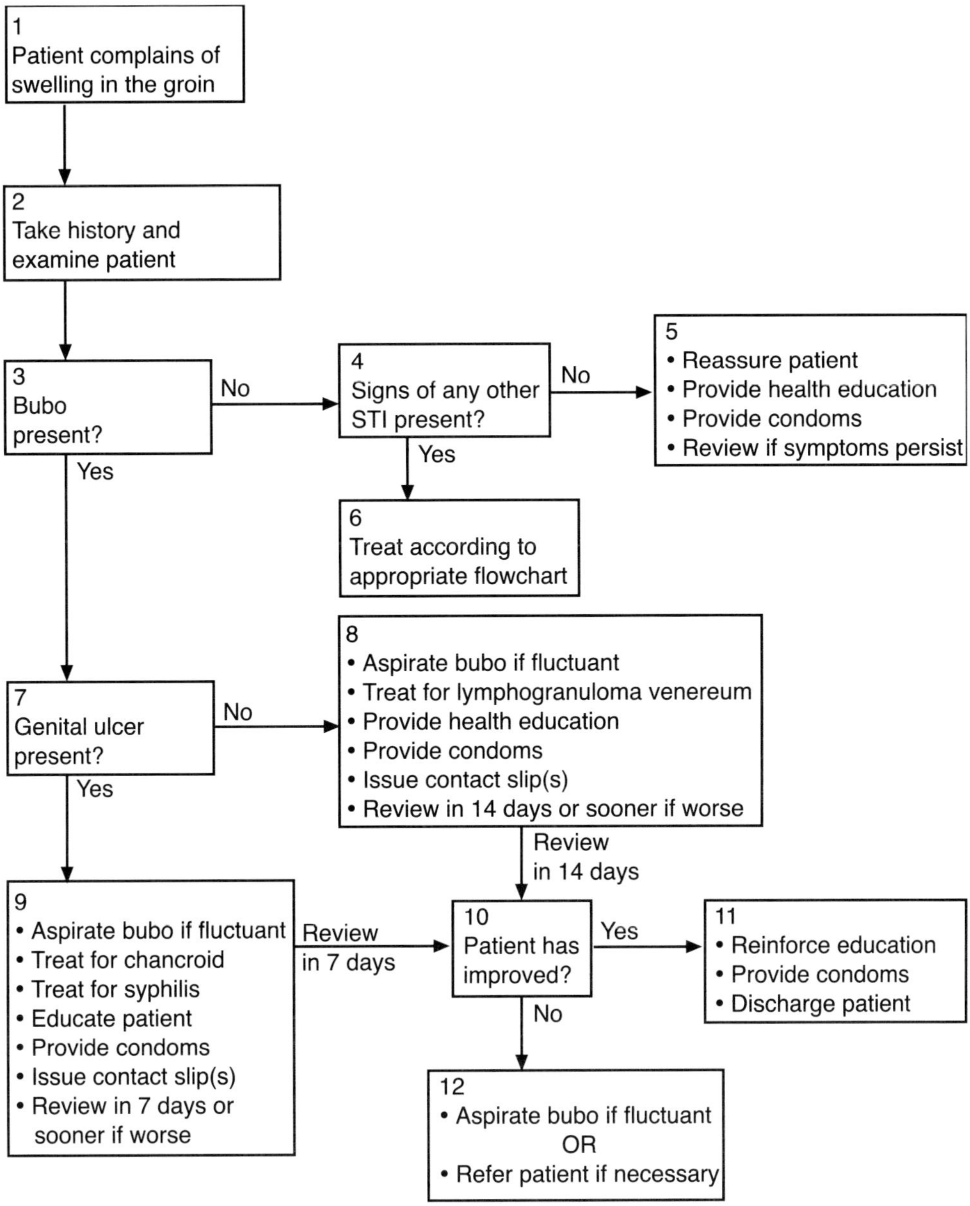

Fig. 10.1.3. Flowchart for the management of bubo in males and females.

aspirated with a wide bore needle attached to a syringe. The aspiration may need to be carried out every 2 or 3 days. When aspirating the bubo, the bubo should be entered through the surrounding normal skin.

- The formation of an abscess after initial treatment does not mean that treatment failure has occurred.

Scrotal swelling

A serious complication of gonococcal urethritis and chlamydial urethritis is infection of the epididymis which becomes swollen, hot and excruciatingly painful. The testis often is also involved. If early effective therapy is not given, the inflammatory process will resolve and healing occurs with fibrous scarring of the epididymis and destruction of testicular tissue. This will render the patient subfertile. Other causes of acute epididymo-orchitis include the mumps virus and infection with the bacterium *Escherichia coli*; the latter may occur as a complication of urinary tract infection. Other conditions which can cause acute testicular pain and/or swelling include torsion of the testis, traumatic haematocoele and testicular tumour. A swollen scrotum may be the result of inguinal hernia, hydrocoele or varicocoele.

Patients with acute swelling of the scrotum should be managed according to the guidelines laid out in Fig. 10.1.4. Clinicians are instructed to take a history from the patient and carry out a physical examination. Those patients suspected of having a surgical condition, e.g. torsion, trauma or tumour, need to be referred, while those that have epididymo-orchitis are treated for gonococcal and chlamydial infection. Infection is strongly suspected if the patient also has evidence of urethritis or gives a history of recently having had urethral discharge or dysuria. Specific antimicrobial therapy for gonococcal and chlamydial infection is listed in Box 10.1.2.

Balanitis/balanoposthitis

Balanitis is defined as inflammation of the glans penis while balanoposthitis is defined as inflammation of the foreskin and the glans penis. Balanitis and balanoposthitis may occur as a result of infection, chemical irritation, hypersensitivity reaction, skin disease or autoimmune diseases (see also Chapter 11.5) The condition is infrequent in circumcized men.

One of the common causes is poor hygiene. Persons who do not regularly wash the glans penis, which requires retraction of the foreskin, develop an accumulation of smegma which is a good medium for bacterial growth.

An equally common cause is fungal infection, especially *C. albicans* which occurs more frequently and more severely in persons with glycosuria (e.g. diabetes mellitus) and in those with immunosuppression due to drugs or HIV infection. The patient may experience irritation, a rash or redness of the glans penis. The glans penis is inflamed and often covered with tiny red papules or a white exudate (see Chapter 8.1). The inner surface of the prepuce may have a similar appearance and the edge may be fissured and swollen. The oedematous prepuce may become phimosed and difficult to retract (check urine for sugar if the glycosuria status is unknown).

Balanoposthitis may be caused by *Trichomonas vaginalis*. The patient will complain of itchiness of the foreskin and the glans penis and may have erythema of the glans penis and occasionally a subpreputial discharge. Itchiness may lead to excoriation of the foreskin.

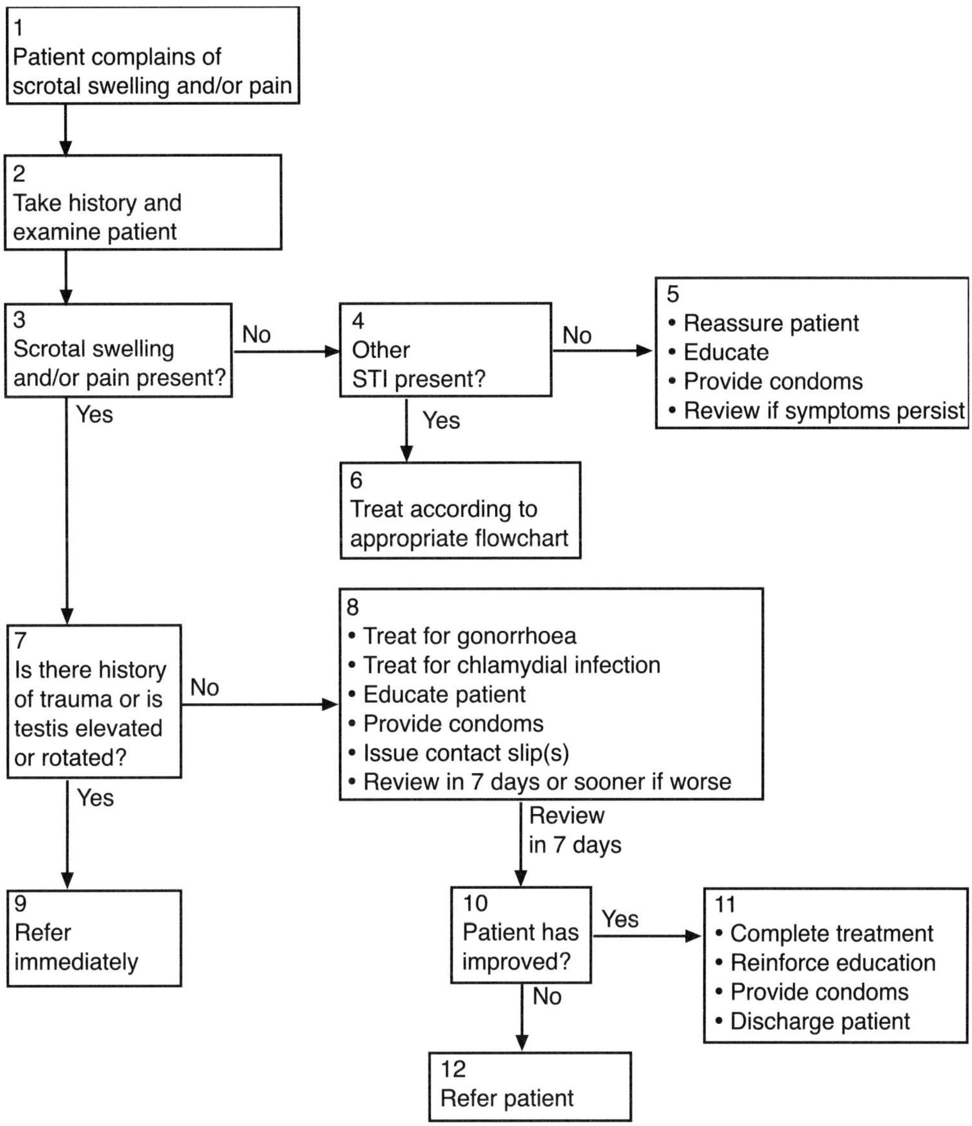

Fig. 10.1.4. Flowchart for the management of acute scrotal swelling.

Occasionally balanoposthitis is caused by fusospirochaetes which tend to invade the subpreputial space, especially in persons with poor genital hygiene and a tight and long foreskin. These organisms are spirochaetes but are not related to the spirochaete that causes syphilis, and they are often associated with anaerobes, especially *Bacteroides* spp. The patient may complain of itchiness/soreness of the foreskin and glans penis as well as a smelly discharge. On examination, preputial oedema, a subpreputial discharge and a number of superficial erosions will be found on the glans penis and the inner surface of the foreskin, i.e. erosive balanoposthitis. The subpreputial discharge will need to be differentiated from urethral discharge (see Chapter 7.4).

The flowchart (Fig. 10.1.5) instructs clinicians to take history and examine patients for genital ulcers or other STI. Patients found to have genital ulcers should be managed according to the genital ulcer disease flowchart (Fig. 10.1.2). If no genital ulcers are found, the patient should be treated for fungal infection in the first instance. If this fails, then treat for trichomoniasis and anaerobic bacterial infection, and treat the sexual partner as well.

The treatment of fungal infection is as follows: gentian violet, 1% aqueous solution applied to the glans penis twice daily for 3 days, *or* nystatin or clotrimazole cream, applied to the glans penis twice daily for 7 days, *plus* (for prevention) provide advice on local hygiene to wash the glans penis and underneath the foreskin regularly with soap and water, but to avoid excessive washing with soap.

The treatment for trichomoniasis and anaerobic bacterial infection is as follows: metronidazole, 2 g in a single oral dose. Give the sexual partner the following treatment: metronidazole, 2 g in a single oral dose, *or* 200 mg orally three times daily for 7 days, *plus* either nystatin pessaries, 100,000 units intravaginally daily for 14 days *or* clotrimazole, 500 mg pessary intravaginally to be inserted at night as a single dose.

Note: do not use metronidazole or avoid it in high dose in the first trimester of pregnancy and breastfeeding.

Vaginal discharge (see also Chapter 10.2)

The problem-oriented management of women presenting with vaginal discharge is not as straightforward as that of urethral discharge in men. Apart from being physiological, vaginal discharge is commonly caused by *T. vaginalis* and anaerobic bacteria, and sometimes by *C. albicans*. These agents are all causes of vaginitis/vaginosis and do not produce serious sequelae. However, other more serious causes of vaginal discharge are *Neisseria gonorrhoeae* and *C. trachomatis*; both these agents cause a cervicitis which in turn may lead to ascending infection resulting in pelvic inflammatory disease (PID) which is a serious consequence of infection. Therefore, cervicitis needs to be treated effectively as quickly as possible. A simple solution to the management of vaginal discharge in the PHC setting would, therefore, be to treat all women with vaginal discharge for all five infections. This, however, would mean unacceptable overtreatment, and therefore some methods should be developed to distinguish between vaginitis and cervicitis. Since PHC facilities do not usually have the manpower and equipment necessary to make a laboratory diagnosis, methods to distinguish between vaginitis and cervicitis should be simple and not laboratory-dependent.

It is known that the symptom of vaginal discharge is neither sensitive nor specific for any of the five causes of vaginitis or cervicitis. Additionally, as mixed infections occur frequently, it is not possible to exclude cervical

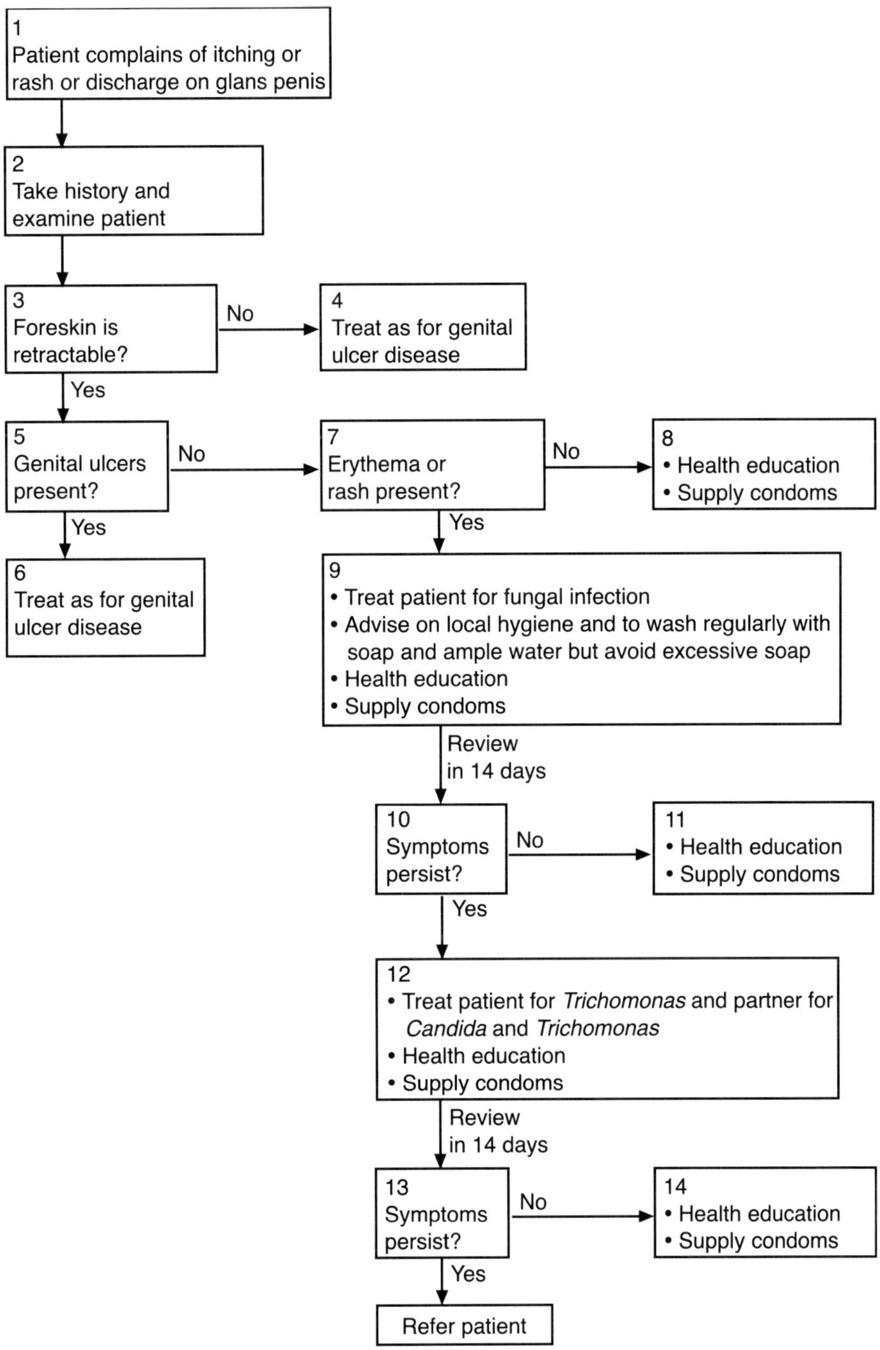

Fig. 10.1.5. Flowchart for the management of balanitis and balanoposthitis.

infection on a clinical basis. Laboratory tests are necessary to exclude the causes of cervicitis confidently. The tests that currently are available can only be performed in sophisticated laboratories which have trained personnel and equipment to carry out bacterial culture and ELISA tests or fluorescent microscopy.

Recent studies carried out in a number of countries have shown that an assessment of risk may help in distinguishing between cervical and vaginal infection. Thus, in women presenting with the symptom of vaginal discharge, cervical infection is assumed to be present if *either* the patient's partner is symptomatic, i.e. she says that her partner has urethral discharge or genital ulcers *or* if the patient falls into any two of the following categories: age less than 20 years, single marital status, more than one sexual partner in the preceding 3 months, new sexual partner in the preceding 3 months.

It is, therefore, recommended that a risk assessment for 'cervicitis' be carried out in any woman who complains of vaginal discharge, and if the risk assessment is positive then she is treated for both cervicitis and vaginitis, but if the risk assessment is negative she is treated for vaginitis only.

For the protocol for the management of vaginal discharge at the PHC level, see Chapter 10.2.

Lower abdominal pain in women

Lower abdominal pain is common in women and may reflect minor or serious illness such as PID (see Chapter 10.3). All women presenting with lower abdominal pain should be examined carefully to exclude conditions such as ectopic pregnancy, abortion or any other cause of acute abdomen requiring immediate referral for specialist attention.

The clinical diagnosis of PID may be difficult to make, and can only be confirmed by laparoscopy or laparotomy. However, the condition should be suspected in all women who complain of lower abdominal pain and who have irregular menstruation, vaginal bleeding, dyspareunia, pelvic pain, vaginal discharge and fever, and in whom a clinical examination reveals pelvic tenderness, cervical excitation tenderness or a tubo-ovarian mass. The treatment of PID should include treatment for gonococcal, chlamydial and anaerobic bacterial infection (see Chapter 10.3).

For the protocol for the management of lower abdominal pain at the PHC level, see Chapter 10.3.

Ophthalmia neonatorum

Ophthalmia neonatorum is defined as purulent conjunctivitis occurring in a baby less than 1 month of age. The common STI-related causes are *N. gonorrhoeae* and *C. trachomatis*, the infection having been acquired at the time of birth during passage through the birth canal. Other causes include *E. coli*, *Staphylococcus aureus* and *Streptococcus pneumoniae*. Ophthalmia neonatorum is an important condition as firstly, if it is caused by *N. gonorrhoeae* it can lead to blindness, and secondly, the condition is entirely preventable.

Gonococcal infection, which is usually a superficial epithelial infection (conjunctivitis), can lead to infection of the cornea (keratitis) if not treated effectively. The keratitis eventually resolves with scarring of the cornea and the cornea becomes opacified. This leads to blindness. Hence it is recommended that all neonates with conjunctivitis are treated for gonorrhoea in the first instance. If in 48 h the infection does not show signs of resolution, then treatment for chlamydial infection is given.

The flowchart for the management of ophthalmia neonatorum is shown in Fig. 10.1.6. When obtaining a history from the mother, the following points should be noted: age of baby, method of delivery, place of delivery, whether ophthalmia prophylaxis was instituted, and whether the mother or the baby's father have any symptoms.

The baby is then examined to determine whether there is purulent conjunctivitis. Remember that often newborn babies have blocked lacrimal ducts and tear production is excessive. The mother might be worried about this alone.

If on examination purulent conjunctivitis is confirmed, the baby is treated for gonococcal ophthalmia neonatorum (Box 10.1.2) while the mother and father are treated for gonorrhoea and chlamydial infection as described previously. (Tetracycline and the tetracycline analogues should not be used in pregnant and lactating women; instead erythromycin should be used.) If, however, purulent conjunctivitis is not found, then the mother is reassured and advised to return with the baby if symptoms persist.

The baby is seen in 48 h and if the conjunctivitis has resolved or is much better, no further treatment is necessary unless the conjunctivitis re-starts. If the eyes are still sticky, the baby is treated with erythromycin orally and tetracycline eye ointment topically. The specific antimicrobial therapy of gonococcal and chlamydial ophthalmia neonatorum is listed in Box 10.1.2.

Prevention of ophthalmia neonatorum

All babies should have ophthalmia prophylaxis carried out as follows:

- As soon as the baby is born, mop both eyes with dry clean cotton wool.
- Then instill 1% tetracycline eye ointment into the lower conjunctival sacs of both eyes.
- The baby's eyes are usually swollen soon after birth and may be difficult to open; therefore the eyes should be opened and the eye ointment instilled carefully so that it is placed in the lower conjunctival sacs and not on the eyelids.

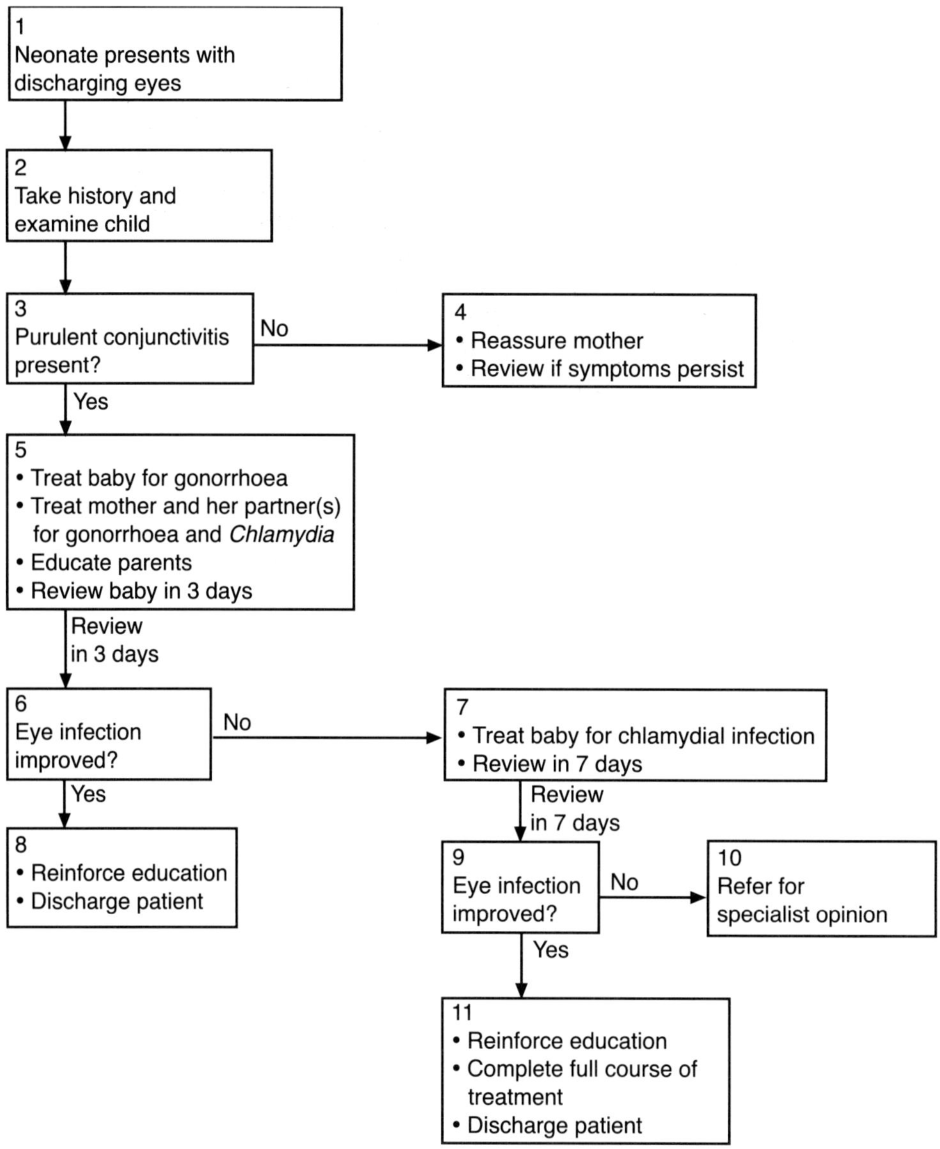

Fig. 10.1.6. Flowchart for the management of ophthalmia neonatorum.

Generalized lymphadenopathy

Generalized lymphadenopathy may occur in a large number of infectious and non-infectious diseases. These include tuberculosis, syphilis, cytomegalovirus infection, HIV infection, toxoplasmosis, Epstein–Barr virus infection, cryptococcosis, histoplasmosis, septic skin conditions, leukaemias, lymphomas and Kaposi's sarcoma. The commonest clinical manifestation of HIV infection is symmetrical generalized lymph node enlargement which occurs fairly early during the course of the infection. The enlarged lymph nodes are most easily palpated in the groins, neck, axillae and in the submental area, and are generally painless, firm, mobile and rubbery. On clinical examination, the lymphadenopathy of HIV infection is not distinguishable from that in secondary syphilis. Other features of each infection should always be looked for. Persons with secondary syphilis may have a healing genital ulcer, condylomata lata, moist papules or non-pruritic macular, papular or squamous rashes. The patients with HIV infection may have fever, night sweats, weight loss, pruritus, skin rash, cough, headache, oral hairy leukoplakia, hyperpigmented nails and oral or genital herpes.

The flowchart in Fig. 10.1.7 gives guidance on the management of persons with generalized lymphadenopathy. The patient should have a history taken and then be examined carefully. In the history, the patients should be asked the duration of the swellings and whether they have had a genital ulcer in the previous 3 months. The clinician ought to confirm that the swellings are in fact lymph nodes. The distribution and size of the lymph nodes should be noted. All patients should be examined for signs of HIV infection and syphilis. In persons with generalized lymphadenopathy, the important conditions to exclude are syphilis, tuberculosis and HIV infection.

If the patient with generalized lymphadenopathy is found to have a genital ulcer or gives a history of having had a genital ulcer, then secondary syphilis should be strongly suspected. Persons with genital ulcers should be treated for both syphilis and chancroid according to the flowchart for the management of genital ulcer disease. All patients, regardless of whether or not they have features of syphilis, should have blood tests to exclude syphilis. Patients requiring referral include those with evidence of Kaposi's sarcoma anywhere on the skin or in the mouth, those in whom there is asymmetric enlargement of lymph nodes or in whom a lymph node measures more than 3 cm in diameter, and those in whom tuberculosis is suspected. Such patients need investigation in a centre where facilities for chest X-ray and biopsy are available.

If the patient has generalized lymphadenopathy and none of the other features described in the flowchart, he/she should be referred to a centre where investigations for syphilis, HIV infection and other conditions may be carried out. Once a specific diagnosis has been made, the patient should be managed accordingly.

Genital warts

Genital warts are caused by the human papillomavirus (HPV). Both overt and subclinical infections occur. Genital warts usually affect sexually active young adults. The infection is spread by direct sexual contact. The average incubation period is about 3 months but may be as long as 9 months. HPV also causes the common skin warts and flat warts. The transmission of the virus strain that causes skin warts (through skin abrasions) is not related to sexual activity. The strains of HPV that cause genital warts are known as the 'genital strains',

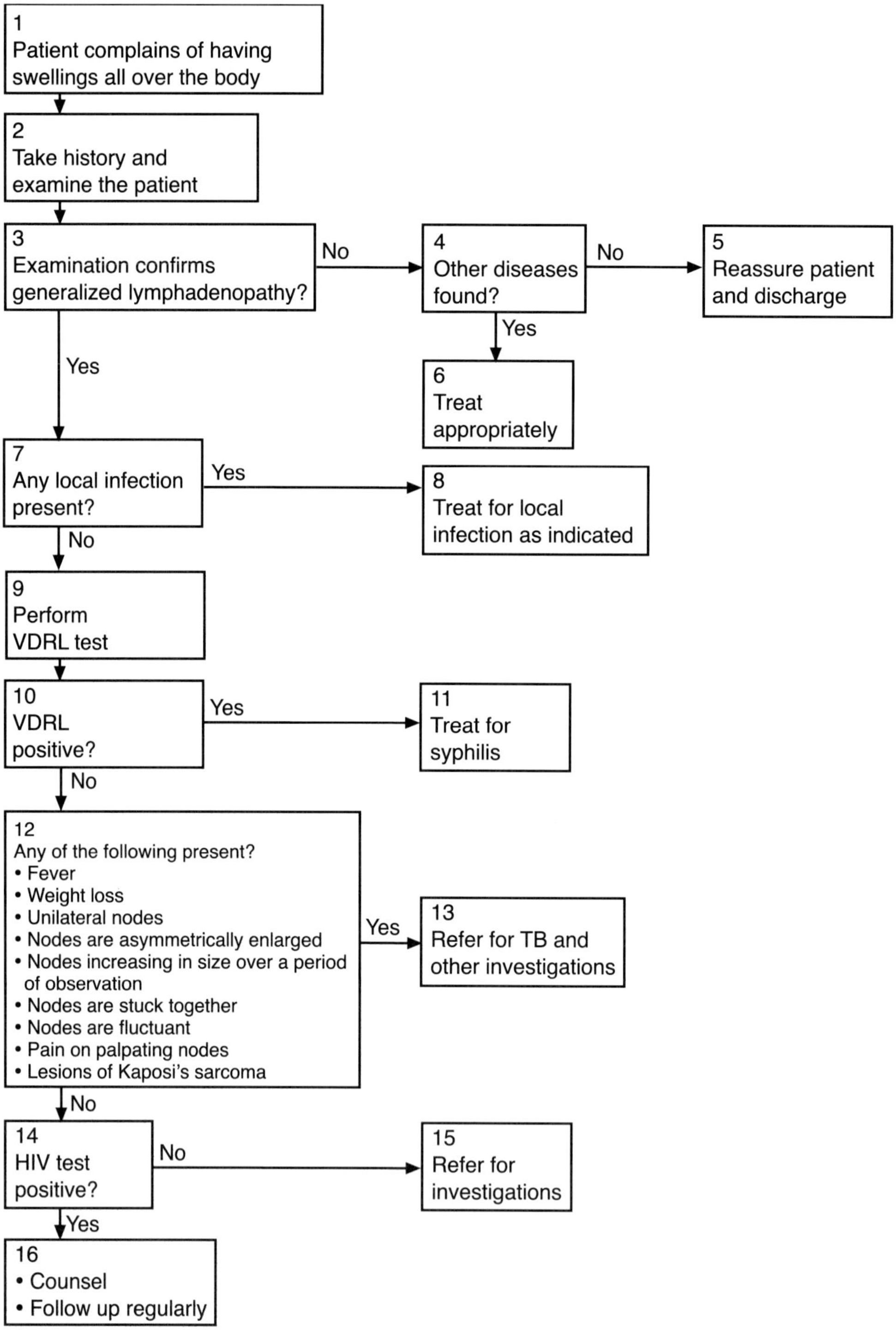

Fig. 10.1.7. Flowchart for the management of generalized lymphadenopathy.

while the strains that cause warts in sites other than the genital region are commonly referred to as the 'non-genital' strains. It is known that the 'genital strains' can infect non-genital sites such as the anus and perianal areas. Anal warts are commonly found in men and women with genital warts. Infants born to mothers with genital warts can develop oral and laryngeal papillomas, infection having been acquired during birth while passing through the birth canal.

There are a number of different strains of HPV. Some strains cause oral lesions, others cause genital warts, while other cause cervical cancer (see Chapters 6.5 and 11.3).

Warts in men are usually of the exophytic type and are known as condylomata acuminata. These are large and fleshy. They often appear first on the frenum of the glans penis, the coronal sulcus, the glans penis and the inner surface of the foreskin. They can also appear on the shaft of the penis, the scrotum and around the anus or inside the anus. Genital warts may also appear in the urethral meatus. Wart lesions are usually multiple.

Men may also develop flat warts which usually appear on the glans penis. They are difficult to see but become prominent after the application of 5% acetic acid to the mucosal surface. They are also multiple.

In women, exophytic warts may be found anywhere on the external genitalia, on the perineum, in the perianal area, inside the anus, and inside the vagina and on the cervix. Flat warts can be found on the cervix, and show up as white flat patches with the application of 5% acetic acid.

Management of genital warts

The patient should have history taken, be examined carefully to confirm warts and checked for any other condition. Comprehensive case management should be given to all patients with genital warts. The treatment of exophytic warts is to remove them by chemical or physical means. Flat warts should be cauterized.

Chemical destruction

Podophyllin 25% in tincture of benzoin is applied carefully to the warts, allowed to dry, and then covered with talcum powder. After 2–4 h this is washed off with soap and water. This treatment is applied twice a week. If there is no improvement in 6 weeks, the treatment modality should be changed or the patient referred to a higher medical centre.

Podophyllin should not be used on the cervix, urethra or anus, and should not be used during pregnancy.

Alternatively, trichloracetic acid 90% (a caustic agent) is carefully applied to the warts, then covered with talcum powder, once a week, It may be effective for small warts and is safe in pregnancy. If there is no response after six applications, the treatment should be changed or the patient referred.

Physical destruction

Warts may be excised surgically or may be removed by electrocautery or cryotherapy.

Chapter 10.2
Vaginal discharge

V. Chandeying
Department of Obstetrics and Gynaecology, Prince of Songkla University, Hat Yai, Thailand

Vaginal discharge is one of the most common complaints in women. Vaginal discharge may be considered to be abnormal if it is excessive at times other than pre- and post-menstruation, or if it is malodorous, creamy, yellow or purulent. It must be emphasized that many women who are harbouring STI agent(s) neither experience nor show any abnormal discharge.

Aetiology

Box 10.2.1 shows the common causes of vaginal discharge.

General considerations

1. The symptoms and appearance of vaginal discharge may suggest a cause but are not reliable for accurate diagnosis.
2. The confirmation of diagnosis depends on the demonstration of the aetiologic agent(s) or other criteria as in the case of bacterial vaginosis.
3. Not infrequently, cervicitis coexists with vaginitis, i.e. concurrent infections are common. Thus gonococcal/chlamydial/infections of the cervix, non-gonococcal non-chlamydial mucopurulent cervicitis, trichomoniasis, bacterial vaginosis and candidiasis may occur in various combinations.
4. The treatment, in the absence of laboratory facilities, may, therefore, need to take the possibility of concurrent infections into account. Knowledge of the local frequency of various combinations will determine the cost-effective treatment regimen(s). Drug safety must also be paramount.
5. The treatment regimen may include therapy for gonorrhoea with efficacy of not less than 95%.
6. Drug acceptability influences compliance and hence the outcome of treatment. The single or short duration oral drug regimens are preferable to injections.
7. Prompt treatment of sexual partner(s) prevents ping-pong infection, reduces transmission of disease and decreases the frequency of occurrence of adverse sequelae of infection.

Box 10.2.1. Causes of vaginal discharge.

Physiological
Puberty, menstrual cycle, sexual arousal, pregnancy

Pathological
Non-infective:
Chemical vaginitis: antiseptics, bath additives, deodorants, douches, spermicides
Foreign body: intrauterine contraceptive device, retained tampons, retained condoms, etc.
Gynaecological: tumours, fistulae, etc.

Infective:
Cervical infections: *Chlamydia trachomatis, Neisseria gonorrhoeae,* herpes simplex virus
Vaginal infections: *Candida* spp., *Trichomonas vaginalis,* bacterial vaginosis (BV) organisms

8. It is recommended that all patients return for evaluation of the outcome of the treatment. The outcome may be classified as: (i) cure or complete response, i.e. resolution of symptoms and signs and elimination of the diagnostic markers(s), (ii) partial response, i.e. asymptomatic carrier state, and (iii) failure or resistance to therapy, i.e. persistence of symptoms, signs as well as the diagnostic marker(s). When the outcome is partial response or failure, the patient needs re-treatment (or referral) and follow-up for re-assessment.

Approaches to diagnosis and management at the PHC level

The observations and recommendations that follow are based on the author's experience in Thailand. As a result, the protocol suggested may not be appropriate in other situations, where it should be evaluated and modified if indicated.

Speculum examination and microscopy possible

Any foreign body in the vagina such as a retained tampon or condom, etc. (Plate 118) will be obvious and should be removed. In the absence of any other cause of vaginal discharge, no further treatment is required.

Antiseptics should not be applied to the vaginal speculum for vaginal examination. The quality and quantity of vaginal discharge and the state of the vaginal walls are assessed, followed by measurement of the pH of the vaginal fluid and the amine test (see Chapter 4). Vaginal secretion for microscopy can be sampled from the speculum blade. All medical attendants should be able to perform microscopy which has the following advantages:

- The result is available immediately.
- The delay incurred as a result of sending the specimen to the laboratory may adversely affect the demonstration of the motility of *Trichomonas vaginalis.*
- Learning by doing helps to correlate the clinical and laboratory findings, thus enhancing the clinical acumen.

Wet preparation and Gram stain

A drop of the vaginal secretion is mixed with a drop of saline. This preparation may be warmed for a second on a spirit lamp in order to increase the motility of trichomonads. The sensitivity of a wet preparation to detect *T. vaginalis* and *Candida* spp. is about 80%. Clue cells are also identified readily in a wet film. However, if the medical attendant is inexperienced or if the specimen has to be sent to a distant laboratory or has to be examined later, then Gram stain is an appropriate option for the diagnosis of bacterial vaginosis.

See also the protocol for the management of vaginal discharge at the PHC level (Fig. 10.2.1) and Chapters 7.8, 8.1 and 9.1 for treatment of bacterial vaginosis, candidiasis and trichomoniasis.

An important step in the evaluation of vaginal discharge is exclusion of cervical infection which is more serious than vaginal infections.

Cervical appearance, specimens and infections

The cervix is inspected after the ectocervix is wiped clean of vaginal material. Any ectopy, oedema, warts, ulcer(s), etc. are noted and the quality of endocervical secretion is assessed.

The term ectropion, sometimes interchanged with the term ectopy, has also been used to describe the patulous parous cervix which gapes and exposes the endocervical columnar epithelium as the blades of the vaginal speculum are opened. There is also confusion between cervicitis and simple ectopy, the latter being associated with changes in the cervix over the reproductive period and during the menstrual cycle. Ectopy *per se*, i.e. not associated with congestion/oedema and/or mucopurulent exudate, is a normal finding and requires no therapy.

Mucopurulent cervicitis may be associated with infection due to *Chlamydia trachomatis, Neisseria gonorrhoeae* and HSV. The last may, in addition, manifest as superficial erosions of the ectocervical squamous epithelium. In some cases, no cause is found. Whereas an experienced eye can often correctly identify cervical mucopus, it does not always prove to be so when subjected to microscopy. A yellowish colour of the pus as compared with the white colour of the swab may sometimes help. With regard to the number of polymorphonuclear leukocytes (PMN) per high power field to define cervicitis, unfortunately, and unlike urethritis in men, there is no agreed cut off point between a normal and abnormal number of PMN in a cervical smear. Both the sensitivity and specificity of these features to diagnose chlamydial and gonococcal infection are unacceptably low (see Table 10.2.1). Further research is needed to unravel more accurate predictors for these conditions.

For the present, if Gram-negative intracellular diplococci suggestive of gonococcal infection are found in a Gram-stained endocervical smear (sensitivity < 65%), or if the partner recently has been treated for gonorrhoea, a treatment regimen effective against gonococci as well as chlamydial infection should be used (see Chapters 7.4 and 7.5, and Box 10.1.2). Chlamydial infection should always be suspected in women with mucopurulent cervicitis (or if the partner recently has been treated for urethritis) whether or not intracellular diplococci are found. Thus the treatment regimen for such women

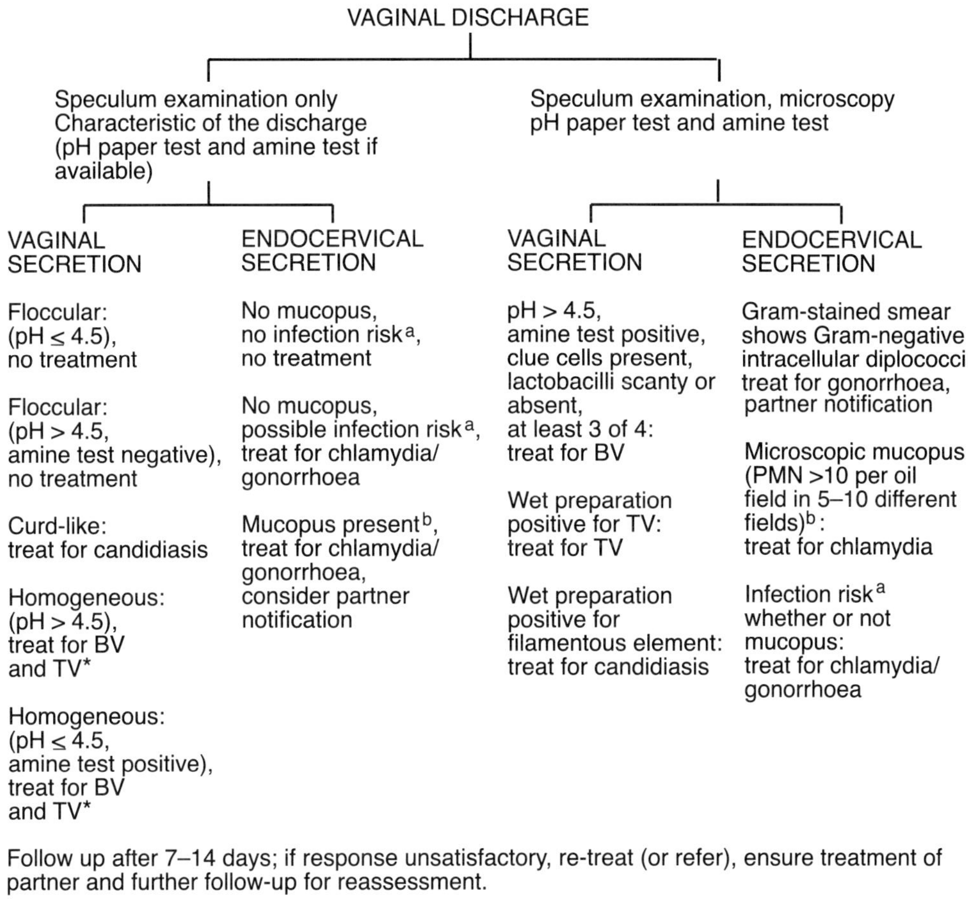

Fig. 10.2.1. Management of vaginal discharge at the PHC level. [a]'Infection risk' means history of unprotected sex with a partner with presumed gonorrhoea or NGU; [b]sensitivity and specificity low (see text); BV, bacterial vaginosis; TV, *T. vaginalis* infection; *metronidazole will cover both BV and TV; treat partner if response unsatisfactory.

should include an antimicrobial active against chlamydial infection. However, if mucopurulent cervicitis persists, as may happen in an occasional case of 'non-specific' cervicitis, an alternative treatment regimen may be prescribed or the patient referred to a higher medical centre.

Speculum examination only possible

In the setting where microscopy is not possible, the diagnosis has to be based on clinical assessment, which requires speculum examination. Obviously, the clinician needs to possess considerable experience in identifying the various clinical features. Vaginal discharge may be classified as floccular (normal), curd-like and homogeneous, and the endocervical discharge as mucopurulent or non-mucopurulent. The sensitivities and specificities of these discharges with respect to the specific infections, supported by comprehensive laboratory testing at a district teaching hospital, are shown in Table 10.2.1. Whereas the sensitivity and specificity of the 'mucopurulent discharge' in the endocervix for the diagnosis of chlamydial and gonococcal infections are unacceptably low (see above), the diagnosis of baterial vaginosis would improve if pH and amine tests are available. The observations in Table 10.2.1 form the basis of the 'speculum examination only' section of the protocol (Fig. 10.2.1). In view of the difficulty in excluding cervical infection, some experts have suggested the use of 'risk assessment' described in Chapter 10.1.

Non-infectious leukorrhoea

Some patients may complain of excessive, usually white, non-smelly vaginal discharge. Clinical examination is normal with an abundance of lactobacilli in the vaginal smear and no known cause is found. The patient should be reassured, and, if appropriate, advised about perineal hygiene. If there is no response, the patient should be re-assessed.

Perineal hygiene

In the female, the position of the urethral orifice, the entrance of the vagina and the anus are all close together. This proximity can result in infection of the former with faecal bacteria and/or secondary spread of *N. gonorrhoeae* from the cervix via the vagina to the anus and rectum. Therefore, cleanliness around the sex organs is important and the following suggestions may be considered for patient education:

1. After defaecation and sexual intercourse, wash the area with water and dry thoroughly before putting on underwear.
2. After defaecation, wipe and wash from front to back or from vagina to anus to avoid faecal entry into the vagina. If underwear is soiled, it should be changed.

Table 10.2.1. Sensitivity and specificity of vaginal and cervical discharge/cervicitis in relation to a definitive diagnosis.

Type of discharge/indicator	Diagnosis	Sensitivity (%)	Specificity (%)
Floccular	Normal	81	90
Curd-like	Candidiasis	72	100
Homogeneous	Bacterial vaginosis/ trichomoniasis	94	88
Visible endocervical mucopus	Chlamydial and/or gonococcal infection	36	86
Microscopic endocervical mucopus (>10 PMN per oil field in 5–10 different fields)	Chlamydial and/or gonococcal infection	64	69

Taken from Chandeying *et al.* (1998).

3. Avoid wearing nylon and rayon underwear which allow moisture to be retained for longer than is the case with cotton underwear. Synthetic materials should also be avoided by those allergic to them.
4. In hot weather, underwear needs changing more frequently.
5. After washing, underwear should preferably be hung in the sun, so that they are thoroughly dry before re-use.
6. The vagina should not be spray-washed as it may allow the carriage of bacteria from the vagina into the uterine cavity. If necessary, the vagina can be cleaned with the fingers. The finger nails should be kept short to avoid risk of trauma.
7. Vaginal douching with antiseptics is unnecessary and may cause irritation, and damage the vaginal epithelium.
8. When there are symptoms indicating the possibility of vaginal infection (e.g. an unusual discharge, smell, irritation, difficult or frequent urination, ulcers), then it is advisable to seek medical attention.

Further reading

Chandeying, V., Skov, S., Kemapunmanus, M., Law, M., Geatar, A. and Rowe, P. (1998) Evaluation of two clinical protocols for the management of women with vaginal discharge in Southern Thailand. *Sexually Transmitted Infections* 74, 194–201.

Syndromic Approaches to STD Management. *Sexually Transmitted Infections* (1998) 74 (Suppl. 1), S1–S178.

World Health Organization (1991) *Report of a WHO Study Group: Management of Patients with Sexually Transmitted Diseases*, WHO Technical Report Series No. 810, World Health Organization, Geneva.

CHAPTER 10.3
Pelvic inflammatory disease and perihepatitis

V. Chandeying

Department of Obstetrics and Gynaecology, Prince of Songkla University, Hat Yai, Thailand

Pelvic inflammatory disease (PID) is a clinical syndrome associated with ascending infection of the female upper genital tract. The syndrome covers a wide range of disorders which include: endometritis, parametritis, salpingitis, oophoritis, salpingo-oophoritis, pelvic peritonitis, pyosalpinx, tubo-ovarian abscess and pelvic abscess. The infection may also spread to the liver to cause perihepatitis (Fitz–Hugh–Curtis syndrome) described below.

Epidemiology

The incidence of PID in developing countries is unknown. However, prevalence rates of chlamydial and gonococcal infections which are the most important causes of PID, of around 10% among gynaecology, antenatal and family planning clinic attenders in urban areas, as well as in population-based studies in rural areas, have been widely reported in sub-Saharan Africa (see also Chapter 1). Many of these women remain untreated mainly because of lack of appropriate health care facilities, also because of ignorance and poverty. Of these women, 10–20% will develop PID, which is a very common cause of hospital admission in these countries. A proportion of those affected will develop recurrent episodes. Some of these women are likely to be re-infected by their male partners who often acquire infection from (or exchange infection with) sex workers.

In addition, postpartum infection as a result of primitive midwifery and induced abortions are not uncommon, serving as important risk factors for PID with or without the presence of concurrent chlamydial or gonococcal infection.

Thus there is a considerable potential for a significant proportion of women to be exposed to the risk of PID and the resulting sequelae such as infertility, ectopic pregnancy and chronic pelvic pain.

Aetiology

The aetiology includes exogenous sexually transmitted pathogens such as *C. trachomatis*, *N. gonorrhoeae*, and possibly also *M. hominis*, *U. urealytium* and HSV (STI-associated PID), and endogenous flora of the lower genital tract (Table 10.3.1).

Other exogenous risk factors include iatrogenic infection associated with gynaecological procedures such as dilatation and curettage, hysterosalpingography, primitive midwifery, induced abortion and insertion of an intrauterine contraceptive device (IUCD). All of these may also serve as predisposing factors for STI-associated PID if the patient is already harbouring sexually transmitted pathogen(s) which had remained undetected. In this context, IUCD-associated risk is thought to be confined to the first 20 days following insertion.

Other risk factors are young age, age at first sexual intercourse, multiple sex partners, the presence of bacterial vaginosis, vaginal douching and history of STI. Oral contraceptives seem to decrease the risk of infection ascending to the upper genital tract possibly by: (i) progesterone effect on the cervical mucus which becomes more dense and (ii) decreasing the uterine muscular activity.

Some patients, especially if not very ill, may be infected with a single pathogen such as *N. gonorrhoeae* or *C. trachomatis*. In many patients with PID, however, multiple organisms are isolated from the upper genital tract. In about 20% of cases, no cause is found.

Pathogenesis

The organisms ascend into the upper genital tract by canalicular spread, resulting in endometritis and endosalpingitis. The fallopian tubes are swollen; there is mucosal congestion and redness of the serosal surface. There are marked inflammatory changes in all the layers of the fallopian tubes. (In PID

Table 10.3.1. Aetiology of pelvic inflammatory disease.

Sexually transmitted pathogens	Other pathogens	Endogenous flora[a]
Chlamydia trachomatis	*Campylobacter fetus*	*Actinomyces israelii*
Neisseria gonorrhoeae	*Haemophilus influenzae*	*Bacteroides fragilis*
Herpes simplex virus	*Mycobacterium tuberculosis*	Other anaerobes
	Streptococcus agalactiae	*Gardnerella vaginalis*
	Streptococcus pneumoniae	*Mycoplasma hominis*
	Streptococcus pyogenes	*Ureaplasma urealyticum*
	Enterobius vermicularis	*Escherichia coli*
	Filarial worms	Other coliforms
	Schistosoma spp.	*Staphylococcus aureus*

[a]Some are sexually transmissible.

following abortion and puerperium, the infection spreads via lymphatics and veins of the uterine wall, resulting in exosalpingitis; prognosis as regards further pregnancy in these cases is more favourable than in those with endo-salpingitis.)

In some cases, the tissue damaged by STI agents (such as *C. trachomatis* and *N. gonorrhoeae*), may subsequently be invaded by the endogenous flora of the lower genital tract.

Further progression of tubal infection may result from escape of purulent exudate from the fimbrial ends of the fallopian tubes, leading to pelvic peritonitis and tubo-ovarian abscess. In later stages, the abdominal ostia of the tubes may become occluded, resulting in pyosalpinx or hydrosalpinx. Spread of infection along the paracolic gutters may cause perihepatitis.

The late sequelae include infertility due to tubal occlusion, ectopic pregnancy, chronic pelvic pain due to pelvic adhesions, and menstrual disorders. After one episode of PID, over 10% may develop tubal infertility, this risk doubling after each subsequent attack.

Pelvic infection in pregnancy

Salpingitis can occur in early pregnancy, i.e. before the chorioamnion obliterates the uterine cavity at about the fourth month.

Clinical manifestations

Symptoms

The clinical spectrum of PID ranges from asymptomatic to a life-threatening condition. However, the pathological process may be quite advanced even in asymptomatic patients. *N. gonorrhoeae*-associated PID is thought to be clinically more severe than *C. trachomatis*-associated disease.

Subacute lower abdominal pain is the most common presentation in clinical practice. The pain is usually dull, bilateral and frequently increases with movement and sexual intercourse. The patient may give a history of pain starting a few days after the last menstrual period.

Other symptoms include fever, vaginal discharge, irregular menstrual bleeding, dysmenorrhoea, dysuria, nausea, vomiting, pain in the right hypo-chondrium (possibly due to perihepatitis), and symptoms of proctitis (painful defaecation, frequency of stools, blood or mucus in stools). More severe symptoms are generally associated with the involvement of endogenous flora.

Almost all of the above symptoms are non-specific and may occur in other genitourinary and gastrointestinal tract diseases.

Signs

On examination, the patient may look ill and mildly febrile. A patient with acute pelvic pain may be anxious, pale, sweating and visibly exhausted. There may be generalized lower abdominal tenderness. Rebound tenderness associated with muscular rigidity, guarding, decreasing bowel sounds and distension, are signs of peritonitis.

There may be signs of urethritis. The vulva and vagina may appear normal, or, vaginal examination may be uncomfortable and there may be evidence of concurrent conditions such as trichomoniasis- or bacterial vaginosis-type discharge. The cervix may look normal or congested with or without mucopurulent discharge.

Pelvic examination may reveal tenderness on manipulation of the cervix to either side, as well as on manipulation of the uterus and adnexa. In severely ill patients, involuntary muscle guarding may preclude adequate palpation. Adnexal involvement is usually bilateral, although one side may be more tender than the other. About 15% of patients may reveal an adnexal mass on bimanual examination. Pelvic examination should be carried out with care. Forceful bimanual examination may in itself be painful, thus eliciting a misleading false-positive tenderness. It may be necessary to perform the examination with only one finger inserted into the posterior and then the lateral fornices, and the palm of the other hand gently pressing the lower abdomen for evaluation of uterine and adnexal tenderness. The cervical excitation is carried out by attempting to displace it anteriorly and posteriorly and then from side to side, and then the uterus is palpated bimanually. If the patient complains of pain (or shows this in her facial expression) in one area, it is preferable to start the examination in a different location.

Differential diagnosis

The differential diagnosis is usually from ectopic pregnancy, torsion of an ovarian cyst, endometriosis, appendicitis, diverticulitis, cystitis, and possibly also may include other conditions such as filariasis, schistosomiasis, tuberculosis, amoebiasis, etc.

Diagnosis

There are no specific symptoms, physical findings or laboratory tests that are pathognomonic for PID. Although clinical criteria have been established to facilitate diagnosis, they have not been standardized. Especially in the outpatient situation, a patient with a previously recorded PID is likely to be labelled with the same diagnosis again when she returns with pain. This can be potentially dangerous because other possibilities are not considered and hence a serious condition may be missed.

It is generally agreed that the minimal criteria for a clinical diagnosis of PID should include lower abdominal tenderness, cervical motion tenderness and adnexal tenderness. Although laparoscopy will confirm PID in only two-thirds of such women, this low threshold approach will lead to treatment of many genuine cases (at the cost of some overtreatment) at an early stage.

Addition of one or more fairly simple tests, such as temperature above 38°C, evidence of lower genital tract infection (inflammatory cells in greater numbers than the other cellular elements in a wet mount of vaginal fluid), elevated erythrocyte sedimentation rate (ESR) and leukocytosis of more than 10,000 mm^{-3}, and elevated C-reactive protein in serum, are reported to increase the sensitivity of the above-mentioned diagnostic criteria. Some experts would consider PID to be unlikely in the presence of a normal wet mount of vaginal contents. Clearly, the diagnosis of PID based on clinical criteria will be associated with false-positive and false-negative results.

Laparoscopy

Laparoscopy is the 'gold standard' for the diagnosis of PID because it provides visual confirmation of salpingitis (hyperaemia of the tubal surface, oedema of the tubal wall, and a sticky exudate on the surface and from the fimbrial ends). It also helps to collect specimens directly from the upper genital tract. However, laparoscopy, possible only in large hospitals, is firstly not feasible as a routine procedure, and secondly may miss a milder form without macroscopic evidence of salpingitis. Nevertheless, visualization of the pelvis by laparoscopy is strongly indicated in the differential diagnosis of problem cases.

Endometrial biopsy

This, providing histopathological evidence of endometritis, has been reported to have a high predictive value in the diagnosis of PID.

Ultrasonography

Ultrasonography techniques such as vaginal ultrasound, may aid in the diagnosis of adnexal mass as well as in the follow-up to assess resolution after treatment. This technique can be performed in an outpatient clinic, but requires expensive equipment and expertise.

Other investigations

Depending on the facilities available, tests are carried out to find the infecting organism(s). Examination of the male partner, who is often asymptomatic, and in whom the diagnosis of STI is relatively easy, may provide a clue to the cause of PID.

The investigations include: appropriate tests from the vaginal contents for bacterial vaginosis, candidiasis and trichomoniasis; appropriate specimens for *N. gonorrhoeae* and *C. trachomatis* from the urethra, endocervix, and possibly also from the endometrium and fimbrial ends of the fallopian tubes, and, after proper explanation, for *N. gonorrhoeae* only from the rectum and pharynx. (Isolates from sites other than fallopian tubes do not necessarily reflect the nature of tubal infection.) Gram-stained smears are examined for Gram-negative intracellular diplococci.

Antibody studies, e.g. chlamydial IgG and IgM antibodies in serum, may be useful especially if seroconversion can be demonstrated, but the result may come too late to be of any practical use. Besides, seroconversion is demonstrable rather infrequently.

A full STI screen should always include serology for syphilis, hepatitis B and HIV infection after appropriate information and explanation.

Treatment

(For management at the PHC level, see Fig. 10.3.1.)

The therapeutic goals in the management of PID include the prevention of the sequelae. The patient should be admitted into hospital if severely ill, if pelvic abscess is suspected, if there is evidence of pelvic peritonitis, if the diagnosis is in doubt, if the patient is pregnant, if oral treatment is not possible or if the response to out-patient treatment is unsatisfactory.

If the patient is to be treated at home, appropriate antibiotics and analgesics are prescribed and the patient is advised to rest and avoid coitus until the infection is resolved.

If an IUCD is present, it should be removed a day or two after commencing treatment. The patient will need appropriate contraceptive counselling. Whether or not the removal of IUCD results in any benefit with regard to the current episode of PID or the prevention of recurrence is unknown.

For severely ill hospitalized patients, although resuscitation is seldom needed, the patient would benefit from intravenous fluids and parenteral analgesics.

The choice of therapeutic agents

As the aetiology in many cases is polymicrobial, a combination of therapeutic agents, which should cover the most likely organisms, is used. This choice will also be determined by bed availability, costs, patient acceptance, local antimicrobial susceptibility and the physician's experience and preference. The treatment should commence before the laboratory results are to hand and may need to be revised after the results become available.

Box 10.3.1 shows examples of recommended regimens on an out-patient and in-patient basis. Mild or moderately ill patients, not requiring hospitalization, and considered to be STI associated, are likely to be infected with one or more STI agents. Accordingly, the drugs used include a cephalosporin to eliminate *N. gonorrhoeae* (including PPNG strains), and doxycycline (or tetracycline or erythromycin) to combat *C. trachomatis*. In addition, some experts include continuous anti-anaerobe therapy even for the mildly ill patients, while others consider it necessary only if the patient has concurrent BV or has had a previous episode of PID or if the condition was preceded by instrumentation. Moderately severe cases who are febrile with or without a palpable adnexal swelling may need to be hospitalized and should, in addition, receive metronidazole to cover for anaerobes. Severely ill patients (febrile, toxic

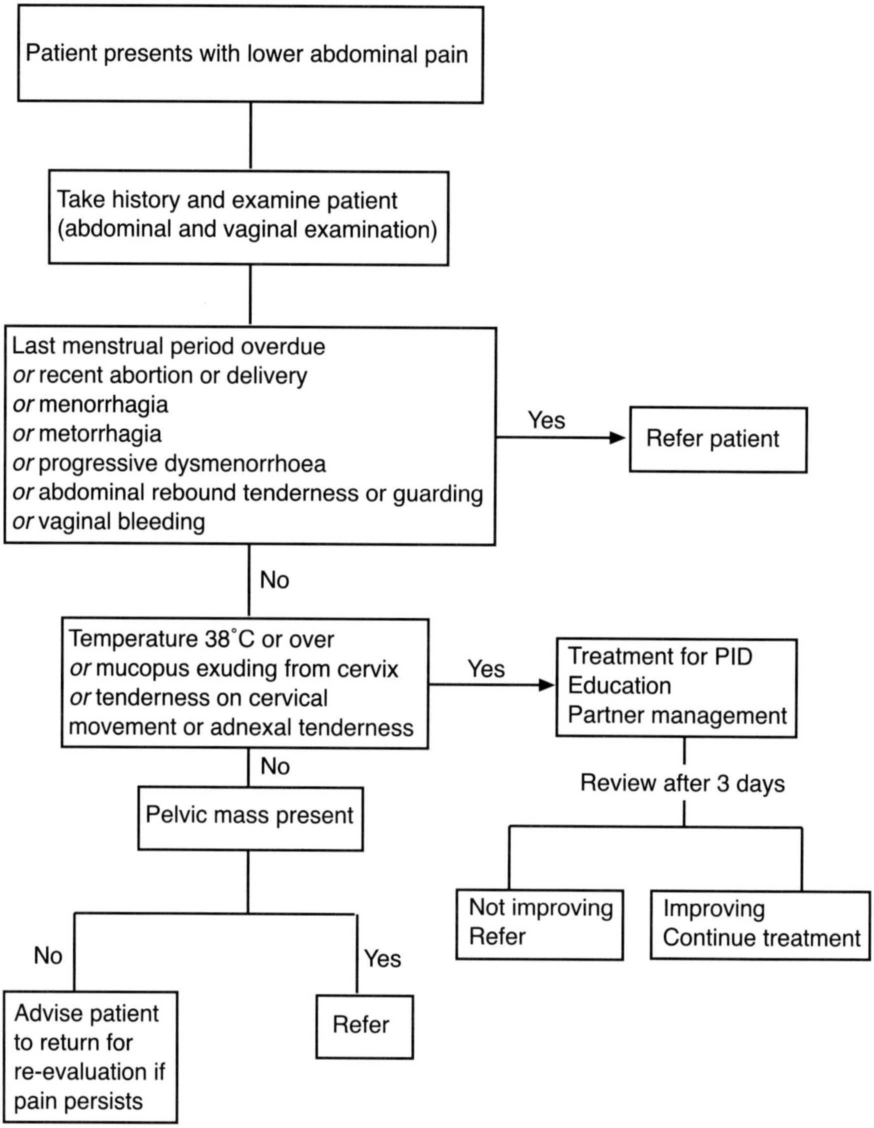

Fig. 10.3.1. Management of lower abdominal pain in women at the PHC level (speculum and bimanual examination possible). Adapted from World Health Organization (1991); *Management of Patients with Sexually Transmitted Diseases*, WHO Technical Report Series, 810, WHO, Geneva, Algorithm 7, p. 24.

with adnexal swelling, peritonitis) will need hospitalization and parenteral treatment which should cover STI agents as well as anaerobes.

It is expected that some of the newer drugs, notably azithromycin which is a macrolide and highly effective for uncomplicated chlamydial and gonococcal

Box 10.3.1. Outpatient and inpatient treatment for PID.[a]

Out-patient therapy

Regimen A (mild cases)

Cefoxitin, 2 g i.m. plus probenecid, 1.0 g by mouth in a single dose,
or ceftriaxone, 250 mg i.m. once,
plus either doxycycline[b], 100 mg orally twice daily for 10–14 days,
or tetracycline[b] hydrochloride, 500 mg by mouth every 6 h daily for 14 days.
(See text regarding the use of metronidazole.)

Regimen B (moderately severe cases not requiring admission: see text)

Regimen A *or* Ofloxacin, 400 mg orally twice daily for 14 days[b]; *plus* metronidazole, 500 mg orally twice daily for 10 days (avoid alchohol).

In-patient therapy (severely ill patients)

Regimen I

Cefoxitin, 2 g i.v. every 6 h, *or* cefotetan 2 g i.v. every 12 h,
plus doxycycline[b], 100 mg i.v. *or* orally every 12 h.

Continue for at least 24 h after the patient has responded satisfactorily. After this, the patient may be discharged and continue with doxycycline, 100 mg orally twice daily plus metronidazole as in regimen B above for up to a total of 14 days.

Regimen II

Clindamycin, 900 mg i.v. every 8 h *plus* gentamicin, 2 mg kg^{-1} of body weight i.v. or i.m., followed by 1.5 mg kg^{-1} of body weight every 8 h.

Continue for at least 24 h after satisfactory initial response. After discharge from hospital, continue with doxycycline[b], 100 mg orally twice daily, or clindamycin (if tuboovarian abscess is suspected), 450 mg orally four times a day for up to a total of 14 days.
Regimen II provides optimal activity against anaerobes and facultative Gram-negative rods, but may not provide optimal activity against *C. trachomatis* if doxycycline is not used.

[a]Adapted from Centres for Disease Control and Prevention (1998) *Guidelines for Treatment of Sexually Transmitted Diseases.*
[b]Avoid in pregnancy.
Doxycycline/tetracycline should be avoided during pregnancy when erythromycin can be used.

infections in a single oral dose, may have the potential of significant application in PID. However, the drug is very expensive at the present time.

Follow-up

The post-treatment assessment may be classified as: (i) initial response, 48–72 h after starting treatment, and (ii) final response at the end of treatment. In a severely ill patient, if the response is unsatisfactory after 3 days' treatment, the diagnosis may need to be reviewed. A patient with, for example, pelvic abscess may require surgical intervention. The out-patients should also be reviewed to ensure compliance and to assess the initial response.

Those found to be harbouring *N. gonorrhoeae* should be re-swabbed 3 (if possible) and 7 days after the start and 14 days after the completion of treatment, and swabs for *C. trachomatis,* if initially positive, should be repeated 4 weeks after the completion of treatment.

Sexual partners

Management of women with STI-associated PID is inadequate unless their sexual partners, who might be asymptomatic, have been evaluated and treated with appropriate regimens for chlamydial and/or gonococcal infection. Failure to treat sexual partner(s) places a woman at risk of re-infection.

HIV infection and PID

The information on any significant differences with regard to PID between women with HIV infection and those without is limited. Anecdotal evidence suggests those with HIV infection may develop severe and repeated attacks. At the very least, the patients should be assessed and managed as described above.

Perihepatitis (Fitz–Hugh–Curtis syndrome)

Perihepatitis occurs mainly in women, in a small proportion of those with chlamydial or gonococcal salpingitis. *C. trachomatis* has been isolated from the liver surface more frequently than *N. gonorrhoeae*. The infection reaches the subphrenic space by transabdominal spread from the fallopian tube along the peritoneum and paracolic gutters. Retroperitoneal lymphatics and haematogenous spread are other suggested routes. There is an inflammation of the liver capsule and the adjacent connective tissue.

The symptoms include fever, nausea and vomiting, but mainly pain in the right hypochondrium referred to the right shoulder and aggravated on deep breathing. On examination, there is tenderness in the right hypochondrium and usually also signs of pelvic infection. Laparoscopy may show inflammatory exudate on the liver surface or violin string adhesions between the anterior surface of the liver and the anterior abdominal wall.

The conditions for the differential diagnosis may include cholecystitis, subphrenic abscess, liver disease, pneumonia, pleurisy, pyelonephritis, pancreatitis and perforated peptic ulcer. Laboratory investigations include swabs for *C. trachomatis* and *N. gonorrhoeae* and other tests as described above for PID.

Treatment is the same as for pelvic infection.

Further reading

Brabin, L., Kemp, J., Obunge, O.K., Ikimola, J., Dollimore, N., Odu, N.N., Hart, C.A. and Briggs, N.D. (1995) Reproductive tract infections and abortion among adolescent girls in rural Nigeria. *Lancet* 345, 300–304.

Centres for Disease Control and Prevention (1998) Guidelines for treatment of sexually transmitted diseases. *Morbidity and Mortality Weekly Report* 47 (No. RR-1), 79–86.

Weström, L. and Mårdh, P.A. (1990) Acute pelvic inflammatory disease (PID). In: Holmes,

K.K., Mårdh, P.A., Sparling, P.F., Wiesner, P.J., Cates, W., Jr, Lemon, S.M. and Stamm, W.E. (eds) *Sexually Transmitted Diseases,* 2nd edn. McGraw-Hill, New York, pp. 593–613.
Weström, L. and Wölner-Hanssen, P. (1993) Pathogenesis of pelvic inflammatory disease. *Genitourinary Medicine* 69, 9–17.

CHAPTER 10.4
Management of HIV-related illnesses at the primary health care level

A.S. Latif
Department of Medicine, University of Zimbabwe, Harare, Zimbabwe

With the ever-increasing size of the HIV epidemic globally, primary health care (PHC) providers throughout the world are faced with a large number of patients presenting with symptoms related to infection with HIV. In developing countries where facilities for specialized laboratory investigations and antiretroviral therapy are not available, even at tertiary care centres, patients need to be managed adequately at the health facilities to which they first present. In countries where the prevalence of HIV infection is high, HIV-related illnesses are among the ten commonest conditions for which patients seek care at the PHC level. In this chapter, guidance is given for the management of persons with HIV infection and related illnesses. Despite the fact that there is no cure for HIV infection and that most persons with HIV infection will develop AIDS and die from it, patients can be treated for many of the illnesses that occur during the course of the infection and thus can be offered a better quality of life.

The spectrum of clinical presentation of HIV infection is very broad and it will not be possible to cover the management of every clinical presentation. It is intended here to give guidance on the management of common conditions and those for which acceptable care may be provided at the PHC level.

Stages of HIV infection

A person with HIV infection may have no symptoms at all; the asymptomatic phase may last many years. Symptoms may occur with the initiation of an immune response against the infection, or with the development of immune suppression. Depending on the degree of immune suppression, the patient may develop illnesses ranging from minor, self-limiting infections to severe life threatening conditions. The stages of HIV infection and the clinical manifestations are shown in Box 10.4.1. All health workers should manage patients as they see them. However, if the patient needs additional attention or investigations that are not available at the PHC level, then the health worker should have no hesitation in referring the patient to a level where such facilities are available.

Box 10.4.1. Stages of HIV infection.

A. Asymptomatic infection

1. There are no symptoms and signs of infection.

2. The diagnosis is made when a person is screened for HIV infection, for instance, if he/she is a blood donor, a contact of person known to be HIV positive, a parent of a child with HIV infection, or if he/she has been tested voluntarily.

B. HIV-related illness

1. Symptoms related to immune mechanisms directed against HIV:
- Acute infection syndrome.
- Generalized lymphadenopathy.
- Urticaria, pruritic dermatoses.

2. Symptoms related to minor immune suppression
- Fever, diarrhoea, weight loss.
- Skin infections.
- Herpes zoster, persistent or recurrent herpes simplex.
- Oral thrush, hairy leukoplakia, genital warts.

C. AIDS

1. Opportunistic infections.

2. Kaposi's sarcoma, non-Hodgkin's lymphoma.

When to suspect HIV infection

In regions where the prevalence of HIV infection is high, clinicians should keep the diagnosis in mind at all times. The common clinical manifestations of HIV infection in adults in developing countries are shown in Box 10.4.2, and the diagnosis should be suspected in patients presenting with any of these symptoms/signs.

Any patient who is sexually active and has engaged in risky sexual behaviour may have HIV infection. Risky sexual behaviour implies having unprotected penetrative sexual intercourse with someone who is not the patient's regular and faithful partner. HIV infection should be suspected if the patient gives a history of having had STI in the past, the patient's sexual partner is known to be HIV infected, the patient is a parent of a child with HIV infection, or if the patient's partner or child has died recently.

Management of HIV infection at the PHC level

In this chapter, the clinical management at the PHC level of the following clinical conditions is discussed: fever, headache, diarrhoea, weight loss, oral thrush, respiratory conditions and skin conditions.

Fever

Fever is a common symptom in many conditions. In persons with HIV infection, fever may be the only clinical manifestation of the illness or may

Box 10.4.2. Common clinical manifestions of HIV infection in adults.

Weight loss
Certain respiratory conditions including tuberculosis
Herpes zoster
Oropharyngeal candidiasis
Generalized dermatitis
Herpes simplex
Generalized lymphadenopathy
Persistent fever
Chronic or recurrent diarrhoea
Severe and persistent STI/genital ulceration
Neurological symptoms
Kaposi's sarcoma

Box 10.4.3. Causes of persistent fever in persons with HIV infection.

1. Infections
Bacterial: pneumococcal, mycobacterial, streptococcal, staphylococcal, rickettsial, *Salmonella* infections.
Viral: cytomegalovirus, Epstein–Barr virus, HIV itself.
Fungal: *Cryptococcus neoformans*, *Pneumocystis carinii*
Protozoal
Infection with *Toxoplasma gondii*, *Plasmodium* spp.

2. Malignancies
Kaposi's sarcoma, lymphoma.

3. Other conditions
Rheumatoid arthritis, sarcoidosis, systemic lupus erythematosus, drugs.

occur as a result of any of the conditions listed in Box 10.4.3. Accordingly, other symptoms and signs may also be present.

Clinical management

A history should be taken and a full physical examination be carried out. Specific points in the history include whether the patient has other symptoms such as headache, cough, difficulty in breathing or swallowing, skin rashes, weight loss or diarrhoea. In addition, it is important to find out whether the patient lives in a malaria endemic area or has recently visited such an area. The axillary temperature is measured and the patient examined for features of dehydration and for features of HIV infection, such as lymph node enlargement, oral thrush, hairy leukoplakia, wasting, skin lesions, anaemia, chest signs, hepatosplenomegaly and neck stiffness.

If the patient has been in a malaria endemic area, a blood slide should be taken and the patient started on the first line recommended treatment for malaria together with an antipyretic agent. In addition, the urine should be examined for blood, protein and white blood cells using a simple dip-stick method. Occasionally it is necessary to treat the patient empirically with cotrimoxazole in order to cover for a respiratory or urinary infection. Patients should always be reviewed in 3 days and, if they have improved, the course of medication may be continued. If the patient is still febrile 3 days after starting malaria treatment or broad-spectrum antibiotics, he/she should be referred to a facility where further investigations may be carried out.

Headache

Headache is an extremely common symptom. The entire population at some time will have suffered from it, needing treatment in the form of analgesics. Persistent, severe and rapidly increasing headache, which does not respond to the drugs commonly used for pain relief, needs to be investigated further. The common causes of headache not related to HIV infection include migraine, tension, sinusitis, dental disorders, anaemia, refractive disorders and hypertension. However, one should always consider the possibility of the headache being related to HIV infection. Therefore, keep in mind the following causes: tuberculous meningitis; cryptococcal meningitis; neurosyphilis; encephalitis caused by HSV, cytomegalovirus and HIV; toxoplasmosis; intracranial lymphoma; and the use of drugs. Patients with headache may also have the associated symptoms of dizziness, nausea, vomiting and drowsiness.

Clinical management

A history should be taken from all patients, including whether the patient is under stress, whether he/she has had headaches previously, whether there is a history of migraine or hypertension, and whether the patient is on medication. All patients should be examined thoroughly. The general physical examination should include level of consciousness, temperature, neck stiffness, anaemia, blood pressure, dental caries and pain on tapping over the sinuses. In addition, the following neurological signs should be looked for: loss of memory, speech impairment, blindness, deafness, hemiplegia, paraplegia and sensory neuropathy. Facial nerve paralysis is a fairly common neurological abnormality associated with HIV infection. Unilateral or bilateral facial nerve paralysis occasionally may be associated with ascending polyneuropathy of the Guillain–Barré syndrome.

The patient with any of the common causes of headache, e.g. nervous tension, migraine, dental caries, sinusitis, anaemia or hypertension, should be managed appropriately. Patients with HIV infection in whom any form of neurologic abnormality is found should be referred to a health centre where further examination and investigations may be carried out. If no neurological abnormality is found, then the patient may be treated with analgesics and referred only if the headache persists.

Diarrhoea

Diarrhoea commonly occurs during the course of HIV infection. Diarrhoea may be intermittent with acute exacerbations or may be chronic in nature. Chronic diarrhoea is defined as passing more than three liquid stools daily for

3 weeks out of each month. The causes include: HIV enteropathy; intestinal parasitic conditions such as cryptosporidiosis, isosporiasis and strongyloidiasis; and bacterial infection of the gut as in salmonellosis, tuberculosis and tropical sprue. Chronic diarrhoea may also occur in a number of other conditions such as malabsorption syndrome and intestinal lymphomas. The patient with chronic diarrhoea may be dehydrated, anaemic and may have the skin and hair changes of kwashiorkor. In advanced AIDS, the chronic diarrhoea, together with other HIV-related factors, leads to severe emaciation commonly termed 'Slim disease'. Such patients may have hypopigmentation of the lips, while the nails may be darkly pigmented.

Clinical management

The most important aspect in the management of diarrhoeal disease is the prevention of dehydration and the treatment of dehydration once it has occurred. A history should be taken from all patients, and all patients should be examined thoroughly. From the history it should be determined whether the patient has chronic or recurrent diarrhoea, or whether the patient has been having short-lived bouts of acute diarrhoea. In addition, the following information should be obtained: duration of illness, consistency, frequency and quantity of stools produced; presence or absence of vomiting; time when last passed urine; and colour of urine.

Clinical examination should include the patient's hydration status, the body temperature, pulse rate, respiratory rate and the skin turgor, the skin colour, and the hydration state of the tongue. The eyes should be examined to determine whether or not they are sunken and the skin felt in order to determine whether it is cold and clammy. Patients who are not dehydrated may be advised about fluid and food intake. A carbohydrate-rich diet should be encouraged. Hydration may be maintained by making sure that the patient takes at least 200 ml of oral rehydration solution (ORS) after the passage of every stool. Patients should be taught how to make up the ORS and also be educated regarding the importance of fluid replacement and continuing with a normal diet when they have diarrhoea in the future. If ORS sachets are not available, make up salt and sugar solution by adding six teaspoonfuls of sugar and a quarter teaspoonful of salt to 750 ml of clean water.

If dehydration is present, it should be classified into mild, moderate or severe (Table 10.4.1). Patients who are mildly or moderately dehydrated should be given ORS as follows: 200 ml every 15 m for the first 4 h, followed by 500 ml every hour while the diarrhoea continues, and after the diarrhoea stops to take 5 litres of ORS daily together with 250 ml of ORS after passing each stool. This is continued until the patient is passing normal stools and is taking a normal diet.

If the patient is severely dehydrated or if the patient is unable to take oral fluids because of vomiting, give fluids intravenously as follows: 1.5 litres of Ringer–lactate or half-strength dextrose in Darrow's solution intravenously in the first hour, and, if tolerated, 500 ml of ORS every hour. Continue intravenous fluids so that the patient receives 2 litres in the next 12 h and then 3 litres every 24 h together with ORS as described above.

Table 10.4.1. Classification of dehydration.

	Dehydration		
Clinical features	Mild	Moderate	Severe
General condition	Weak	Weak	Restless, irritable, cold, sweaty, peripheral cyanosis
Pulse	Normal	Slight tachycardia	Rapid, feeble
Respiration	Normal	Normal	Deep and rapid
Skin elasticity	Normal	Pinch retracts slowly	Pinch retracts very slowly
Eyes	Normal	Sunken	Deeply sunken
Mucous membranes	Slightly dry	Dry	Very dry
Urine flow	Normal; urine dark	Reduced amount; dark amber in colour	No urine flow, empty bladder

All patients with diarrhoea should be encouraged to take potassium-containing foods such as fruit and vegetables, and particularly over-ripe bananas. Some experts feel that all patients with HIV infection and chronic diarrhoea should also receive a 10-day course of cotrimoxazole two tablets twice daily orally; and those patients who do not improve on cotrimoxazole should be given a 7-day course of metronidazole, 400 mg orally three times a day.

Weight loss

The weight loss is often severe in the more advanced stage of HIV infection. The condition is then known as 'HIV-associated wasting syndrome', or 'Slim disease'. The cause of the wasting is not clear. It is known that patients with AIDS lose weight as part of the chronic debility. Some other reasons for the weight loss include chronic and recurrent diarrhoea, malabsorption, HIV-induced myopathy and intestinal parasitic infestations. None of these factors have been substantiated as the exact cause of the severe weight loss. Slim disease is often associated with chronic diarrhoea and recurrent or persistent fever.

The patient complains of involuntary weight loss, loss of appetite with or without fever and diarrhoea. The patient is usually so debilitated that he/she can no longer cope with work. Examination reveals an ill and emaciated patient who may be feverish and dehydrated. The skin is usually dry and there may be evidence of a rash. Examination of the mouth may reveal plaques of oral thrush and hairy leukoplakia. The patient may be anaemic and usually has cheilitis and hyperpigmented nails. Depending on how advanced the HIV infection is, the patient may, in addition, have other manifestations of AIDS, such as oesophageal thrush, Kaposi's sarcoma, tuberculosis and other respiratory conditions, and features of neurologic involvement as well.

Clinical management

All persons with HIV infection should take a balanced diet which should be high in calories and should have both carbohydrate and protein. The diet should be made calorie rich by adding oil and sugar to the staple base of maize, sorghum or rice. Protein-rich foods include milk and milk products such as cheese or sour milk, eggs, beans, groundnuts, meat, fish and soya beans. Fat-containing foods include cooking oil, groundnuts, milk and milk products, meat, fish and soya beans. Patients should also take fruit and vegetables such as cabbage, spinach, rape leaves, bean leaves and pumpkin leaves.

In patients with severe stomatitis and difficulty in chewing or swallowing, the diet should be made into a palatable liquid or porridge. Ill patients may prefer to take sour milk together with the staple made into a porridge. Very ill patients may be given a high-energy supplement made of soya bean meal, sunflower oil and sugar. This is made up into a soft liquid porridge and the patient is fed this frequently. Soya bean milk may not be affordable by all patients and hence a high-energy drink may be made up at home by adding 50 g of sugar and 20 ml of cooking oil to 500 ml of milk. This high-energy milk could be fortified further by beating up one egg into the mixture if eggs are available and are tolerated. An adult should drink 500 ml of high-energy milk daily until he is able to take a full normal diet. Usually patients with 'Slim disease' have lost more than 15% of their body weight. Attention should be paid to nutrition and vitamin supplementation. They should receive one to two tablets of vitamin B complex daily.

Any treatable infection should be identified. Such patients often have tuberculosis which should be actively sought. Persons found to have tuberculosis and those strongly suspected of having tuberculosis should be treated adequately. The patients with a neurologic abnormality or suspected malignancy should be referred to an appropriate higher level.

Oral thrush

Thrush is caused by the fungus *Candida albicans*, and hence the condition is termed candidiasis. The organism, which is a yeast, colonizes most body cavities and often does not produce symptoms. Oral thrush is seen commonly in neonates and infants. Up to one-third of all normal women carry *C. albicans* in the vagina. The gastrointestinal tract of both men and women, and the genital tract in women, are the sites most commonly colonized by the fungus. The condition occurs more frequently in persons with certain predisposing factors which include pregnancy and use of oral contraceptives, use of broad-spectrum antibiotics and systemic steroids, glycosuria/diabetes mellitus, congenital or acquired immune deficiencies, a chronic debilitating condition, malnutrition, cancer and chemotherapy or radiotherapy for cancer.

The common manifestations of thrush are vulvovaginal and oral infection.

Women with vaginal candidiasis may develop a vaginal discharge and vulvovaginal pruritus. Genital thrush occurs in males as well and, in this situation, infected symptomatic men will develop balanitis or balanoposthitis and will complain of a subpreputial discharge and itchiness of the penis and foreskin. Elsewhere in the body, *C. albicans* can infect the skin and cause a pruritic dermatitis. Depending on the level of immune suppression, oral infection may extend to involve the oesophagus. Rarely, bronchial infection may occur, and, even more rarely, disseminated infection occurs.

Clinical aspects

Oral thrush includes infection of the buccal mucosa, tongue, oropharynx, gums, and the hard and soft palate. Patients may have no symptoms at all or may complain of burning in the mouth when eating food. Some patients may complain that they have noticed sores or white patches in the mouth. If the thrush has extended into the oesophagus, then patients may complain of pain on swallowing food, retrosternal pain or excessive salivation. Examination of the oral cavity will reveal redness and inflammation of the mucosa and in some areas there will be small patches of white plaques. The palate, the throat, the gums, the tongue and the inside of the cheeks may look inflamed. When the tongue is affected, it may be smooth and red, and the papillae normally found on the tongue may be absent. In a person with poor oral hygiene, white flakes are also seen, but these are loose particles of food. Also, such patients will have a coated tongue. This should be distinguished from the adherent plaques of thrush (see also Chapter 11.5).

A number of conditions other than oral thrush may be seen in the mouth of persons with HIV infection.

GINGIVITIS. Gingivitis is inflammation of the gums. The gums are usually swollen and red, and tend to bleed easily.

PYORRHOEA.. In pyorrhoea, pus accumulates between the gums and the teeth. The condition is usually associated with gingivitis.

APHTHOUS ULCERS. These are painful punched out ulcers on the mucosal surface. They are usually covered with a purulent exudate and tend to bleed when touched.

ORAL HERPES. Oral herpes is caused by the herpes simplex virus. The infection usually leads to the development of superficial painful ulcers which appear in a small group anywhere in the mouth. Lesions of herpes simplex may also be seen in the skin of the lips and around the nose.

STOMATITIS. Stomatitis means inflammation of the mucosa in the oral cavity. It is often associated with poor oral hygiene and bacterial invasion with anaerobic bacteria.

ORAL HAIRY LEUKOPLAKIA. Its aetiology has been linked to Epstein–Barr virus. Lesions appear as fine, white, linear warty growths on the edge of the tongue (see also Chapter 11.5).

KAPOSI'S SARCOMA. Lesions are often seen on the hard palate and occasionally on the tongue, throat, tonsils and gums. Sometimes the lesions may be large and pedunculated. The lesions are papules which are purple in colour and are usually painless (see also Chapters 11.3 and 11.5).

Clinical management

Patients with oral thrush should be examined for other features of HIV infection. Attempts should be made to exclude oesophageal infection clinically. However, the diagnosis of oesophageal candidiasis can only be confirmed by direct visualization of the oesophageal mucosa through an endoscope. This investigation will not be available at most PHC facilities, therefore a good history should be taken from all patients. Symptoms suggestive of oesophageal thrush are difficulty or pain on swallowing food and retrosternal chest pain. In all patients with HIV infection, even those with obvious oral thrush, the oral cavity should be examined carefully for other lesions including pyorrhoea, herpes, aphthous ulcers and Kaposi's sarcoma.

Oral thrush may be managed with local or systemic antifungal agents. Patients may be treated initially with applications of a 1% aqueous solution of gentian violet twice daily to the oral cavity for 7 days. Failing this, the patient may be given nystatin tablets, 500,000 units to suck 6-hourly for 7 days. The patient should also receive advice on oral hygiene, i.e. to gargle the mouth with warm salty water (made up by adding one teaspoonful of table salt to a tumblerful of warm water) after every meal and to brush the teeth at least twice daily. Ketoconazole, 200 mg orally twice daily for 10 days, is effective in treating oesophageal candidiasis. This drug may, however, not be available at the primary care level, and patients who do not respond to first line treatment should be referred.

Patients with gingivitis, pyorrhoea and aphthous ulcers may be treated with metronidazole, 400 mg orally twice daily for 7 days, *or*, erythromycin, 500 mg orally four times a day for 7 days, together with good oral hygiene practices. Patients with suspected Kaposi's sarcoma need to be referred for specialist management.

Respiratory conditions

Respiratory problems in persons with HIV infection are many and varied. They range from minor recurrent viral upper respiratory tract infections to life-threatening bacterial, viral and fungal pneumonias. Respiratory failure resulting from severe pulmonary infection is probably the commonest cause of death in adults and children with HIV infection. Early in the course of HIV infection, patients may present with bacterial pneumonias which respond readily to antibiotics. Later, and with the onset of immunosuppression, patients may develop opportunistic pulmonary infections, one of the most important and common of which is pulmonary tuberculosis. As cell-mediated immunity becomes severely depressed, patients may develop life-threatening opportunistic infections which include *Pneumocystis carinii* pneumonia and severe pulmonary infection with certain fungi and viruses.

Box 10.4.4 summarizes the pulmonary manifestations of HIV infection. In immunosuppressed persons, tuberculosis may occur as a result of reactivation of an old healed focus of infection, or as a result of re-infection. However, as a result of the poor immune status, dissemination of infection to other parts of the body frequently occurs. Box 10.4.5 gives a summary of the spectrum of the presentation of tuberculosis in persons with HIV infection.

Tuberculosis responds well to the standard antituberculosis treatment regimens. However, care should be taken as some of the drugs used may cause serious adverse reactions.

Clinical aspects

Remember that cough and shortness of breath may be due to asthma and congestive cardiac failure, and these conditions should always be kept in mind in persons with HIV infection. Patients with respiratory problems will present with a history of cough, shortness of breath (dyspnoea) or chest pain. It is important to obtain information regarding the following from the history: the duration and severity of symptoms, whether the cough is productive of sputum, the presence or absence of blood in the sputum, whether the chest pain is pleuritic in nature, the nature and severity of dyspnoea, and whether dyspnoea is experienced at rest or on lying flat in bed.

Box 10.4.4. Pulmonary manifestations of HIV infection.

Bacterial infections
- Pneumococcal pneumonia
- *Klebsiella* pneumonia
- Staphylococcal pneumonia
- Tuberculosis
- Lung abscess
- Emphysema

Viral infections
- Cytomegalovirus infection
- Herpes simplex virus infection

Fungal infections
- Cryptococcosis
- Histoplasmosis
- *Pneumocystis* pneumonia

Other conditions
- Kaposi's sarcoma
- Pleural effusion
- Pericardial effusion
- Pneumothorax
- Strongyloidiasis hyperinfection syndrome

Box 10.4.5. Tuberculosis in persons with HIV infection.

Pulmonary tuberculosis
- Typical presentation: cavitation
- Atypical presentation: widespread broncho-pneumonia

Extra-pulmonary tuberculosis
- Pleural effusion
- Lymphadenopathy
- Miliary TB
- Tuberculous meningitis
- Tuberculous pericarditis and peritonitis
- Spine and bone tuberculosis
- Renal and genital tract tuberculosis

On examination, note the general condition of the patient, i.e. is the patient comfortable lying in bed, does he/she need to be propped up, is he/she able to talk without becoming short of breath? Note whether the patient is having difficulty in breathing. Measure the pulse and respiratory rates. Examine the mouth in order to determine the presence of central cyanosis. Determine whether the patient is in respiratory distress. The signs of respiratory distress are central cyanosis, tachycardia (>120 beats per min), rapid respiratory rate (>30 per min) and severe dyspnoea (strenuous effort required to breathe).

Clinical management

The history and clinical examination are most important in assessing a patient with respiratory problems. The following should always be considered:

- The patient may be in respiratory failure and this can lead to death.
- The patient may have a straightforward pneumonia which may be easily treated.
- The patient may have tuberculosis.

All patients with severe symptoms should be referred to a facility where the following are available: a broader range of drugs, facilities to perform chest X-ray and laboratory tests, and specialist medical care. When transferring such patients to a hospital, give supportive care as detailed below:

- Administer oxygen by mask
- If the patient has asthma, give him/her oxygen by mask, intravenous hydrocortisone, 200 mg, and give inhaled salbutamol before referring the patient.
- If the patient has cardiac failure give him/her oxygen by mask, prop him/her up in bed and give frusemide, 80 mg intravenously slowly before referring the patient.
- Before transferring the patient, it may be advisable to commence the patient on antibiotics as well.

At the primary care facility, all patients who have respiratory problems and who do not require immediate referral should be given either amoxycillin, 500 mg 8-hourly orally, *or* cotrimoxazole (trimethoprim 80 mg/sulphamethoxazole 400 mg), two tablets orally twice daily. If the patient is improved on this treatment when reviewed in 72 h, then the antibiotic should be continued for a full 10 days. If the patient fails to respond to amoxycillin or cotrimoxazole, arrange for referral for further investigations and management.

Skin conditions (see also Chapter 11.5 and other relevant chapters and plates in the book)

The range of skin conditions that occur in persons with HIV infection are very broad and include all the skin conditions encountered in persons who do not have HIV infection plus those that are related to HIV infection and to immunosuppression. Skin involvement in persons with HIV infection may be the result of a direct effect of the virus on the skin, the effect of the body's immune mechanisms directed against HIV, opportunistic and non-opportunistic skin infections and other dermatoses.

Possible direct effect of HIV on skin

Although the exact pathogenesis is not clear, the following skin conditions probably occur as a result of the direct effect of HIV on the skin.

PAPULAR PRURITIC DERMATOSIS. This is a common clinical problem. Adults with papular pruritic dermatosis usually complain of severe pruritus associated with a follicular or papular rash. The rash usually has a generalized distribution, sparing the face.

SEBORRHOEIC DERMATITIS. This is a common skin manifestation of HIV infection. The rash is scaly in nature and usually appears on the face, particularly around the nostrils and on the chin. The rash may sometimes also be found on the chest, abdomen and upper arms.

GENERALIZED ERYTHRODERMA. This is an erythrosquamous generalized eruption which affects mainly adults. The skin is reddish in appearance and looks hyperpigmented and scaly. The rash is similar in appearance to that of eczema.

Immune-mediated rashes

Some rashes develop as a result of the body's immune mechanisms being directed against HIV.

URTICARIA. Early in the course of HIV infection, usually at the time of development of antibodies against HIV, some patients develop urticaria. This probably occurs as a result of the antibody reacting against the viral antigen, forming antibody–antigen complexes (immune complexes) that are deposited in the dermis. The deposition of the immune complexes releases histamine which causes the typical flat, itchy wheals and papules of urticaria to appear.

PRURITIC MACULOPAPULAR RASH. A generalized itchy maculopapular rash may appear during the acute illness phase of HIV infection. The rash, the cause of which is unclear, may be seen all over the body, including the face. Like all the other manifestations of the acute illness syndrome, this rash often disappears on its own. It is different from the rash of papular pruritic dermatosis in that the latter often persists for a long period of time.

Skin infections

With the onset of immunosuppression, a number of opportunistic skin infections may occur. Opportunistic infections may be viral, bacterial, fungal or parasitic and may affect adults and children equally.

VIRUSES. Infections with HSV, varicella-zoster virus (VZV), molluscum contagiosum virus (MCV) and human papillomavirus (HPV) often occur in immunosuppressed persons. HSV causes oral and genital herpes, VZV causes shingles and chickenpox, MCV causes molluscum contagiosum, and HPV causes warts.

BACTERIA. Any pyogenic bacteria may infect the skin. In persons with immunosuppression, infection with *Staphylococcus aureus* and *Streptococcus pyogenes* may result in impetigo, furuncles and boils. Bacterial infection of the apocrine glands is encountered fairly commonly in persons with HIV infection; the condition which is known as hidradenitis suppurativa is a chronic one and usually proves very difficult to treat. Tuberculosis of the skin should also be kept in mind in persons with HIV infection.

FUNGI. Cutaneous fungal infections occur more commonly amongst immunosuppressed persons. Fungal infections include candidiasis, dermatomycosis and histoplasmosis.

PARASITES. In persons who are immunosuppressed, scabies follows an atypical course. Lesions are more numerous, more widespread and larger than those found in normally immune individuals.

Other dermatoses

Conditions such as acne, boils, eczema and psoriasis are affected adversely in persons who have HIV infection. All these conditions are common in the general adult population. However, they occur with increasing frequency and are more difficult to treat in immunosuppressed individuals. Boils, skin sepsis and eczema occur frequently in children, but acne and psoriasis are rare in this age group. In addition, the adverse drug reactions, for example to anti-tuberculosis drugs and sulphonamides, etc. occur more frequently in persons with HIV infection. The conditions that occur as a result of side effects of drugs are fixed drug reaction, erythema multiforme, Stevens–Johnson syndrome and toxic epidermal necrolysis. The latter two are serious conditions and may be fatal.

Kaposi's sarcoma (see also Chapter 11.3)

The skin lesions of Kaposi's sarcoma are purple papules that may be found anywhere on the body including the mucosal surfaces. Kaposi's sarcoma occurs uncommonly in children.

Approach to the management of skin conditions

At the primary care level, it is not intended that clinicians be expected to make an exact aetiologic diagnosis of the skin condition. However, there are a number of skin conditions that may be easily managed without need for referral. A small number of skin conditions produce a particular type of skin rash or skin lesion. Therefore, if a clinician is able to identify the type of lesion or skin rash, then the differential diagnosis may be narrowed down to a short list of conditions which a clinician may be able to manage adequately.

Clinical aspects

A history is taken and the patient is examined. From the examination, the health worker should decide on the type of rash the patient has.

The various types are summarized below.

- *Macular rash.* A macule is a flat lesion within the skin and is of a slightly different colour to that of normal skin.
- *Erythematous rash.* An erythematous lesion is red in colour. Over a period of time, the lesion becomes brown and looks slightly more hyperpigmented than normal skin.
- *Papular rash.* A papule is an elevated lesion which one can see and feel. It has a distinct margin.
- *Follicular rash.* This rash is made up of tiny papules, the size of hair follicles and skin pores.
- *Purpuric rash.* This rash is a collection of tiny areas of bleeding and is caused by platelet dysfunction or by abnormalities of the capillaries.
- *Haemorrhagic rash.* Any rash in which bleeding occurs is known as a haemorrhagic rash.
- *Vesicular rash.* A vesicle is a small superficial lesion which contains fluid. Larger lesions with fluid are blisters or bullae.
- *Pustular rash.* A pustule is a small lesion (3–5 mm in diameter) containing pus.
- *Papillomatous rash.* A papillomatous lesion is a warty lesion.
- *Squamous rash.* A squamous rash is a scaly rash.

The identification of the type of rash is necessary to facilitate appropriate care. Most rashes of importance in clinical practice are made up of one or more of five types, i.e. papular, warty, vesicular, pustular or squamous. These types of skin rashes are easy to recognize provided that the patient is examined in a well lit room. These are now described in detail

Papular or maculopapular skin eruptions may occur in secondary syphilis when they are usually non-pruritic. The lesion produced by the molluscum contagiosum virus is a papule that has a central umbilication; the lesion looks like a vesicle but, when it is pierced, fluid is not obtained but a white cheesy substance exudes out. The lesions of scabies are also papules; they are extremely itchy and, usually when a person has scabies, a large number of excoriated lesions will be seen. Pruritic papular dermatosis is a condition which occurs during the course of HIV infection; itchiness is the dominant symptom. Papular lesions, which are usually excoriated, appear all over the body; at times the lesions are scaly as a result of the itchiness. The lesion of Kaposi's sarcoma is also a papule which is purplish in colour, is not painful and feels firm to touch.

Warty skin lesions and genital warts are caused by HPV. Warts are recognized by their appearance: on the skin, they are hard and dry and are made up of thick keratinized epithelium; on the mucous membrane, they are of a lighter colour and are firm and usually moist.

Vesicular skin eruptions may be caused by HSV and VZV. The former produces oral, labial and genital herpes, while the latter produces shingles (zoster) and chickenpox (varicella). Vesicles may also occur as part of a drug reaction.

Pustular skin eruptions may occur in varicella and zoster and pustules may be found in persons with acne, pyoderma, impetigo, boils and furunculosis.

Squamous skin eruptions are scaly, dry rashes. In squamous rashes, the skin overlying the lesions becomes loose and is shed. Squamous eruptions are found in eczema, seborrhoeic dermatitis, pruritic papular dermatosis, fungal skin infections, late secondary syphilis and in drug reactions.

Clinical management

At the primary care level, persons with HIV infection who present with skin rashes may be managed according to the type of rash that is found.

Papular rash

SECONDARY SYPHILIS. The rash of secondary syphilis is classically a maculopapular erythematous rash. The rash is not itchy and is found all over the body, including the face and palms. Papules may be found on mucous surfaces in the mouth and on the genitals. The patient may have a healing ulcer on the genitals. Other features of secondary syphilis, such as condylomata lata, may also be present. Manage patients with suspected secondary syphilis as follows:

1. Take blood for a syphilis serology if possible
2. Give the patient benzathine penicillin, 2.4 mega units by intramuscular injection; for persons allergic to penicillin, give doxycycline, 100 mg orally twice daily for 14 days, *or* erythromycin, 500 mg orally four times a day for 14 days for pregnant women allergic to penicillin.
3. Educate the patient regarding the nature of syphilis, the mode of transmission of the infection, the possible complications of infection, the need for changing sexual behaviour, the need to engage only in safer sexual acts, and on how to use condoms.
4. Advise the patient with regard to the treatment of sexual partner(s).
5. Give the patient a supply of condoms.

MOLLUSCUM CONTAGIOSUM. The lesions of molluscum contagiosum are papules with a shiny surface and central depression, and may look like vesicles. Lesions usually measure no more than 1–3 mm in diameter. However, in immunosuppressed persons, large lesions measuring more than 5 mm in diameter may be found. Lesions may be found anywhere on the body, including the face and genitalia. One way of treating this condition is to bore the centre of the lesions with a pointed matchstick dipped in phenol or strong iodine solution.

SCABIES. The lesions of scabies are itchy, elongated papules found mainly in the finger webs on the dorsal aspect of the hands. The papules may also be seen along the ulnar margins of the forearms, around the umbilicus, on the buttocks, the upper thighs and the genitalia. The patient and all household and sexual contacts are treated as follows: after taking a bath, the patient should apply to the whole body either a 25% emulsion of benzyl benzoate, *or* 1% gamma-benzene hexachloride in liquid paraffin and leave it on for 24 h in adults and for 8 h in children before having another bath to wash off the medicine.

PRURITIC PAPULAR DERMATITIS. The patient presents with a generalized papular rash which is extremely itchy. The rash may affect any part of the body. There will be signs of scratching and there may be lichenification of some lesions. Occasionally there will be signs of skin sepsis as a result of secondary bacterial infection. The treatment of pruritic papular dermatosis is with topical application of 1% hydrocortisone ointment. In addition, patients may require oral antihistamines.

KAPOSI'S SARCOMA. Lesions are hyperpigmented papules and macules. They are a dark brown to black colour on the skin and a purple colour on the mucous membranes. As Kaposi's sarcoma is a lymphatic disease, there is often lymphoedema of the legs. Lymph nodes in the groins, neck and axillae may be large and hard. Kaposi's sarcoma occurs uncommonly in children. All patients with suspected Kaposi's sarcoma should be referred for expert opinion and management.

Warts

SKIN WARTS. Touch the lesion only with a silver nitrate stick. This is done once or twice a day until the wart falls off.

GENITAL WARTS. Apply 20% podophyllin compound once weekly. Make sure that the podophyllin does not touch normal skin. Podophyllin should not be used on the cervix nor inside the urethra.

Vesicular rash

If the patient has varicella or zoster, no specific treatment is given. The patient is advised to keep the area clean and dry. Analgesics in the form of paracetamol, 1 g 8-hourly orally, may be given for pain. All patients who have extensive zoster and all those with zoster affecting the eye should be referred for specialist opinion and further management. In patients who have a high persistent fever or extensive infected lesions, a 5-day course of flucloxacillin, 250–500 mg 6-hourly, *or* erythromycin, 500 mg 6-hourly, may be given.

If the patient has labial, oral, genital or anal herpes, no specific treatment is necessary. Analgesics in the form of paracetamol, 500 mg 8-hourly orally, may be prescribed for pain. If the ulcers are large, extensive or very painful, the patient should be referred for specialist opinion and further management.

Antiviral agents such as aciclovir will probably not be available at the primary care level. Aciclovir and similar agents have been shown to be beneficial in the management of varicella, zoster and herpes virus infections.

If the patient has a drug reaction, the offending drug should be discontinued and the patient should be referred to the next level for advice on further management and for the need to continue with an alternative drug.

Pustular rash

CHICKENPOX. Chickenpox is a generalized skin condition. Lesions start as vesicles but soon become pustules which crust over and then scab. In a person with chickenpox lesions, all four stages will be seen. The skin around the vesicle is usually erythematous. Lesions of chickenpox may also be seen on the mucous membranes in the mouth.

ACNE. Acne produces tender inflammatory lesions. Some lesions have a black head while others have frank pus and are superficial abscesses. Lesions are usually found on the face and the upper back. The adult with acne is treated with a 5-day course of tetracycline, 500 mg orally 6-hourly; after the initial 5 days, tetracycline is continued in a dose of 250 mg orally twice daily for 4–6 weeks. Alternatively, doxycycline, 100 mg daily for 4–6 weeks may be used. Erythromycin (dosage regimen similar to tetracycline) may be prescribed for those who cannot tolerate tetracycline.

IMPETIGO. These are superficial large blisters which become infected and contain pus. The lesions may be found anywhere on the body, including the face. Lesions rupture easily and tend to ooze serum and pus which crusts at the edges of lesions. If the patient has impetigo (bullae and infected bullae), they should be given a 7-day course of phenoxymethylpenicillin, 500 mg orally 6-hourly, *or* flucloxacillin, 250–500 mg 6-hourly, *or* erythromycin, 500 mg orally 6-hourly, *or* cotrimoxazole (trimethoprim 80 mg/sulphamethoxazole 400 mg), two tablets twice daily.

BOILS. These are abscesses found in the skin. They sometimes occur as a result of coalescence of the pustular lesions of acne. Usually they are caused by staphylococci. The patient with boils should be treated with a 7-day course of tetracycline, 500 mg orally 6-hourly, *or* erythromycin, in the same dose, *or* doxycycline, 100 mg orally twice daily.

Squamous rash

ECZEMA. In eczema, there is scaling, inflammation and itchiness of the skin. The rash usually affects the antecubital or the popliteal fossae, but may occur anywhere on the body, including the face, hand and legs. The condition causes severe pruritus and, after scratching, lesions will ooze serum (weeping eczema). Over a long period of scratching and inflammation, lesions can become thick and lichenified. The treatment of eczema is with topical application of emulsifying ointment or 1% hydrocortisone ointment twice daily.

SEBORRHOEIC DERMATITIS. There is thickening, crusting and scaling of the skin in seborrhoeic dermatitis. Areas affected mainly are the scalp, the skin around the nostrils, and on the chin, upper back and upper arms. The treatment of seborrhoeic dermatitis is with topical application of 1% hydrocortisone ointment.

DERMATOMYCOSIS. Fungal skin infections may appear anywhere on the body, including the limbs, the trunk, the back, the face, the groin, hands and feet. Usually the lesions are circular with slightly elevated margins and scaling in the centres. The lesions may be itchy. The treatment is with topical application of clotrimazole cream.

CHAPTER 11
Special topics

CHAPTER 11.1
STI in pregnancy and children

O.P. Arya
Department of Medical Microbiology and Genitourinary Medicine, University of Liverpool, Liverpool, UK

The interactions between STI and pregnancy include the effects of pregnancy on STI and of STI on pregnancy. The latter is more important because STI may affect the outcome of pregnancy resulting in fetal damage, illness of the infant or even death. Several recent surveys in tropical countries have confirmed a very high prevalence of STI and HIV in pregnant women, over a quarter of the women in some settings having at least one STI, signifying a very great risk to the fetus *in utero* and to the newborn (see also Chapter 1). In many cases, the adverse outcomes, especially when associated with classical STI, can be eliminated or reduced if appropriate action is taken in time as described elsewhere in this book.

Mode of transmission of infection to fetus, infant and older child

The infection may occur: (i) *in utero* by way of ascending infection across the amnion or haematogenously across the placenta; (ii) intrapartum during delivery; or (iii) postpartum by direct contact or breast milk. The presence of STI in older children may suggest the possibility of sexual abuse or voluntary sexual activity.

Bacterial STI in pregnancy and children and their management including prevention

Syphilis. Chapter 7.1.
Gonorrhoea. Chapter 7.4.
Chlamydial infection. Chapter 7.5.
Bacterial vaginosis. Chapter 7.8.
Post-abortion and postpartum endometritis due to *Neisseria gonorrhoeae*, *Chlamydia trachomatis* and *Mycoplasma hominis*. Chapter 10.3.

Viral STI in pregnancy and children and management aspects

HIV infection and AIDS. Chapter 6.2.
Herpes simplex virus infection. Chapter 6.3.
Cytomegalovirus infection. Chapter 6.4.
Human papillomavirus (HPV) infection. Chapter 6.5.
Hepatitis. Chapter 6.7.

Fungal infections in pregnancy and children and management

Candidiasis. Chapter 8.1.

Protozoal infections in pregnancy and children and management

Trichomoniasis. Chapter 9.1.

Arthropod infestations

Scabies and pediculosis. Chapter 9.2.

Other organisms/infections

Several other organisms which are frequent colonizers of the female genitourinary tract and sexually transmissible have been reported, albeit in certain circumstances, to be associated with chorioamnionitis, prolonged rupture of membranes, pre-term delivery and/or low birthweight. They include group B. *Streptococcus*, *Ureaplasma urealyticum*, *Escherichia coli*, *Haemophilus influenzae* and anaerobic organisms. The significance of their role in adverse pregnancy outcome and/or the prevention of such outcomes remains problematic even in industrialized countries.

Treatment in pregnancy

Some drugs can have harmful effects on the pregnant women and/or on her fetus, and are, therefore, to be avoided in pregnancy. Some treatment regimens may need to be modified or become less effective, e.g. a pregnant woman may not tolerate erythromycin, 500 mg orally four times daily, because of gastro-intestinal side effects; a decreased dose, however, may fail to eradicate the infection. The common problems relating to treatment in pregnancy have been addressed in the relevant pages of the treatment sections in the book. The readers are also advised to consult their national formularies for guidance.

Further reading

Nageswaran, A. and Kinghorn, G.R. (1993) Sexually transmitted diseases in children: herpes simplex virus infection, cytomegalovirus infection, hepatitis B virus

infection and molluscum contagiosum. *Genitourinary Medicine* 69, 303–311.
Robinson, A.J. and Ridgway, G.L. (1994) Sexually transitted diseases in children: non viral including bacterial vaginosis, *Gardnerella vaginalis,* mycoplasmas, *Trichomonas vaginalis, Candida albicans*, scabies and pubic lice. *Genitourinary Medicine* 70, 208–214.

CHAPTER 11.2
STI in homosexual men

O.P. Arya
Department of Medical Microbiology and Genitourinary Medicine, University of Liverpool, Liverpool, UK

There is a paucity of data on STI in homosexual men in tropical countries. One reason is that homosexuality is taboo in many areas and, therefore, remains hidden. This concealment is detrimental to STI/AIDS control. In industrialized countries, the barriers have been largely broken, allowing continued participation of all concerned in STI/AIDS prevention and control programmes. Homosexuality seems to be less frequently practised in black Africa than in the other tropical regions.

Homosexual practices and infections which are principally sexually acquired

Homosexual practices include mutual masturbation, body rubbing, kissing, insertive and receptive anal intercourse, active and passive penile–oral contact (fellatio, oral sex), and active and passive oroanal contact (anilingus, rimming). Mutual masturbation, body rubbing and social kissing are relatively safe unless there are obvious lesions. The other practices, however, especially when unprotected, expose the partners to considerable risk of acquiring STI including AIDS, herpes simplex virus (HSV) infection, HPV infection, hepatitis B, syphilis, chancroid, gonorrhoea, chlamydial infections including lymphogranuloma venereum, and granuloma inguinale. All of these conditions with regard to their symptoms and signs involving genital and extragenital structures along with their management have been described elsewhere in the book.

History, examination and taking specimens (see also Chapter 4)

It must be emphasized that infections of the pharynx, anus and rectum are often asymptomatic. Therefore, if undetected and untreated, these patients may continue to spread the infection and develop complications. Thus, the importance of obtaining an accurate history as regards sexual orientation and sexual practices is obvious. The relevant questions should be asked in a non-judgemental and frank manner. An appropriate explanation for the need for this information will usually prompt correct responses and facilitate examination and obtaining specimens. The clinical examination should include a general physical examination, examination of the external genitalia and visualization of the throat, anus and rectum. The specimens should be obtained from all of the appropriate anatomical sites as well as sample(s) of blood for serological tests for syphilis, HIV, hepatitis B and others as indicated.

Enteric infections

In addition to the infections which are principally sexually acquired described above, certain practices, such as oral–anal contact and fellatio of a faecally contaminated penis, may expose the patient to the risk of acquiring enteric organisms which are traditionally known to be transmitted via contaminated food and water supply. These organisms include:

- Viruses: hepatitis A
- Bacteria: *Campylobacter* spp., *Salmonella* spp., *Shigella* spp.
- Protozoa: *Entamoeba histolytica, Giardia lamblia, Cryptosporidium parvum, Microsporidium* spp., *Isospora belli.*
- Helminths: *Enterobius vermicularis, Strongyloides stercoralis.*

The above infections are briefly described.

Clinical features

See Chapter 6.7 for information regarding hepatitis A.

Many patients infected with enteric organisms are asymptomatic. There is a considerable overlap in symptoms and signs. The common pathology is proctocolitis and/or enteritis. The symptoms in varying severity include abdominal discomfort, diarrhoea, flatulence, tenesmus and fever. The patients with severe illness due to *Shigella* spp. or pathogenic strains of *E. histolytica* may pass blood, mucus and pus in stools. Those harbouring only the cyst forms of *E. histolytica* may be completely asymptomatic.

In many normal immunocompetent persons, some infections, notably salmonellosis, shigellosis and cryptosporidiosis, are self-limiting diarrhoeal illnesses. However, in an immunocompromised patient, *Salmonella* infections may result in persistent bacteriaemia, and cryptosporidia may cause severe gastrointestinal disease and spread to other mucus planes such as the bile ducts and respiratory tract.

Giardiasis is suspected in the presence of pale, greasy, foul-smelling and explosive stools. Pruritus ani is the main symptom of threadworm infection. A patient with *S. stercoralis* infection may experience urticarial eruptions, and the infection may become widespread involving several organs in an immunocompromized individual.

Intestinal spirochaetosis

In some, the lower intestinal tract may be colonized with spirochaetes other than *Treponema pallidum.* A small proportion of these individuals may develop diarrhoea.

Differential diagnosis

The differential diagnosis includes all of the enteric infections mentioned above. Persistent intestinal symptoms will necessitate consideration of other conditions such as Crohn's disease, ulcerative colitis, HIV enteropathy, *Mycobacterium avium-intracellulare* and cytomegalovirus (CMV) colitis in a patient with HIV infection, neoplasms such as Kaposi's sarcoma (KS), etc. As for pruritus ani, which is a common symptom in homosexuals, the other causes include anal warts, haemorrhoids, fungal infection, anal fissure and poor hygiene.

Diagnosis

The diagnosis is confirmed by the detection of the pathogen concerned.

- For *Campylobacter*, *Salmonella* and *Shigella*, the diagnosis is made by the isolation of the organism by culture of the stool specimen on an appropriate medium
- For *E. histolytica* and *G. lambia,* freshly passed stools are examined for cysts and trophozoites.
- For *Cryptosporidium* and *I. belli*, the diagnosis is confirmed by examination of a stool specimen stained by safranin methylene blue, auramine phenol or a modified Ziehl–Neelsen stain.
- For *Microsporidium* spp., the diagnosis is made by staining stool specimens with trichrome or by electron microscopy of jejunal biopsies.
- For *E. vermicularis*, the worms may be seen crawling around the anus or obvious on rectal examination. More frequently, however, the diagnosis is made by the microscopic examination of a cellophane tape which had been applied to the perianal skin preferably in the morning before the patient has defaecated. The ova, if present, adhere to the sticky surface of the cellophane tape.
- For *S. steroralis*, the diagnosis is confirmed by finding the larvae in a stool specimen.
- For *intestinal spirochaetosis*, the diagnosis is made by darkfield microscopy and H & E stain of the rectal biopsy specimen.

Treatment

The dehydrated patient will require fluid and electrolytic replacement.

Campylobacter enterocolitis

The treatment is with erythromycin, 500 mg orally four times daily for 7 days, *or* ciprofloxacin, 500 mg orally twice daily for 5–7 days.

Salmonellosis and shigellosis

Antibacterial therapy is usually not indicated. Severely ill patients, however, may be treated with ciprofloxacin, 500 mg orally twice daily for 5–7 days.

Amoebiasis

The treatment is metronidazole, 800 mg orally three times daily for 5 days, and followed by diloxanide furoate (active against the cysts), 500 mg orally three times daily for 10 days. Some experts do not consider it necessary to treat patients who excrete only the cyst forms.

Giardiasis

Treatment is with metronidazole, 2 g orally daily for 3 days, *or* metronidazole, 400 mg orally three times daily for 5 days, *or* mepacrine hydrochloride, 100 mg orally three times daily for 5–7 days.

Cryptosporidiosis

Treatment is mainly supportive.

Microsporidiosis

Albendazole, 400 mg orally twice daily may help to control diarrhoea associated with species of *Encephalitozoon* and *Septata,* but it is ineffective for *E. bieneusi.*

Isosporiasis

Cotrimoxazole may alleviate symptoms but may not eradicate the organisms.

Enterobiasis

The treatment is mebendazole, 100 mg orally as a single dose, *or* pripsen one sachet of oral powder (piperazine phosphate 4 g/sennosides 15.3 mg) stirred into a small glass of milk or water and drunk immediately, and repeat after 14 days.

Strongyloidiasis

The treatment is thiabendazole, 25 mg kg^{-1} (maximum 1.5 g) every 12 h orally for 3 days.

Spirochaetosis

Only the symptomatic patients need be treated with metronidazole, 400 mg orally three times daily for 10 days.

Prevention

Preventive measures include attention to personal hygiene, safer sexual practices, avoidance of oral–anal contact, boiling of drinking water, and public health measures to improve sanitary facilities and food hygiene.

CHAPTER 11.3
STI, AIDS and malignancy

H.D.L. Birley
Department of Medical Microbiology and Genitourinary Medicine, University of Liverpool, Liverpool, UK

Microorganisms can cause the cellular genetic changes that result in malignancy in a number of ways, e.g. activation of oncoproteins or loss of tumour suppressor genes, loss or mutation of differentiation markers or inappropriate activation of angiogenesis. To this may be added the specific mechanism of impairment of immune surveillance by which HIV may indirectly act as a carcinogen. Some of the oncogenic mechanisms of some sexually transmitted pathogens are becoming understood. In others, such as syphilis and many bacterial infections, an association with malignancy, if any, seems to be related to prolonged inflammation rather than to a specific action of the microorganism itself. An analogy may be drawn with the development of squamous cell carcinoma following a long-standing cutaneous ulcer. In yet other instances there is an association between non-infective genital conditions such as lichen sclerosus et atrophicus (LSA) and malignancy. Such conditions are not strictly within the remit of this chapter since no sexually transmitted cause is known to underlie them. Recently, a number of malignant and proliferative diseases have been shown to be caused by the previously unknown virus, Kaposi's sarcoma-associated herpes virus (KSHV)/HHV-8. There is mounting evidence that this virus may be sexually transmitted and it often causes tumours in individuals infected with sexually transmitted HIV. It is by no means impossible, therefore, that conditions such as LSA may be shown to have an infective cause which also contributes to their malignant potential. For the present, however, this chapter will focus on two viruses in which sexual transmission is well established and some understanding of the mechanism of oncogenesis exists. These are human papillomavirus (HPV) and KSHV (HHV-8). In addition, hepatitis B virus, EBV and HIV are described briefly.

Human papillomavirus and carcinoma of the cervix

Carcinoma of the uterine cervix is the commonest cancer of women in many developing countries; in developed countries, it is much less common, as well as being less frequent than some other cancers, e.g. breast, lung and colon. The discovery of HPV as an aetiological agent of cervical cancer (and of other anogenital malignancies) has prompted a great deal of interest in the biology and oncogenicity of this virus, including large-scale epidemiological surveys comparing HPV and other possible causative agents between areas of high and low incidence of cervical carcinoma. Sexual practices, parity, diet, smoking, other diseases including STI, and immunogenetic characteristics may all play a contributory role in the development of cervical carcinoma. These factors may be independent of each other and of association with HPV infection. Age-standardized rates of cervical cancer differ very markedly worldwide – from 5.6 per 100,000 in Pakistan, the lowest reported incidence, to 96.5 per 100,000 in Recife, Brazil. In general, rates are lower in developed countries (see Fig. 11.3.1).

Papillomaviruses

Papillomaviruses are classified within the family *Papovaviridae*. All are small unenveloped viruses with a circular double-stranded DNA genome approximately 8 kb in length which utilize all three forward reading frames. The genome is transcribed and differentially spliced to produce early proteins (E1–E7) and two late proteins (L1 and L2). The early gene products are non-structural proteins which control viral replication and, in some cases, oncogenicity. The late gene products are structural proteins making up the

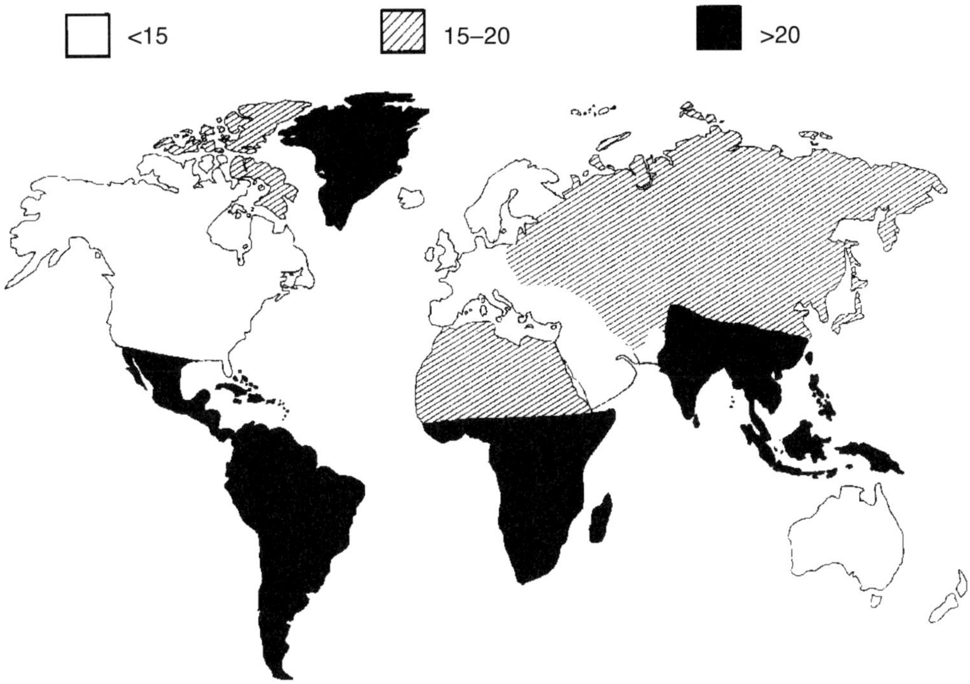

Fig. 11.3.1. Worldwide incidence of cervical cancer (cases/100,000 women). Adapted from Parkin, D.M., Pisani, P. and Ferlay, J. (1993) Estimates of the worldwide incidence of eighteen major cancers in 1985. *International Journal of Cancer* 54, 594–606.

virus capsid (see Chapter 6.5). Over 70 human types have been differentiated by DNA sequence analysis. Different types often display tropisms for different epithelial surfaces. About 20 HPV types characteristically infect mucosal epithelia, usually those of the genital tract.

Most papillomaviruses (and all HPV genotypes) can only infect epithelial cells. HPV does not lyse the epithelial cell which, however, must undergo its normal maturation for productive HPV infection. Thus, progeny virions are produced only near the mucosal surface, and little, if any, viral protein is produced in the basal layers of an infected epithelium. In view of the ubiquity of papillomaviruses amongst human and other vertebrate species, this fundamental strategy would seem to have evolutionary advantages. It may be that the expression of viral protein only in the distal epithelium helps to hide antigen from immune surveillance.

Equally, production of new infectious virions at the epithelial surface creates opportunities for transmission. The antigenically quiet cycling of the viral genome in basal epithelial cells may underlie the capacity of the virus for long periods of clinically silent, latent infection. Most papillomavirus infections are trivial to their hosts, but papillomavirus-associated malignancy is well known in several animal models, for example in cattle and cotton-tail rabbits.

The dependence of the virus on epithelial cell differentiation has had an important consequence for its study, namely the difficulty of growing HPV *in vitro*. Although investigators recently have produced virions, by using 'organotypic rafts' on which keratinocytes are induced to mature, there is no easy system for diagnostic culture or for infectivity or neutralization assays. In consequence, with the exception of some studies using live animals, all studies involving the detection of papillomaviruses or their pathogenic mechanisms have tended to use molecular biological techniques. In general, these have been nucleic acid based because of the difficulty of separating closely related types antigenically when pure antigens are so hard to produce. The classification of different papillomavirus types based upon DNA sequence heterogeneity is a prime example of this.

Mechanisms of oncogenesis

Over the last 30 years, techniques of DNA detection have led to discovery of HPV DNA in carcinomas of the cervix, in cell lines derived from them as well as in other anogenital malignancies. Epidemiological evidence had long suggested that a sexually transmissible agent might be related to carcinoma of the cervix. However, some STI tend to be risk factors for cervical carcinoma and therefore confound each other. Over the last 20 years, it has been established that DNA from HPV of certain oncogenic genital types (principally types 16 and 18) is present in nearly all cells derived from cervical cancers as well as in a proportion of anal, vulval and penile carcinomas. Viral DNA in a benign HPV infection such as a wart is episomal and remains circular, but viral DNA in malignant cells is usually truncated, linear and integrated into the host chromosomal DNA. Such DNA cannot support a productive infection since the reading frames for structural proteins are lost. However, certain early proteins are overexpressed, and the interaction between these and host proteins is intimately involved in the transformation to malignancy.

Two viral proteins, E6 and E7, bind to and inhibit two key cellular anti-oncogenes, p53 and the retinoblastoma protein (Rb). In normal cells, p53 and Rb regulate cell cycling and apoptosis, and their deletion in cell lines leads to immortalization. Only E6 and E7 from oncogenic HPV such as types 16 and 18 seem to have high affinity for binding these anti-oncoproteins. E6 and E7 proteins from types 6 and 11, the viruses commonly found in benign anogenital warts, cannot bind or do so only with low affinity. These types are almost never found in malignant carcinomas. Furthermore, transfection of human keratinocytes with the genes for E6 and E7 alone from HPV16 immortalizes these cells and renders them tumorigenic in nude mice after passage. More recently, it has been shown that another viral protein, E5, prevents the presentation of peptides by HLA class 1 by inhibiting TAP, a precursor protein. This may underlie the mechanism by which cervical carcinoma cells invading subepithelial tissues avoid immune recognition even when expressing foreign (viral) protein.

Epidemiology

Most epidemiological studies have used DNA detection methods (PCR being the most sensitive), since serological methods which will identify HPV types with high sensitivity and specificity have yet to be developed. The findings of various studies may be summarized as follows:

1. A high prevalence (up to 50%) of HPV in sexually active young women which rapidly declines with age beyond 55 years to less than 4%.
2. A strong association between: (i) age at first sexual intercourse and (ii) lifetime number of sexual partners and HPV positivity. There is a less consistent association with lifetime number of pregnancies/live births.
3. When HPV (especially HPV16 and -18) positivity is taken into account in multivariate analyses, the association between other factors which have been linked to cervical intraepithelial neoplasia (CIN) (such as smoking, race, social class, oral contraceptive use, other STI) disappears. This suggests that such factors are only risks for CIN in as much as they are risks for HPV infection.
4. A small residual effect of higher parity, earlier age of first sexual intercourse and more lifetime partners on cervical carcinoma persists independently of HPV infection.

The above findings tend to support both the sexual transmission of HPV and the causality of HPV in pre-malignant cervical dysplasia. More striking support has come from longitudinal cohort studies. The risk of developing CIN 2–3 (moderate to severe dysplasia) was significantly higher with HPV types 16 or 18 than in women who had only 'benign' HPV types (e.g. 6 or 11) or who remained HPV negative. Intriguingly, CMV and *Chlamydia trachomatis* antibody positivity also conferred an independently increased risk.

It would seem that the risk of developing cervical cancer may be more closely related to the inability of individuals to lose oncogenic HPV infection than to the risk of acquiring infection in the first place.

Cofactors

One of the most important factors which may account for persistence of HPV in some individuals or in some populations rather than in others is immunosuppression. Patients who are iatrogenically immunosuppressed, such as renal transplant recipients, are prone both to cutaneous and to genital HPV infection as well as to HPV-related malignancy. The classification of cervical cancer as an AIDS-defining diagnosis recognizes the influence of HIV-related immunosuppression upon HPV disease. It is very likely that, in the developing world where HIV is spreading most rapidly, this coinfection will further worsen the high incidence of cervical and other HPV-related malignancies.

Other cofactors which have been postulated to increase the oncogenicity of HPV infection include smoking, nutrition and oral contraceptive use. Nicotine and cotinine are found in the cervical mucus of smokers and may contribute to epithelial transformation. Amongst HPV-positive subjects, smoking seems to increase cancer risk. Vitamin deficiency, especially folate deficiency, is a logical cofactor since women are often deficient during pregnancy. Hypovitaminosis A is particularly associated with severe viral disease of mucosal surfaces (e.g. measles). Treatment with retinoids can reverse pre-malignant epithelial conditions in humans and animals. Although no firm evidence links cervical cancer with oral contraceptive use independently of HPV infection, there is experimental evidence that progesterone may enhance HPV16 oncogenicity. Such hormone–viral interactions may also be related to the association of cervical cancer with increased parity.

Strategies for cervical cancer prevention

Knowledge of the significant cofactors which enhance HPV oncogenicity suggests public health strategies which, despite formidable cultural obstacles, are probably the most practical ways to reduce the community burden of HPV-related malignancies, especially in developing countries. Many are appropriate general and sexual health measures. Examples are delay in first sexual intercourse/first pregnancy, reduction in pregnancies, reduction in number of sexual partners by both women and men, promotion of barrier methods of contraception, reduction in smoking and appropriate nutrition. Some of these may lead directly to a reduction in the prevalence of oncogenic HPV, but experience in other sexual health campaigns suggests that this will be at best a very slow process.

Besides grand multiparity, the most important risk factor for cervical cancer in women from Mexico, Panama, Costa Rica and Colombia was never having had a cervical smear test. Screening by cytology of cervical smears has long been established as an effective means of prevention of cervical cancer in developed countries. Most programmes have screened adult women at least every 5 years until the age of 65 or so, but even a single smear at age 45 years might reduce the incidence of cervical cancer by 25%, and two smears at ages 45 and 55 years would reduce it by 40–45%. Studies have shown that even simpler methods may detect cervical cancer at a stage when operative treatment is curative; visual inspection alone identified 63%. Such modified programmes would reduce costs, but effective prevention by this means depends critically upon the provision of adequate smear-takers and cytologists as well as expertise and equipment to treat pre-malignant lesions. In order to reduce cervical cancer in a population, it is essential to screen a very high proportion of it. Frequently, the attendance of high-risk women is poor. Cervical screening in developed countries has often failed in one or more of these aspects; the difficulties in developing countries are likely to be greater.

New directions in HPV immunology

Despite the latency of papillomaviruses, which suggests a capacity for immune avoidance, there is histopathological evidence that elimination of infection is achieved through immune mechanisms. The striking reduction in oncogenic HPV prevalence in older cohorts supports this.

A principal difficulty in studying the immune response to HPV lies in the difficulty in obtaining pure antigens. Nevertheless, patients with genital warts have been shown to have significantly increased antibody responses.

New serological tests for HPV are being investigated through the ability to express HPV proteins in eukaryotic cells by using recombinant viruses. Using a recombinant insect baculovirus expressing the outer capsid L1 protein of HPV16, the majority of HPV16-infected subjects can be identified, and seroreactivity seems to be a sensitive marker of the acquisition of infection. If these tests bear out their early promise, a much simpler (and potentially cheaper) method of screening for oncogenic HPV infection may be possible. This might represent a major advance for countries unable to provide cytology-based cervical screening. The multiple types of oncogenic HPV pose a serious problem in vaccine design. Although most cervical cancer worldwide is caused by HPV16, there are areas where HPV18 is as common or more common. Furthermore, the allocation of a papillomavirus to a type does not imply antigenic uniformity. The reported HLA associations with cervical cancer and the ability of HPV to evade the host immune response may complicate matters further (see also Chapter 12.2).

Human herpesvirus type 8 and Kaposi's sarcoma

The classical KS, first described over 100 years ago, is a rare, slowly progressive tumour of elderly males. Lesions are mainly confined to the skin of the extremities. The endemic KS discovered later in Africa has four different clinical variants: (i) benign disease with few lesions reminiscent of classical KS; (ii) aggressive disease mainly localized to extremities with local invasion and destruction; (iii) widely disseminated disease with visceral involvement; and (iv) a lymphadenopathic form with preferential involvement of lymph nodes and visceral organs but minimal mucocutaneous lesions. Such aggressive endemic KS affects women, young adults and children, and not just elderly men. Nowadays, in developed countries, KS most commonly is associated with HIV infection, and this variant, termed 'epidemic KS' is characterized by widely distributed lesions, visceral as well as lymph node involvement, and a rapidly progressive course (Plate 119: see also Chapter 11.5). KS also occurs in iatrogenically immunosuppressed individuals ('iatrogenic KS').

The clinical presentation of KS may be unusual. Often multifocal lesions arise *de novo* in distributions inconsistent with metastatic spread. New KS lesions, particularly, contain multiple cell types which form slit-like vascular spaces lined by flattened endothelial cells. A cellular infiltrate of lymphocytes and plasma cells is often present, and can, when combined with aggregated endothelial cells, contribute to the 'pseudogranulomatous' character of some of these lesions. Later KS lesions are dominated by more uniform spindle-like cells. These observations, together with reports of regression of KS lesions in transplant patients (after withdrawal of immunosuppressive medication), suggest that early KS at least is not a truly malignant lesion but a proliferative one.

The monoclonal cellular nature of individual KS nodules and the fact that 'malignant' cell lines can be established from KS biopsies suggests that the transformation of at least some cells in the KS lesion to a malignant phenotype is possible. Their origin is still controversial. Endothelial cells (either vascular or lymphatic endothelium), cells from venous lymphatic junctions, fibroblasts, smooth muscle cells and dermal dendrocytes have all been proposed as possible progenitors of KS spindle cells. Several growth factors, including platelet-derived growth factor (PDGF), interleukin-1 (IL-1) and IL-6, are produced by KS cells *in vivo* and *in vitro* and may be required for their growth. KS cells related to endothelial cells produce PDGF which is required for the growth of spindle cells exhibiting fibroblastoid characteristics, which suggests the interdependence of cells of different lineages found in a KS lesion.

The epidemiology of KS, most notably its rarity in haemophiliacs as opposed to homosexual men with HIV, strongly suggests a sexually acquired infective cause. The search for such a cause has yielded a plethora of candidate 'KS agents'. Herpesvirus-like particles, cytomegalovirus, C-type retroviruses, papillomaviruses, HHV-6 and *Mycoplasma penetrans* have all been considered with varying degrees of supporting evidence. Recently, DNA of a previously unknown herpesvirus was discovered by 'representational difference analysis' – identifying DNA sequences in KS lesions which are not present in non-diseased tissues taken from the same patient. There is now mounting evidence for the causative association of this virus, KSHV (or human herpesvirus 8) with KS. DNA of KSHV has been found in all varieties of KS and can be found in blood and some tissues and body fluids (including some semen samples) of patients with KS but has not been found in blood from UK blood donors. In asymptomatic HIV-positive patients, detection of KSHV in peripheral blood mononuclear cells (PBMC) predicts subsequent development of KS. The presence of KSHV in semen supports sexual transmission, and a report of the virus in PBMC of an HIV-infected child prior to development of KS suggests that vertically transmitted KSHV could cause childhood KS. KSHV has also been found in AIDS-related B-cell lymphomas, usually, but not always, associated with EBV.

Cofactors

Clearly, other factors besides KSHV must contribute to the development of KS. For example, although common in sexually transmitted AIDS, the tumour is relatively much rarer in women, possibly because of hormonal factors.

Much work is needed to unravel the pathogenesis of Kaposi's tumour and the role of this newly discovered herpesvirus in it. The knowledge thus gained may help in the development of therapeutic interventions and vaccines against this major killer.

Other sexually transmitted and HIV-related tumours

Hepatitis viruses (see also Chapter 6.7)

Hepatitis B virus, which can be sexually transmitted, is a well-established oncogenic virus and a major cause of hepatocellular carcinoma. This tumour is particularly common in Africa and in the Far East, where rates of persistent HBV infection are high. Sexually transmitted HBV, however, is rarely the cause of hepatocellular carcinoma since this tumour rarely occurs in individuals who are not chronic carriers of the virus, usually those who are infected vertically or in early childhood. Hepatitis C is another cause of hepatocellular carcinoma, but although there is some evidence that this agent may be sexually transmitted, this would seem to be unusual. Whether coinfection with both HBV and HIV predisposes to cancer is unknown. Certainly HIV may permit increased viral replication through immunosuppression, but there is good evidence that at least part of the mechanism for HBV-related tissue damage (and oncogenesis) may be mediated via an immune response to infected cells. On the other hand, the lack of substantial numbers of HIV-infected individuals developing hepatocellular cancer may be because they die first from other illnesses.

Epstein–Barr virus (EBV) (see also Chapter 6.4)

HIV may act as a cofactor with other herpesviruses such as EBV, which is extremely common in the 'Burkitt-like' B-cell lymphomas which are a common AIDS diagnosis. Although not exclusively so, EBV may itself be sexually transmitted.

HIV

As well as acting as a cofactor with other viruses, there is evidence that, like some related retroviruses, HIV may be oncogenic in its own right. In addition, HIV may potentiate the action of non-infective carcinogens. Recently, a dramatic increase in the rate of conjunctival squamous cell carcinoma in HIV-infected Ugandan patients has been reported. Although the mechanism of this is not known, it has been suggested that exposure to ultraviolet light may have a role.

CHAPTER 11.4
Interaction between HIV and other STI

O.P. Arya
Department of Medical Microbiology and Genitourinary Medicine, University of Liverpool, Liverpool, UK

HIV and other STI may interact with each other basically in two ways: (i) effects of other STI on HIV; and (ii) effects of HIV on other STI.

Effects of other STI on HIV (see also Chapter 1)

A number of studies have shown or suggested that certain sexually transmitted infections may facilitate transmission of HIV. Based on present knowledge, the situation may be summarized as follows: STI activate T lymphocytes and macrophages which, being target cells for HIV infection, increase susceptibility to HIV infections of a seronegative individual and increase HIV shedding from, and thus infectivity of, a seropositive individual. To prove whether other STI do indeed enhance HIV transmission is fraught with difficulties, the most obvious being the same high-risk sexual behaviour involved in the transmission of these infections as well as the fact that mixed infections do occur anyway. The other confounding factors which need to be controlled include the use of condoms, status of circumcision, menstruation, cervical ectopy, stage of HIV disease, virulence of HIV strain, quality of diagnostic assays used and the various facets of sexual behaviour, etc. Even longitudinal studies, essential to research these interactions, are subject to error especially with regard to sexual history (often unreliable), condom use (subject to reporting bias), time sequence of infection and STI status of the primary source (often difficult to determine). Nevertheless, several studies have shown consistently that ulcerative STI, such as syphilis, chancroid and possibly also others, facilitate HIV transmission. In addition to the presence of activated target cells and increased shedding of the virus, the ulcerative lesions, being open, easily permit contact of virus-infected cells with susceptible host cells. The role of non-ulcerative STI in this respect is not so clear-cut and some studies have produced contradictory results. However, high concentrations of HIV-1 reported in semen of HIV-1-seropositive men with gonorrhoea prompted suggestions that gonorrhoea may thus enhance HIV-1 infectivity and transmission (see also Chapter 7.4)

A randomized controlled trial in Tanzania did indeed demonstrate that interventions against STI reduced the transmission of HIV – thus supporting the cofactor role of STI in HIV transmission. There was, however, no significant impact on the incidence of STI, which may at least partly be due to the inevitable shortcoming of the 'syndromic' approach used in the study.

This facilitating role of STI in HIV transmission has given impetus to urging governments into action to institute STI control measures as an essential component of HIV prevention programmes. This can only do good even though it has been clear that STI, being a major public health problem in many tropical countries, merited a no less intensive control programme in their own right. Obviously, what we need now is an integrated prevention and control programme for STI, HIV and AIDS (see Chapter 12.1).

Effects of HIV on other STI (see also Chapter 1)

The effects of HIV on other STI are due to the immunological abnormalities associated with the former (see Chapters 3 and 6.1). The possible or actual effects include alterations in the clinical presentation and the natural history of STI, the reliability of diagnostic tests, and the response to conventional treatment. These have been described in the individual chapters on the specific infections. In addition, ulcerative diseases and HIV infection may prolong each other's infectiousness synergistically.

Further reading

Cohen, M.S., Hoffman, I.F., Royce, R.A., Kazembe, P., Dyer, J.R., Dally, C.C., Zimba, D., Vernazza, P.L., Maida, M., Fiscus, S.A., Eton, J.J. Jr and the AIDSCAP Malawi Research Group (1996) Reduction of concentration of HIV-1 in semen after treatment of urethritis: implications for prevention of sexual transmission of HIV-1. *Lancet* 349, 1868–1873.

Grosskurth, H., Mosha, F., Todd, J., Mwijarubi, E., Klokke, A., Senkoro, K., Mayaud, P., Changalucha, J., Nicoll, A., Kagina, G., Newell, J., Mugeye, K., Mabey, D. and Hayes, R. (1995) Impact of improved treatment of sexually transmitted diseases on HIV infection in rural Tanzania: randomized controlled trial. *Lancet* 346 , 530–536.

Quinn, T.C. (1996) Association of sexually transmitted diseases and infection with the human immunodeficiency virus: biological cofactors and markers of behavioural interventions. *International Journal of STD and AIDS* 7 (Suppl. 2), 17–24.

Wasserheit, J.N. (1992) Epidemiological synergy: interrelationships between human immunodificiency virus infection and other sexually transmitted diseases. *Sexually Transmitted Diseases* 19, 61–77.

Chapter 11.5
Dermatological manifestations of HIV infection and other STI, and some other dermatological conditions of genitalia encountered in STI clinics

A. Sivayathorn
Department of Dermatology, Siriraj Hospital, Bangkok, Thailand

Dermatological manifestations of HIV infection

Skin and mucous membrane disorders are highly prevalent among persons infected with HIV. In many instances, the presence of a skin disorder is the first manifestation of HIV infection or serves as a clue which leads to the correct diagnosis. It is important to recognize these conditions from the standpoints of diagnosis and treatment, as well as improvement of quality of life of these individuals.

Most of the dermatological manifestations of HIV infection are well documented in the literature, but there are notable differences in disease patterns between tropical and temperate zones. This chapter outlines some of the common and important skin and mucous membrane manifestations of HIV infection seen in the tropics.

Whereas most cutaneous disorders can appear at any stage of HIV infection, they are more persistent, severe and extensive when the $CD4^+$-count falls below 150 cells mm^{-3}. Infective conditions may present in atypical or exaggerated forms because of the underlying immunosuppression, including impairment of the skin immune systems (Langerhans cells of the skin are targets in HIV-1 infection).

Viral infections

Primary HIV-1 infection

Over half of the patients with HIV-1 infection develop an acute clinical illness after an incubation period of 3–6 weeks. This glandular fever-like illness may last from 1 to 2 weeks. Some patients may experience a symmetrical, erythematous, non-pruritic, maculopapular skin rash which may resemble secondary syphilis. The diagnosis requires a high index of suspicion.

Herpes simplex infection

HIV-infected patients often have locally destructive and persistent herpes simplex infection (Plate 120) but rarely generalized manifestations. The majority of these infections are due to reactivation of the latent virus; hence lesions commonly occur at the usual sites, i.e. lips, mouth, genitalia and anus. Untreated, these lesions become large, deep, confluent ulcers which are often covered with necrotic crust. The diagnosis is confirmed by viral culture.

TREATMENT. Treatment is with a course of oral aciclovir, 400 mg five times a day for 7–10 days. In the absence of laboratory confirmation, a therapeutic trial is justified. Newer antiviral drugs, such as famciclovir and valaciclovir, have the advantage of less frequent dosing but their efficacy in the immunocompromised host needs further confirmation. Failure to respond to treatment indicates that these chronic ulcers are either non-herpetic or caused by aciclovir-resistant virus. Aciclovir-resistant infections have been reported to respond to treatment with foscarnet, 40 mg kg^{-1} body weight intravenously every 8 h until the lesions have resolved. To minimize the development of resistance, long-term suppressive therapy with aciclovir should be reserved for patients with frequent attacks.

Herpes zoster

The clinical occurrence of herpes zoster is the result of reactivation of a latent residual varicella-zoster virus (VZV) infection within a sensory ganglion. The cutaneous eruption occurs in a localized dermatomal distribution and is characterized by painful clusters of vesicles.

The possibility of undetected HIV infection should be strongly considered in a young patient (<35 years of age) who presents with severe herpes zoster. The eruption may be bullous, haemorrhagic, purulent, ulcerative or necrotic, filling the whole segment of a dermatome with moderate to severe neuralgia (Plate 121). Occasionally it is multidermatomal, recurrent within the same dermatome, or disseminated. The majority of these patients experience an uneventful recovery. However, atypical clinical courses are not uncommon. Lesions may persist for months, appearing as hyperkeratotic, ulcerated, painful nodules. Scarring from these zoster episodes is usually quite prominent and serves as another marker for HIV infection.

TREATMENT. Treatment of herpes zoster in HIV-infected patients is not clearly defined. Most clinicians will treat these patients with aciclovir, 800 mg orally, five times a day for 7–10 days or until new lesions cease to appear. As in the case of herpes simplex virus, aciclovir-resistant VZV has been isolated from chronic ulcerations and hyperkeratotic lesions. Aciclovir-resistant VZV responds to treatment with foscarnet, 40 mg kg^{-1} body weight intravenously every 8 h for 5–7 days.

Anogenital warts

Anogenital warts frequently become large, confluent and more numerous in immunosuppressed patients.

See Chapters 6.5 and 11.3 for other details including cervical dysplasia.

TREATMENT. Patients with early stages of HIV infection may respond favourably to treatment. As the immunosuppression progresses, treatment becomes increasingly difficult. Because the presence of intact cell-mediated immunity is important in clearing warts, treatment is likely to be prolonged. Podophyllin 25% in tincture benzoin is applied and left on for 4 h, with an increase in exposure time on subsequent treatment depending on the patients' responses. Other destructive methods that have been used include liquid nitrogen cryotherapy, the topical application of 80–90% trichloracetic acid or 5-fluorouracil. Massive condylomata are extremely difficult to treat and may require surgical or laser removal if they cause sufficient discomfort.

Molluscum contagiosum

See below and Chapter 6.6.

Oral hairy leukoplakia

Oral hairy leukoplakia is a specific, viral-induced eruption, a manifestation of epithelial hyperplasia caused by Epstein–Barr virus, with no malignant potential. It occurs almost exclusively in HIV-infected persons and is predictive for the development of progressive immunosuppression. Clinically it presents as a white, corrugated, non-removable patch, usually occurring on the lateral margin of the tongue (Plate 122). The lesion may appear either unilaterally or bilaterally and may also be present on the ventral surface of the tongue. Occasionally the floor of the mouth, soft palate and tonsillar pillar are involved.

TREATMENT. The condition is usually asymptomatic and requires no treatment and may regress spontaneously. In patients with severe symptoms such as pain or burning, administration of high-dose oral aciclovir results in temporary regression of lesions.

Bacterial infections

Pyoderma

Pyogenic bacterial infections are common in HIV-infected patients. Both *Staphylococcus aureus* and *Streptococcus pyogenes* skin infections occur and commonly present as impetigo, ecthyma, furunculosis, abscesses, cellulitis and ulcers. Recurrent infections are common, especially in individuals with nasal colonization by the organisms. Occasionally, cutaneous infections are caused by Gram-negative bacteria or can be polymicrobial. Gram-stained smear and cultures of pus are recommended routinely.

TREATMENT. Treatment is usually with flucloxacillin, 250–500 mg orally four times daily. Prolonged treatment may be required. Severe cases should be hospitalized. If there is no clinical response, the antibiotics should be changed according to the results of sensitivity tests. Rifampicin, 300 mg orally once daily for 10 days, may facilitate cure and the elimination of chronic carrier state.

Syphilis

There is increased prevalence of syphilis in HIV-infected persons and vice versa. Clinical features of syphilis in some HIV-infected patients may be atypical. Generalized papulosquamous lesions with central necrosis, vesicular eruption of the palms and soles, hyperpigmented lesions of the flexures, and multiple oral ulcerations have been reported as presenting signs of secondary syphilis in patients with concurrent HIV infection.

See Chapter 7.1 for further details on syphilis–HIV interaction and management.

Fungal infections (see also Chapter 8.2)

Candidiasis

Oral candidiasis is the most common oral opportunistic infection seen in patients with HIV infection and occurs in more than 90% of HIV-positive patients at some point during their disease. These patients also commonly have angular cheilitis and pharyngeal and oesophageal infections. Intertrigenous infections can involve the groin, axillary vault or inframammary areas. A hallmark of candidal intertrigo is the presence of satellite pustules. Candidal paronychia is also common.

Several clinical variants of oral candidiasis exist. Thrush or pseudomembranous candidiasis is the most obvious type. Clinically, it appears as white plaques that are removable by scraping, leaving an erythematous surface with superficial erosion, commonly occurring on the buccal mucosa, the palate or the dorsal surface of the tongue (Plate 123). Erythematous candidiasis shows red macular patches on mucosal surfaces. This clinical variant is seen most commonly in HIV-infected individuals and is rarely seen in normal people. Hyperplastic oral candidiasis occurs often on the buccal mucosa and has white plaques that are unremovable by scraping. Angular cheilitis is characterized by fissures and ulceration at the corners of the mouth. Organisms can usually be demonstrated from the scraped material by Gram stain.

See Chapter 8.1 for vulvovaginitis and balanitis due to *Candida* spp.

TREATMENT. Topical therapy should be tried initially. Clotrimazole 10 mg oral troche dissolved slowly in the mouth five times a day for about 1 week is an effective treatment, but relapses are common. Clotrimazole can also be used as a cream for the treatment of angular cheilitis. Systemic treatment is required in cases with widespread disease or when topical therapy has failed.

Ketoconazole is recommended at a daily dosage of 200–400 mg. Fluconazole, 100 mg daily or itraconazole, 200 mg daily, are less toxic with better efficacy and fewer drug interactions, but are more expensive. Infections due to *Candida* spp. other than *C. albicans* are becoming increasingly important, and such yeasts are reported to be much more resistant to antifungals.

Dermatophytosis

Tinea cruris (often with truncal involvement), tinea pedis and tinea corporis frequently occur in patients with HIV infection, whereas tinea capitis and tinea faciale are less common. These conditions are usually similar in appearance to the diseases in non-HIV-infected persons but are more widespread. They are also caused in most instances by the same organisms that cause disease in non-HIV-infected patients. Clinical diagnosis should be confirmed by the KOH examination of skin scrapes.

TREATMENT. Most forms of dermatophytosis in HIV-positive patients respond well to topical antifungal agents, even in patients with a profound reduction in $CD4^+$ T-cell count. If the disease is extensive, orally administered antifungal medications may be necessary. Griseofulvin, 500 mg orally once or twice daily, should be tried initially, but resistance to this drug is common.

Ketoconazole, 200 mg orally daily, can be used in patients who are intolerant or refractory to griseofulvin. Rarely, prolonged treatment with this drug has been reported to result in fatal hepatitis. The absorption of ketoconazole requires an acidic environment; therefore, patients should be advised to take this medicine with a fruit juice or carbonated beverage to increase the gastric acidity because HIV-positive patients are often achlorhydric.

Itraconazole has less hepatotoxicity than ketoconazole but is more expensive. The usual dose of itraconazole is 100 mg orally daily. Oral terbinafine, 250 mg daily, also holds promise in the management of these infections.

Although superficial mycoses are easily treated, they recur frequently in this immunosuppressed population. Thus the major problem is to prevent recurrences. In addition to local measures, such as keeping the area dry and limiting maceration, it may be necessary to treat these patients long term with a topical or oral antifungal agent.

Onychomycosis

Tinea unguium of the toenails (mostly due to *Trichophyton rubrum*), often with extensive involvement of the dorsal area of the foot, is common in HIV-positive patients. Fungal disease of the fingernails is less common. Proximal white subungual onychomycosis, a classic nail sign of HIV infection, occurs when the fungus spreads under the proximal nail fold, establishes itself in the nail fold and nail bed epithelium, invades the ventral nail plate, and spreads distally.

TREATMENT. Until recently, management of onychomycosis in HIV-positive patients was difficult because griseofulvin lacks efficacy. The response to ketoconazole is somewhat better but requires prolonged therapy. Itraconazole, 200 mg orally daily for 3 months, is highly effective in clearing the nail infection.

Pityrosporum *infections*

Pityriasis versicolor is caused by overgrowth of yeasts of the genus *Pityrosporum*. In dark-skinned people, it appears as hypopigmented patches. Although the disease can be very extensive, especially in HIV-positive patients living in the tropics, its prevalence is similar to that in HIV-negative persons. *Pityrosporum ovale* occasionally can cause a folliculitis in HIV-positive patients. This is characterized by numerous papules and pustules occurring on the upper trunk and proximal arms. KOH preparation of scrapings from the lesions can be performed to confirm the diagnosis.

TREATMENT. For pityriasis versicolor, conventional topical treatment, such as clotrimazole cream, should be tried first. Both pityriasis versicolor and pityrosporum folliculitis will repond to a 10–14-day course of ketoconazole, 200 mg daily.

Cryptococcosis

Cutaneous dissemination occurs in about 10% of HIV-negative patients with cryptococcal disease but may be more common in HIV-positive patients who often develop cryptococcosis. Erosions, ulcerations and, less frequently, vesicles, papules and nodules may be cutaneous signs of cryptococcosis in patients with HIV infection. Systemic symptoms include malaise, headache and fever. Papules associated with disseminated cryptococcosis can usually be distinguished from those of molluscum contagiosum by the evidence of crusting in the former. Molluscum lesions usually do not crust unless they have been excoriated or treated. Results of the India ink test are positive in most patients with AIDS with cryptococcal meningitis, as are CSF antigen test and cultures. Appropriate biopsy specimens are required to isolate the fungus from skin lesions.

TREATMENT. Amphotericin B is the standard treatment for cryptococcosis. It is administered by slow intravenous infusion daily at the dosage of 0.3–0.6 mg kg^{-1} body weight for 6–8 weeks or until a total dose of 2 g is achieved. The current treatment regimen consists of an induction course with amphotericin B followed by maintenance treatment with fluconazole, 200 mg orally daily. Itraconazole is also effective in cryptococcal meningitis. There are on-going studies comparing the efficacy of fluconazole and itraconazole. Ketoconazole is not effective in AIDS patients.

Histoplasmosis

Histoplasma capsulatum infections are difficult to diagnose in patients with AIDS because they can have numerous, non-specific symptoms and signs, including fever, weight loss, abdominal pain, diarrhoea, hepatic and splenic enlargement, skin lesions, adrenal insufficiency, and gastrointestinal, pulmonary and blood diseases. The cutaneous lesions may mimic molluscum contagiosum infection or cellulitis. However, any uncharacteristic lesions should be biopsied. The diagnosis is confirmed by performing a culture. Bone marrow produces the highest yield, followed by blood and sputum.

TREATMENT. Clinical experience with amphotericin B in the treatment of histoplasmosis has been disappointing. Preliminary results with itraconazole (400 mg daily for 12 weeks) suggest that it may be more effective than ketoconazole and amphotericin B in the primary treatment of histoplasmosis. Itraconazole is also effective in prevention of relapse.

Penicilliosis

Penicillium marneffei is an unusual dimorphic fungus that can cause human infection in compromised hosts and rarely in healthy subjects. This systemic mycosis is endemic to countries of Southeast Asia and the southern part of China. The prevalence of *P. marneffei* infection has increased substantially during the last few years. This increase has occurred exclusively among patients with the advanced stage of HIV infection and is currently considered as an AIDS-defining disease.

Cutaneous manifestations occur in about 75% of the cases. The characteristic eruption is a generalized papular rash with predilection for the face, upper trunk and arms. The papules have central necrotic umbilication resembling lesions of molluscum contagiosum (Plate 124). A direct stained smear (Wright's stain) from the lesion and/or a skin biopsy usually reveals clumps of yeast cells with binary fission. Less frequent skin manifestations of this disease include folliculitis, subcutaneous nodules and chronic ulcers. Systemic symptoms include fever, weight loss, anaemia, cough, lymphadenopathy, hepatosplenomegaly and diarrhoea. In cases without skin lesions, early diagnosis can be made on the basis of characteristic septate yeast-like cells in Wright's-stained bone-marrow aspirate or a touch smear of lymph node biopsy specimens.

The mortality rate of patients with *P. marneffei* infection is very high and is mostly due to failure to make a timely diagnosis. Early diagnosis and treatment thus greatly improve survival.

TREATMENT. A useful treatment regimen comprises induction treatment with amphotericin B for 2 weeks followed by oral itraconazole, 200 mg orally twice daily for 6 weeks. After that, suppressive treatment with itraconazole, 200 mg orally daily, is continued indefinitely.

Non-infectious skin manifestations

Seborrhoeic dermatitis

Seborrhoeic dermatitis is a benign dermatosis of unknown cause with a prevalence of 1–3% in the general population and 3–5% in young adults. The erythematous, scaling plaques are most often seen on the scalp, ears and seborrhoeic areas of the face, including the eyebrows, beard and nasolabial regions. It may also occur less commonly in other hair-bearing areas of the body such as the axillae, groins, anterior aspect of the chest, and the genitalia.

Seborrhoeic dermatitis often appears early in HIV infection. Indeed, HIV infection should be suspected in any young person from an 'at risk' group who develops severe inflammatory seborrheic dermatitis.

Between 30 and 80% of patients with AIDS have seborrhoeic dermatitis. The patients often have thick, greasy, scaly papules and plaques on the face, without much scalp involvement. Frequently, the upper chest, upper back and the pubic region are also involved. Lesions of seborrhoeic dermatitis in HIV-infected patients are more erythematous and papular than in HIV-negative patients (Plate 125). Often the lesions are psoriasiform in appearance.

The pathogenesis of seborrhoeic dermatitis in HIV infection is still unknown. Studies on the role of *Pityrosporum* yeasts have shown conflicting results.

TREATMENT. Topical antifungal agents such as ketoconazole cream and shampoo should be tried first. Patients refractory to antifungal treatment should be treated with twice daily applications of a non-fluorinated topical steroid such as 1% hydrocortisone cream. Some patients may require fluorinated steroid especially in the presence of lichenification.

Psoriasis

Psoriasis may be the first manifestation of HIV infection. The development of explosive psoriasis or a sudden flare of pre-existing psoriasis in potential AIDS candidate should raise the possibility of an underlying HIV infection.

HIV-associated psoriasis is often atypical in distribution or may present with more generalized scaling than noted in classic psoriasis. Prominent involvement of the groin, axillae and scalp may occur (Plate 126). Palmoplantar keratoderma is common.

TREATMENT. Zidovudine, 1200 mg daily may improve or clear psoriasis in some cases. If there is no response, etretinate or acitretin (neotigason), 0.5 mg kg^{-1} body weight daily may be tried. These drugs are teratogenic and should be used under specialist supervision. Ultraviolet B phototherapy has also been reported to be effective. Methotrexate is contraindicated in HIV-associated psoriasis because it may enhance immunosuppression. A low-potency topical steroid or calcipotriol are useful adjunctive therapies.

Pruritic papular eruption (PPE)

PPE is a common feature in HIV infection in the tropical climate. Clinically, it appears as pruritic, symmetrical, discrete, red or skin-coloured papules, some with central pitting, which involve the trunk, extremities or face to varying degrees (Plate 127). Chronic lesions, as a result of intense itching and oozing, become excoriated and hyperpigmented. The patient may feel stigmatized. The cause of this peculiar condition is unknown. PPE appears to be less common in patients with AIDS in Europe and the USA. The apparent geographic restriction of these pruritic eruptions to tropical area suggests an environmental factor such as insects or an allergic phenomenon. Increased antibody titres to mosquito salivary gland antigens have been reported in some patients. Because of the high prevalence of PPE in HIV-infected patients in tropical areas, it has become a useful marker for HIV infection. Any high-risk person who suddenly develops unexplained widespread pruritic papular eruption should be urged to undergo counselling for HIV testing. PPE runs a chronic course with waxing and waning of symptoms, which may be exacerbated by heat and sweating.

TREATMENT. Oral antihistamines are of limited help in ameliorating the pruritus, but should be tried. Topical therapy with a potent steroid, such as clobetasol cream, offers partial relief in most cases. Phototherapy (both UVB and PUVA) has been employed when other measures fail.

Drug reactions

Adverse skin reaction to drugs are also more prevalent in HIV-positive individuals. This is most likely to be caused by the increased use of medications and increased risk of drug hypersensitivity in this population. Clinical patterns include morbilliform eruption (80–90%), urticaria, vasculitis, erythema multiforme, Stevens–Johnson syndrome, toxic epidermal necrolysis and exfoliative dermatitis. The most common drugs implicated include sulphonamides, antituberculous drugs (isoniazid, rifampicin), phenytoin and antibiotics.

Some drugs used for treating HIV infection have been reported to cause characteristic skin reactions which make them more easily recognizable. These reactions include pigmentation of the nail plate and dermatomyositis-like syndrome caused by zidovudine, ulceration at a pentamidine injection site, painful oral and genital ulceration following foscarnet administration, cyanosis associated with the use of dapsone, and dapsone syndrome (morbilliform eruption and toxic hepatitis), and gyrate erythema at the granulocyte-stimulating factor injection site.

TREATMENT. The clinical management of a drug eruption includes avoidance of the offending drugs. Patients with *P. carinii* pneumonia who are allergic to trimethoprim–sulphamethoxazole should be switched to pentamidine treatment or desensitization. Administration of antihistamine is of benefit in a mild reaction. Patients with severe reaction may require treatment with a short course of systemic steroid.

Skin tumours (see also Chapter 11.3)

KS is an endothelial tumour with widespread mucocutaneous and systemic involvement. In Western countries, KS is the most common cutaneous neoplasm in HIV-infected patients. In contrast, KS is rarely associated with HIV infection in Asia. Although the cause of KS is still not definitely known, recent evidence suggests that human herpesvirus 8 (HHV-8) may be the aetiologic agent of KS. Unlike other herpesviruses, HHV-8 is probably not ubiquitous. This might well account for the low prevalence of KS in non-endemic areas of HHV-8 infection.

Clinical lesions of KS vary from small erythematous papules to tumourous, haemorrhagic, ulcerated lesions. Treatment modalities include cryotherapy, chemotherapy, surgical excision, irradiation and interferon.

Other skin tumours reported in patients with HIV infection include lymphomas, squamous cell carcinoma, basal cell carcinoma, and dysplastic nevi.

Skin manifestations of certain STI

Specific dermatologic syndromes are manifestations of or associated with a number of STI. This section considers some of these conditions. Others are described elsewhere in the book.

Molluscum contagiosum (see also Chapter 6.6)

Molluscum contagiosum is caused by a pox virus and is transmitted by close body contact. It is most prevalent in children, and lesions are usually found on the body. In adults, however, the disease is mainly sexually transmitted, with a predilection for the genital area. The incubation period is 2–3 weeks.

A typical lesion of molluscum contagiosum is a pearly dome-shaped papule with central umbilication. In HIV-infected patients, lesions are usually numerous, appear in unusual sites or become grotesque (Plate 128). Diagnosis is usually clinical. However, identification of characteristic intracytoplasmic inclusion bodies in either histological or cytological specimens under the microscope confirms the diagnosis.

TREATMENT. The treatment modalities include curettage, removal with comedone extractor, application of 50–90% trichloroacetic acid, cryosurgery with liquid nitrogen, or simply scraping off the lesion with an orange stick followed by application of tincture of iodine to the denuded area. Molluscum contagiosum in HIV-infected patients is recalcitrant to therapy, but it is possible to decrease the number of lesions with intensive topical treatment. Treatment should be tailored to the individual patient because of variable responses in each person. Sexual partners may also have lesions, and should be checked for any other STI and treated accordingly.

Reiter's syndrome

See Chapter 7.5.

Balanitis (see also Chapters 8.1, 9.1 and 10.1)

Balanitis is an inflammatory disease of the glans penis. In uncircumcized men, the inflammatory process also involves the inner surface of the overlying prepuce causing balanoposthitis. Aetiology includes infections (some of which may be sexually acquired), poor hygiene, chemical factors (e.g. local deposit of sugar in glycosuria, use of strong antiseptics) and hypersensitivity reactions to drugs. Humid climate, a long prepuce, phimosis, physical trauma, smegma accumulation and the resulting irritation may all predispose to secondary infection.

Infective agents which may be associated with balanitis/balanoposthitis include *C. albicans*, anaerobes such as *Bacteroides* spp., *Treponema pallidum*, non-syphilitic spirochaetes, other bacteria such as *S. aureus* and group B streptococci; protozoa including *Trichomonas vaginalis* and *Entamoeba histolytica*; and viruses such as herpes simplex and HPV.

Other conditions and special forms of balanitis include psoriasis, Reiter's syndrome (Chapter 7.5) balanitis xerotica obliterans, balanoposthitis of zoon, erythroplasia of Queyrat and other non-venereal genital dermatoses (see below). In some cases, no cause is found.

CLINICAL FEATURES. The patient may present with a rash, redness, soreness, irritation (focal or diffuse) of the glans penis and swelling, and limited and painful retraction of the prepuce, discharge and ulcers. *Candida* balanitis associated with glycosuria (such as in diabetes) may be very severe, with a reddened glazed glans penis covered with white exudate, and oedema and fissuring of the foreskin which may be difficult to retract. Anaerobic balanitis is usually associated with ulcers on the glans penis and adjacent prepuce, and preputial oedema and offensive subpreputial discharge. Inguinal lymph glands may be enlarged and tender.

DIAGNOSIS. Diagnosis is based on history, and careful clinical examinations and should be confirmed by laboratory investigations where applicable (e.g. wet film, darkfield examination, Gram stain and culture, if indicated, of material from the glans penis and subpreputial sac, and urine for sugar). Blood tests should be carried out and repeated after 3 months to exclude syphilis.

In psoriasis, the rash is rather dry and scaly and there may be typical lesions of psoriasis elsewhere on the body. Circinate balanitis is self-evident and is usually a manifestation of Reiter's syndrome (Chapter 7.5) but can also occur alone. In a drug reaction, the balanitis usually appears as a painful erosion with desquamation of the mucous membrane, serum oozing and bleeding.

In many cases, the rash may be non-specific, and questioning about the use of condoms, stimulant cream, lubricants, personal products, etc., may give clues to the cause of irritants or allergens. The term non-specific balanitis is used in cases where no cause could be found and probably results from poor hygiene or mild non-specific irritation.

PREVENTION AND TREATMENT. Men who are not circumcized should wash the glans penis and the inner surface of the prepuce daily with water. Those with recurrent balanitis and phimosis may benefit from circumcision.

Appropriate treatment depends on the cause, for which the reader may refer to the relevant section of this book. In general, moist or oozing lesions should be treated with wet compresses to the area for 1–2 days to lessen the inflammation. In mild balanitis, cleaning the glans penis with an emollient non-detergent soap is usually sufficient. In more severe cases, application of a non-fluorinated steroid cream such as 1% hydrocortisone twice daily is very helpful. Candidal balanitis should be treated with topical clotrimazole or miconazole cream twice daily, and trichomonal and anaerobic balanitis with a course of metronidazole tablets. Fusospirochaetal balanitis will respond to an injection of benzathine penicillin (dose similar to that for primary syphilis). Sexual partners should be examined and treated as appropriate, when the condition is recurrent or has an infective aetiology. A patient with glycosuria should be referred for further assessment.

If the condition does not improve within 2 weeks of treatment, an expert opinion should be sought and a biopsy may be necessary.

Non-venereal genital dermatoses

There is a wide variety of local and systemic diseases that produce lesions in the anogenital region. Because genital lesions caused by skin conditions frequently resemble those caused by STI, it is important that practitioners familiarize themselves with these conditions to avoid making an inappropriate diagnosis. Some common genital lesions are described below.

Fixed drug eruption

Fixed drug eruption is a circumscribed drug reaction recurring at the same site. The genitalia and face are sites with special predilection. Erythematous, sharply demarcated patches appear soon after drug exposure, accompanied by itching or burning (Plate 129). The area often blisters and then erodes. If there is no secondary infection, the lesion dries, becoming dark brown, and re-epithelialization occurs within 2 weeks followed by complete healing. Drugs frequently involved include aspirin, barbiturates, tetracycline, sulphonamides and phenolpthalein. A careful history will usually reveal the offending drug.

Treatment is by drug avoidance and wet compress of eroded lesions.

Contact dermatitis

Contact dermatitis in the anogenital region may result from contraceptives, spermicides, topical antifungals, cosmetics, lubricants, materials used in condoms, clothing, detergents, etc. A wide variety of skin lesions have been reported. They may consist of scaly patches, erythematous papules, or eczematous lesions with oozing and weeping. Diagnosis is made by obtaining a careful medical history of the patient's use of topical medications or cosmetics.

TREATMENT. The offending substances should be removed and future contact avoided. Weeping lesions should be treated with wet compresses with saline or Burow's solution (aluminium acetate 1:40). Dry inflamed lesions should be treated with a mild steroid cream.

Lichen planus

Lichen planus is a common skin disease of unknown aetiology. Characteristic features are violaceous, shiny, flat-topped papules or plaques. A fine white network (Wickham's striae) overlying the papules may be seen. Lichen planus may involve the penis or vulva as part of a widespread eruption (including buccal mucosa) or as a solitary lesion. In the genitalia, the typical papular lesions have a tendency to assume an annular configuration. The clinical course of this disease is variable.

TREATMENT. Genital lesions often respond to application of a mild steroid cream. However, most minor lesions resolve spontaneously in 6–12 months and reassurance is all that is necessary.

Artificial penile nodules

These nodules are implantation of foreign bodies mainly into the skin of the penis in order to improve sexual performance. The materials used range from plastic, polished stones or liquid silicone, to pearls and ivory. Two to five are usually used (Plate 130). The practice is most common in the Orient, and is almost non-existent in the West. In most instances, the practice does not produce symptoms unless the inserts become secondarily infected.

Seborrhoeic keratosis

Seborrhoeic keratoses are common benign skin tumours, generally in older people. These tumours tend to occur on the chest, back, face and neck. Occasionally, they may appear in the anogenital region (Plate 131). The lesions are sharply circumscribed, appear 'stuck to the skin' and vary in size and colour. They can also be flat or minimally raised, with smooth or verrucous brownish to black surfaces. The diagnosis is usually obvious clinically because of the characteristic 'stuck-on' appearance and dark brown granular surface. The diagnosis may be confirmed by biopsy.

Treatment is not necessary, but flat lesions respond well to cryosurgery. Thick and keratotic lesions often require curettage.

Fordyce's spots (see also Chapter 6.5)

Fordyce's spots are ectopic sebaceous glands which appear as streaks or patches of asymptomatic, multiple, small, yellow or white, pinhead-sized spots on the vulva or under the prepuce. They may also affect the lips or buccal mucosa.

Management is by reassurance of the patients.

Pearly penile papules (see also Chapter 6.5)

Pearly penile papules occur in up to 20% of the male population. They are congenital abnormalities that histologically resemble fibromas. The papules are present in one or more rows, usually around the corona. These hypertrophic papillae vary in size from 0.5 to 4 mm and are whitish red to whitish yellow in colour. Occasionally, they may be somewhat brownish and show a filiform configuration. These lesions frequently are confused with genital warts and treated unnecessarily.

Management is by reassurance of the patient.

Angiokeratomas of Fordyce

The angiokeratomas of Fordyce are tiny, superficial, vascular malformations which are characterized clinically as multiple small red papules with slightly verrucous surfaces. They are present mainly on the scrotum of elderly patients (Plate 132). Diagnosis is usually obvious clinically and can be confirmed by a skin biopsy.

Treatment is not necessary. If desired, however, excision, electrodesiccation or laser may be used.

Plasma cell balanoposthitis of Zoon

This is a benign condition of unknown aetiology. The patient may present with a red shiny velvety slightly raised, usually painless lesion of the glans penis, coronal sulcus and adjacent prepuce (Plate 133). It may mimic erythroplasia of Queyrat. Biopsy is essential to confirm the diagnosis and will show plasma cell infiltration of the upper dermis.

The condition resolves after circumcision.

Lichen sclerosus et atrophicus

Lichen sclerosus et atrophicus is a dermatosis affecting the genitalia of both sexes, but is rather uncommon in dark-skinned people. The cause is unknown. The condition is characterized by hyalinization of the dermal collagen, hyperkeratosis of the epidermis in early stages but becoming thin later, followed by loss of subepidermal elastic tissue.

In men the manifestation is termed balanitis xerotica obliterans. The patient may present with tiny white papules or white plaques on the glans penis and prepuce. Careful examination may also show speckled purpura. The lesions may progress to constriction of the terminal urethra and phimosis (Plate 134), The patient may then experience urethral discharge and obstruction in passing urine. A female patient may present with white atrophic plaques of the vulva and perianal region, vulval irritation and lichenification (Plate 135). The labia may fuse and eventually atrophy.

Diagnosis is confirmed by biopsy. The possibility of neoplastic change (in both sexes) necessitates long-term surveillance.

TREATMENT. This is with local application of a potent topical steriod cream or ointment. Additional measures in males include dilatation of the meatus and terminal urethra, meatotomy and circumcision.

Erythroplasia of Queyrat

Erythroplasia of Queyrat represents Bowen's disease of the mucous membrane. It is characterized by moist, red, well-defined plaque that bleeds easily (Plate 136). It commonly involves the glans penis in men, and rarely the labia minora in women. The disease has to be differentiated from other types of balanitis. Diagnosis is by biopsy.

TREATMENT. Erythroplasia of Queyrat can be treated with 5-fluorouracil, cryotherapy or local excision.

Squamous cell carcinoma of the penis

Cancer of the penis usually occurs in middle-aged or elderly men. Uncircumcized men are predominantly affected. The lesion usually starts as a firm mass appearing as a red plaque or nodule which may break down into a destructive ulcer. Later it enlarges and transforms into a fungating mass covered with purulent or bloody exudate (Plate 137). When the lesion metastasizes, inguinal nodes are primarily involved and become stony hard. Diagnosis is established by biopsy.

TREATMENT. Surgical excision is the treatment of choice. The affected inguinal nodes should be removed along with the primary tumour.

Behçet's syndrome

Behçet's syndrome is a subacute or chronic multisystem disease comprising painful genital and oral ulceration (Plate 138), uveites, arthritis and vascular lesions, which may be widespread. The cause is unknown, but immunological and genetic factors are involved. The diagnosis is made mainly on clinical grounds. The genital ulceration may mimic genital herpes or chancroid.

Treatment is with topical and systemic steroids, colchicine and azathioprine.

CHAPTER 11.6
Tropical diseases with genital manifestations

G.B. Wyatt
Liverpool School of Tropical Medicine, Liverpool, UK

A number of tropical diseases may present with genital manifestations which, on occasion, may need to be differentiated from those due to STI. The relevant aspects of some common tropical diseases with genital manifestations are described briefly in this chapter.

Schistosomiasis

Schistosomiasis or bilharzia infection is acquired by infection with cercariae in fresh water penetrating the skin. These cercariae are derived from the intermediate hosts, various aquatic snails in which the parasites multiply. Infection of the snails comes from active miracidia derived from the *Schistosoma* ova shed in urine or faeces from the human host. There are three major varieties of human schistosomiasis: *Schistosoma haematobium* causes urinary schistosomiasis and is also the commonest cause of genital problems, and *S. mansoni* and *S. japonicum* cause intestinal and liver problems. However, there is a considerable overlap in the disease pattern caused by the different *Schistosoma* species.

Schistosoma haematobium

This form of schistosomiasis is found throughout the African continent and also in the Middle East in Syria, Iraq and the Arabian peninsula, as well as on some islands in the Indian ocean. Pairs of male and female worms live in the terminal venules of the bladder and genital organs and produce ova which are excreted in the urine, semen or, occasionally, stools. Female worms may live for 3–8 years, or occasionally much longer. Most of the pathology of schistosomiasis is caused by granulomatous reactions around the ova lying in the tissues. Eggs are deposited in greatest numbers in the bladder, with slightly lower concentrations in the seminal vesicles and fewer still in the prostate. In the bladder, the pathological effects may include small tubercles, 'sandy patches' caused by calcified eggs, polyps and larger granulomatous masses which may occlude the lower ureters, ulceration, squamous metaplasia and carcinomatous change. The heaviest infections in indigenous communities tend to occur at around 5–14 years of age, and haematuria in young boys may be regarded as 'normal' in such communities.

Some people infected with schistosomiasis for the first time develop acute schistosomiasis or 'Katayama fever'. While this is less prominent in *S. haematobium* than in *S. mansoni* or *S. japonicum* infections, it can lead to some months of ill health with fever, urticarial rashes, joint pains and wheezing. The main clue to the diagnosis is marked eosinophilia; ova are usually not found at this stage and serological tests may be negative initially.

Terminal haematuria is the commonest symptom of urinary schistosomiasis. Although usually painless, dysuria or pain felt at the tip of the penis is sometimes present. The symptoms, especially in men, may occasionally mimic those of non-gonococcal urethritis. In addition, infection in men may present with abnormalities of the semen. Some complain of blood in the semen and others of lumpy semen – 'like small pieces of bread'. Painful ejaculation, low backache or perineal heaviness are sometimes symptoms of seminal vesiculitis or prostatitis. Rectal examination may reveal bilaterally enlarged or fibrotic seminal vesicles. The testis and epididymis are rarely involved. Schistosomal involvement of the urethra occurs, but is now rare; in the past fistulas, and a 'watering can' appearance were described. Egg granulomas may also involve the female genital tract. They are not thought to be a common cause of infertility but sometimes present with papillomatous lesions of the vulva especially before puberty. Vaginal ulcers and ulcers involving the cervix may lead to dyspareunia or post-coital bleeding and need to be differentiated from cervical neoplasia.

Diagnosis

The terminal spined eggs of *S. haematobium* should be sought in urine passed between 10 am and 2 pm after centrifugation or sedimentation. The presence of red cells in the urine should lead to a determined search. Filtration methods can pick up small numbers of eggs and quantify the number of eggs. Ova may also be sought in the semen; they are often surrounded by masses of pus cells (Fig. 11.6.1). Rectal biopsy specimens examined after squashing between two glass slides will often show ova. ELISA antibody techniques are useful for diagnosis in expatriates but are of limited value for others since they do not differentiate between active and old infections. Antigen tests are becoming available and should prove useful.

Treatment

Praziquantel is the drug of choice, and a single dose of 40 mg kg^{-1} body weight is often sufficient.

Schistosoma mansoni

This form of schistosomiasis occurs in Africa and parts of South America and the Caribbean. Although *S. mansoni* primarily causes intestinal and hepatosplenomegalic schistosomiasis, the ova are quite often excreted in the urine and sometimes in the semen. Occasionally skin lesions due to this schistosome are found in the perineum.

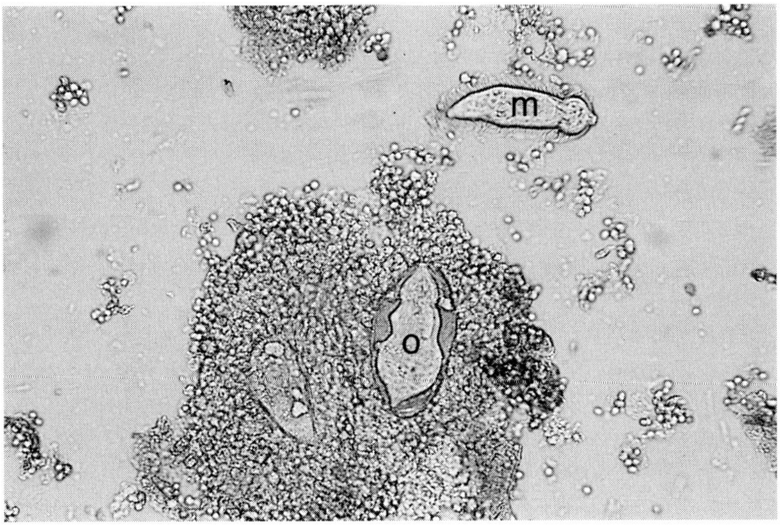

Fig. 11.6.1. A miracidium (m) of *Schistosoma haematobium* in semen above a clump of white cells enclosing an ovum (o).

Filarial infections

The filarial worms which are long string-like tissue nematodes are a frequent cause of problems in the genital area.

Bancroftian filariasis

Wuchereria bancrofti infection is transmitted by the bites of various anopheline and culicine mosquitoes throughout much of the tropics (Central and South America, Africa, Asia and the Pacific islands). *Culex quinquefasciatus* is a mosquito that breeds in polluted water; it is an effective vector of *W. bancrofti* and has led to an upsurge of filariasis in urban areas. Adult *W. bancrofti* develop in the lymphatics of humans, and females give rise to active microfilariae which are found in the blood only at night in most geographical areas (nocturnal periodicity). Although many people infected in childhood show no symptoms of disease, there is increasing evidence of lymphatic dilatation and damage even in these 'asymptomatic carriers'. Symptomatic filariasis usually occurs in adults, and the incubation period is usually at least a month but may be much longer.

Acute filariasis

Some infected persons develop attacks of fever with rigors and painful lymphadenopathy. Groin lymph nodes are most often affected, with tender enlargement and sometimes lymphangitis which typically spreads from the centre to the periphery (unlike streptococcal lymphangitis). Lymphatics in the spermatic cord are often inflamed (funiculitis) and an epidydimo-orchitis may develop which has to be distinguished from bacterial (including gonococcal and chlamydial) infections, mumps and testicular torsion. Attacks of lower abdominal pain may be caused by inflammation of intra-abdominal lymphatics. Rarely lymph nodes may break down to form a filarial abscess. Attacks of fever, lymphadenitis and lymphangitis may recur over several years.

Chronic filariasis

Recurrent episodes of inflammation caused by reactions to secretory products of the adult worms or by secondary bacterial infection lead on to lymphatic obstruction and lymphoedema. The commonest presentation of this obstructive stage in East Africa and some other areas is hydrocoele. If the incidence of hydrocoele is high in a tropical district, filariasis should always be sought. Lymphatic varices akin to varicose veins may also be found affecting the groin or the scrotum. Such varices are sometimes mistaken for a hernia. Sometimes varices rupture to release protein-rich fluid. Secondary bacterial infection of a 'lymph scrotum' can be unpleasant and difficult to treat. Elephantiasis, the overgrowth of subcutaneous tissues secondary to lymphatic obstruction, is the other common late presentation. Although elephantiasis most often affects the lower leg, the scrotum, penis, vulva, arm or breast can also be involved (Plate 139). Swelling is at first caused by fluid accumulation, pits on pressure and goes down after elevation of the part. As elephantiasis progresses there is an overgrowth of subcutaneous soft tissues with fissuring, darkening and warty excrescences of the overlying skin. Scrotal elephantiasis may grow to an enormous size, weigh several kilograms and cause major disability. Elephantiasis is often made worse by repeated episodes of bacterial, usually streptococcal, infection. Not all elephantiasis is caused by filariasis as anything that destroys lymphatics can present in the same way. Lymphogranuloma venereum, tuberculous adenitis and neoplasms including KS should be excluded. Elephantiasis confined to the foot and lower leg is also caused by alumino-silicates entering the lymphatics of barefoot agricultural workers on volcanic soils.

Chyluria is the passage of milky lymph in the urine. It is caused by the rupture of varicose obstructed lymphatics into the urinary tract, and bancroftian filariasis is the commonest underlying cause. The patient usually first passes bloody urine but this quickly becomes milky, and the urine, if allowed to settle, will show an upper fatty layer with yellow urine below. Chyluria is usually intermittent and settles with bed rest, but severe chyluria can lead to wasting. Chylous ascites are also encountered occasionally.

Diagnosis

In the early stages of filariasis there is a marked blood eosinophilia, but this is no longer present in the late obstructive stages. In most geographical areas, microfilariae should be sought in blood taken between 10 pm and 4 am by examining thick blood films, or examining anticoagulated blood by filtration though a nucleopore filter or in a counting chamber. Where there is clinical doubt between filarial and bacterial lymphangitis, appropriate antibiotic treatment should be given. Microfilariae are not usually demonstrable in the late obstructive stages. Adult worms can sometimes be demonstrated within lymphatics by ultrasonography. Antibody tests such as the filarial complement fixation or ELISA tests are usually strongly positive in the late stages of disease but are not very specific in endemic areas. Antigen-detecting tests, such as the rapid immunochromatographic test, are easy to perform and appear specific.

Treatment

Diethylcarbamazine (DEC) quickly kills microfilariae and also kills adult with prolonged or repeated courses. DEC is given in divided doses of 6 mg kg^{-1} day^{-1} for 12 days or longer. Small hydrocoeles or early elephantiasis may resolve after repeated treatment. Surgical treatment is appropriate for larger hydrocoeles or elephantiasis of the scrotum. Strict cleanliness and washing with soap and water is very important to prevent secondary infection which exacerbates elephantiasis.

Brugian filariasis

This is caused by *Brugia malayi* and is an important cause of leg elephantiasis in Southeast Asia but rarely involves the scrotum or genitalia.

Onchocerciasis

Onchocerca volvulus is another filarial worm found only in tropical Africa, Yemen and in small foci in Central and South America. Adult worms live in human subcutaneous tissues and are often encapsulated by host fibrous tissue to form subcutaneous nodules. Microfilariae spread through the skin and infect the eyes. Microfilariae are taken up from the skin by biting black flies (*Simulium* spp.) usually in the vicinity of their breeding sites in fast-flowing rivers. After development in the flies, the parasite is ready for transmission by bite to other people. The chief symptoms of onchocerciasis are caused by immunological reactions to dying microfilariae in the skin or eyes. Severe skin itching is most frequent, but eye involvement ranging from conjunctivitis to blindness from sclerosing keratitis or optic atrophy is most feared. Groin lymph node enlargement is a common feature and the nodes may become inflamed from secondary infection after scratching of the legs or during treatment when large numbers of microfilariae are killed. Sometimes the coexistence of gross lymphadenopathy and the skin atrophy which is a feature of late onchocerciasis leads to a hanging groin (Fig. 11.6.2) with folds of skin containing the nodes forming a sort of apron. Hernia is a differential diagnosis but may also accompany this condition. Subcutaneous nodules in Africa are most often found lying over bony prominences around the pelvis such as the pelvic brim, the sacrum or the greater trochanter. Patchy depigmentation with spots of hyperpigmentation (the leopard skin appearance) is most often seen over the shins in late onchocerciasis but may be encountered also over the pelvis. Minor degrees of scrotal elephantiasis are also sometimes found in this disease.

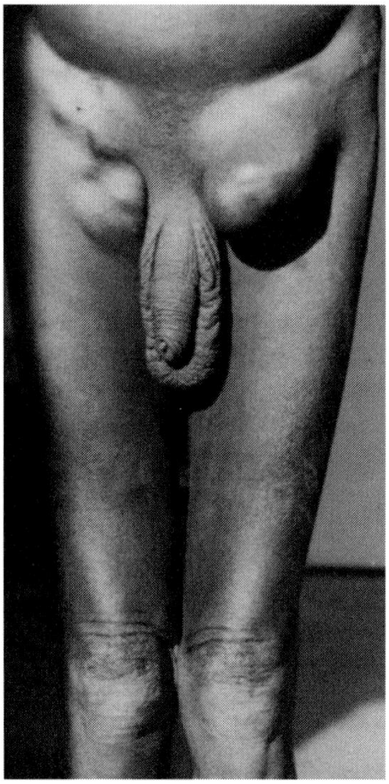

Fig. 11.6.2. Hanging groin in onchocerciasis.

Diagnosis

Microfilariae can often be demonstrated by bloodlessly removing small slivers of skin from around the pelvis with a needle and razor blade and allowing the active worms to emerge in a drop of saline. Microfilariae may also be found in the eye with a slit lamp or adult worms found in excised nodules. Differential diagnosis is especially from scabies.

Treatment

Ivermectin at a dose of 150 μg kg^{-1} body weight as a single dose is the drug of choice for killing microfilariae without causing serious side effects but it does not kill adult worms and, therefore, repeated doses may be required every 6–12 months for 5 years or more.

Leprosy

Mycobacterium leprae spreads chiefly by inhalation of bacilli derived from patients with lepromatous or near lepromatous (multibacillary) disease who harbour myriads of bacteria in their nasal mucus. Most infected people do not develop clinical disease and those who do often have an incubation period measured in many years. The type of disease that develops depends upon the degree of specific cell-mediated immune reaction of the individual. Those with reasonably effective immune responses develop tuberculoid disease with few bacteria to be found (paucibacillary). Those with very poor cell-mediated immunity develop lepromatous disease. Borderline leprosy lies between these two polar types. Because *M. leprae* grows best at around 30–33°C, those parts of the body with a lower temperature are especially likely to be attacked; these include the skin and the testis. Superficial nerves are also invaded, preferentially and it is nerve damage that is the most important pathology in leprosy.

Leprosy often involves the skin of the buttocks and, less commonly, that of the scrotum or vulva. Non-itching chronic skin lesions whether single or multiple with alteration in texture, sweating or pigmentation should be considered suspicious in any person who has lived in a developing country. Remember to feel for enlarged cutaneous nerves and to test skin lesions for loss of sensation to heat and light touch; both features are likely to be present in paucibacillary leprosy. Slit skin smears should also be taken from the edges of suspicious skin lesions with a small scalpel blade, avoiding contamination with blood; these smears are then examined for acid-fast bacteria and will be positive in multibacillary leprosy. Multibacillary leprosy often invades the testes, causing orchitis and later atrophy and gynaecomastia. The commonest differential diagnosis is from fungal infection of the skin. Dermatophyte infections often itch, and fungal elements can be visualized in skin scrapings mounted in potassium hydroxide.

Leprosy is now a curable disease, and multidrug treatment using rifampicin, dapsone and clofazimine is very effective provided the patient complies with long-term treatment.

Other cutaneous manifestations of tropical disease

Amoebiasis

Amoebiasis rarely causes spreading ulceration around the anus (Plate 140) or on the penis and genitalia in the female (as a result of extension of intestinal lesions or anal intercourse). Ulcers have an irregular undermined edge with a granulomatous base. Once skin invasion is established, it can spread with alarming rapidity. A history of bloody diarrhoea or of anal intercourse with a partner with diarrhoea can be helpful. Active trophozoites of *Entamoeba histolytica* containing ingested red blood cells can be demonstrated on smears from the base of the ulcers and examined immediately under the microscope.

Dermal leishmaniasis

This usually occurs on skin surfaces exposed to the bites of infected sandflies. However, transmission of skin infection by scratching can initiate infections of the genitalia. Such skin lesions evolve over weeks or months from small papules to chronic ulcers with a rolled edge. The diagnosis is confirmed by finding leishmanial amastigotes in smears made from aspirates or, better still, from incisions into the edge of the lesion.

Larva migrans

Larva migrans (Plate 141) is usually caused by contact of bare skin with soil harbouring the larva of dog hookworms. Although the foot is the commonest site of infection, perineal lesions are not uncommon, especially in children. A raised, serpiginous, intensely itchy track elongates at a rate of around 1 cm in 24 h. Multiple lesions also occur.

Larva currens

This is a condition similar to larva migrans caused by migrating larvae of the intestinal nematode parasite *Strongyloides stercoralis.* Once a person is infected with this nematode by the larvae penetrating skin exposed to infected soil, they may remain infected for 50 years because the gut parasite produces living larvae which often penetrate the perianal skin and, after migration, give rise to a new generations of worms. Larva currens lesions quite often appear around the buttocks or perianal area as serpiginous urticarial tracks which progress much faster than those of larva migrans and usually disappear after a few days only perhaps to recur after a few weeks. Rarely, *Strongyloides* worms infect the bladder or genital tract, but the chief importance of this infection is the risk of a life-threatening hyperinfection syndrome if the patient is treated with high-dose corticosteroids or is immunosuppressed.

Tuberculosis

Tuberculosis is extremely common throughout the developing world, and the situation has worsened considerably with the spread of HIV infection which leads both to recrudescence of previous tuberculous infection and to increasing problems with the management of patients. Genital tuberculosis is usually caused by secondary haematogenous spread from pulmonary, lymph node or bone disease. Occasionally it is due to spread from renal lesions or even by sexual transmission. These manifestations often present many years after primary tuberculosis.

In women, tuberculous salpingitis is usually bilateral and involves the outer parts of the tubes more than the uterine ends. It can be an indolent infection but may present quite acutely with pain and fever and be difficult to differentiate from STI-associated and other causes of PID except by laparoscopy and biopsy. An association with peritoneal tuberculosis with ascites and adhesions is frequent, and the condition may be mistaken for spreading ovarian cancer. Treated tuberculous salpingitis is sometimes followed by ectopic pregnancy. Women with tuberculous endometritis may present with irregular or excessive bleeding, amenorrhoea or, most commonly, with infertility. Diagnosis is by curettage with histological examination and culture of the curettings. Tuberculous cervicitis causes an irregular granulomatous ulceration which bleeds easily and looks like a cervical carcinoma, although it is usually softer and typically does not spread to the vaginal vault. Separate tuberculous vaginal ulcers do occur. Vulval tuberculosis can present with granulomatous ulceration, scarring and sinus formation. Clinically, differentiation from lymphogranuloma venereum, donovanosis and schistosomiasis is difficult, and diagnosis is dependent upon biopsy and culture.

In men, tuberculous epididymitis is quite common in developing countries. It is usually haematogenous in origin although sometimes it may result from spread from renal or prostatic disease. It occurs chiefly in young sexually active men who present with a scrotal mass which is sometimes painful. Blood occasionally is seen in the ejaculate (cf. schistosomiasis). Most often the disease is unilateral, with epididymal induration and a beaded vas. In about 40% of cases signs are limited to the globus minor. Sinus formation to the posterior part of the scrotum may be present. The chief differential diagnosis is from chlamydial and gonococcal epidydimo-orchitis, but failure to respond to antituberculous treatment within 6 weeks should warrant surgical exploration to rule out a seminoma.

The penis, urethra, seminal vesicles and prostate can also be infected by tuberculosis, but these are all rare events. Tuberculosis of the kidneys and bladder may cause dysuria, nocturia, frequency, haematuria and loin pain. This form of tuberculosis is much commoner in men than women, and should be suspected in the presence of sterile pyuria (cf. chlamydial infection). Renal calcification and hypertension are sometimes encountered. Culture of early morning urine specimens on three or more occasions and intravenous urography are helpful in making the diagnosis.

Tuberculous inguinal adenitis is frequent in the tropics. In time, nodes become fluctuant, matted together and may form sinuses. Remember also the possibility of a tuberculous psoas abscess arising in the spine and presenting at the groin. The buttocks are a fairly frequent site for implantation tuberculosis of the skin causing concentric, warty, hyperplastic rings.

Modern short course antituberculous chemotherapy is effective in genitourinary tuberculosis but will not reverse sterility.

Further reading

Cook, G.C. (ed.) (1996) *Manson's Tropical Diseases*, 20th edn. Saunders, London.
Husain, I. (ed.) (1984) *Tropical Urology and Renal Disease*. Churchill Livingstone, London.

CHAPTER 12
Control aspects

CHAPTER 12.1
Control of STI, HIV and AIDS

A. Meheus
Department of Epidemiology and Community Medicine, University of Antwerp, Antwerp, Belgium

STI/AIDS – a major public health problem

The epidemiology and burden of STI in developing countries differs greatly from the situation in industrialized nations.

First, prevalence and incidence rates of the various STI are high, both in rural and urban areas. For example, STI are among the top five causes of consultation at health services in many African countries. High rates of infection are found in specific population groups, for example prostitutes and their clients are an important high-risk group for STI/HIV infection and transmission, while male homosexuals are not a significant group.

Second, the incidence of STI complications and sequelae is much higher, because of high infection rates and inadequate management of STI. Major complications and sequelae are neonatal and infant infections, pelvic inflammatory disease, infertility in both sexes, ectopic pregnancy, urethral stricture in males, blindness in infants due to gonococcal ophthalmia neonatorum and in adults due to gonococcal keratoconjunctivitis, and genital cancers, in particular cancer of the cervix uteri and penile cancer.

Third, the epidemiology of the acquired immunodeficiency syndrome (AIDS) remains markedly different from that in industrialized countries: heterosexual contact is the predominant mode of transmission of HIV, which is spreading in the same populations which are already affected by high levels of STI ('an HIV epidemic compounds the STI endemic'). HIV prevalence levels of 20–30% have been documented in adults in some areas of the developing world, which makes AIDS the leading cause of morbidity and mortality in those areas.

Fourth, STI prevention and control has not been a health policy priority for governments and international development agencies due to lack of awareness of the health and socioeconomic consequences of STI, competition for resources with other major health problems and reluctance to deal with diseases transmitted through sex. This situation is now changing as the interactions between 'classical' STI and HIV became evident, in particular the enhancement of HIV transmission by classical STI, presenting as genital ulcers or genital discharges. Due to the commonality of intervention strategies, control programmes are now aiming more and more at HIV and the other STI.

Coordination of STI and HIV/AIDS programmes

As most developing countries did not have a strong STI control programme at the time AIDS appeared, separate and well-resourced HIV/AIDS prevention and control programmes were developed in most countries. However, for optimal effectiveness and efficiency STI and AIDS programmes should be integrated or at least closely coordinated (Box 12.1.1).

Classical STI increase HIV transmission. Another HIV and STI interaction of great significance for control programmes is that immunodeficiency associated with HIV seems to change the natural history of STI in an individual: severity of clinical manifestations may be increased, infectivity increased and prolonged, and response to conventional treatment reduced.

All the above arguments make a combination of AIDS and STI programmes essential and control of classical STI a major intervention in HIV/AIDS prevention and control.

General principles of STI control

STI control has three main objectives: (i) to interrupt the transmission of STI, (ii) to prevent the development of disease, complications and sequelae; and (iii) to reduce the transmission of HIV infection.

These objectives can be achieved through primary prevention measures aimed at reducing the incidence of infection, and secondary prevention aimed at reducing prevalence through shortening the duration of infection and disease and, as a result, reducing the probability of complications and sequelae, and of disease transmission.

Primary prevention activities are essentially the same for HIV and the other STI. They aim at reducing the exposure to infection through health promotion (IEC = information, education and communication), counselling and safer sexual behaviour including condom use. Due to the increasing importance of the incurable viral STI such as genital herpes, HPV infections and, in particular, the fatal condition of HIV/AIDS, primary prevention strategies currently receive much higher priority. STI clinical care offers a major opportunity for primary prevention by education and counselling of STI patients, a group who are by definition at increased risk of STI.

Secondary prevention activities include the provision of adequate diagnostic and treatment facilities for STI patients (curative care), early detection mostly of asymptomatic infection through screening and case-finding, promotion of health care-seeking behaviour particularly of those at

Box 12.1.1. Reasons to integrate STI and HIV/AIDS programmes (WHO/UNAIDS, 1997).

- The predominant mode of transmission of both HIV and other STI is sexual, although other routes of transmission for both include blood, blood products, donated organs or tissue and through an infected woman to her fetus or newborn infant.
- Most of the measures for preventing sexual transmission of HIV and STI are the same, as are the target audiences for these interventions.
- STI clinical services are an important access point for persons at high risk of both AIDS and STI, not only for diagnosis and treatment but also for education.
- There is a strong association between the occurrence of HIV infection and the presence of other STI, making early diagnosis and effective treatment of STI an important strategy for the prevention of HIV transmission.
- Trends in STI incidence and prevalence can be useful early indicators of changes in sexual behaviour and are easier to monitor than trends in HIV seroprevalence.

increased risk of STI/HIV, and partner referral and treatment.

Any primary prevention effort to reduce risky sexual behaviour will have spin-off effects on all STI including HIV. In addition, the traditional interventions of secondary prevention through adequate management of treatable STI will have a threefold effect: first, to reduce the reproductive sequelae of those STI; second, to decrease their transmission in the community; and third, through controlling genital ulcers and discharges, to slow the HIV epidemic.

Failure to control STI

Treatable STI of public health importance, e.g. gonorrhoea, chlamydial infection, syphilis, chancroid and trichomoniasis, have reached an equilibrium at a low level or are still declining in industrialized countries. In developing countries, treatable STI have also reached a 'steady state' but at an unacceptably high level.

Poverty, resulting in health budgets often between US$5 and US$10 per capita per year, is the main reason for the vicious circle of poor STI control. Box 12.1.2 lists a number of factors to be tackled if renewed efforts for STI control are to be effective.

Components of STI/AIDS control

Comprehensive prevention and control programmes are needed in the fight against STI/AIDS. These programmes include intervention strategies aimed at decreasing the incidence and prevalence of STI, and support components which increase the effectiveness of the interventions. In any programme, an adequate balance must be achieved between interventions and support.

The major intervention strategies are: (i) primary prevention mainly through health promotion (IEC); (ii) adequate and comprehensive STI patient management, mainly through curative health services; (iii) early detection of STI through screening and case-finding; and (iv) partner referral and treatment.

Box 12.1.2. Factors contributing to the failure to control STI (WHO/UNAIDS, 1997).

- Low priority has been afforded by policy makers and planners in allocating resources for reasons such as an association of STI with perceived discreditable behaviour; failure to associate the diseases with the complications and sequelae; failure to recognize the magnitude of the problem.
- Control efforts being concentrated on symptomatic patients (usually men) have failed to identify asymptomatic individuals (commonly women) until complications arise.
- Service delivery has often been through specialized STI treatment facilities which provide inadequate coverage and are particularly stigmatizing for women.
- Treatment strategies have focused on unrealistic requirements for definitive diagnosis rather than on practical decision making.
- Ineffective low-cost antibiotics continue to be used for reasons of economy.
- There has been little emphasis on educational and other efforts to prevent infection.
- There has been an absence of authoritative guidance on a rational, practical and well-defined package of activities as a basis for prevention and control programmes.

The support components are: (i) training of all types of personnel involved in STI/AIDS control; (ii) laboratory services supporting diagnosis in symptomatic and asymptomatic individuals; (iii) research: behavioural, epidemiological, clinical and operational; and (iv) STI information systems of which STI surveillance is the principal component.

This chapter deals principally with the intervention strategies.

Primary prevention

Primary prevention activities aim to reduce the incidence of infection and disease. This can be obtained through behavioural interventions, immunization and use of topical microbicides. As behaviour is the major determinant in STI acquisition and transmission, a change in that behaviour is fundamental to control STI. No cure is as yet available for viral STI and, since the advent and spread of HIV/AIDS, behavioural interventions have become a major focus of STI control programmes. An immunization strategy against STI is still highly limited, as the only effective vaccine currently available is hepatitis B vaccine. Topical microbicides are highly effective in the prevention of gonococcal ophthalmia neonatorum through application of Crédé's prophylaxis.

Behavioural interventions

Health promotion

Health promotion activities aim at behavioural changes which decrease exposure to and transmission of STI. Behavioural changes to be effected include delay of onset of sexual intercourse, decrease in the rate of sex partner change, selection of low-risk sex partners, safer sex practices, condom use and faithful monogamy or polygamy. A strategy of IEC can aim to reach the population as a whole or can be targeted to specific audiences. While mass media campaigns were shown to be useful in increasing knowledge and awareness of HIV/AIDS, it is doubtful whether this approach leads to behavioural changes in high-risk behaviour individuals. Priority should be given to health promotion activities targeted at STI core groups. A problem with this strategy is a potential increase in stigmatization and segregation which should be avoided through careful planning. The messages should reflect the demands and needs, and members of core groups should therefore be involved in elaborating and conveying the safer sex and other behavioural strategies. Core groups for targeted health promotion include: (i) political and community leaders including religious leaders, technical experts and advisers; through an impact on decision making they can exercise great influence in the community; (ii) adolescents and school children, for whom the aim is not to develop high-risk behaviours; many children drop out of school and, as illiteracy can be high (especially among girls), appropriate communication methods must be used such as radio, meetings, discussions, drama, songs and pictures; and (iii) core group transmitters, characterized by high-risk sexual behaviour; these include STI/AIDS patients and their sex partners, prostitutes and clients, the military, long-distance truck drivers, etc.

Condom promotion

When used properly, condoms considerably reduce STI transmission, but condom availability and use remain low in most of the developing world, except for East and Southeast Asia. A range of obstacles to the promotion and use of condoms has been encountered, which include personal dislike of condoms by men and women, the association of condoms with sexual promiscuity, the lack of negotiating power of women, religious opposition, misconceptions on the effectiveness of condom use, the link between sexual risk-taking behaviour and alcohol and other substance abuse, and low availability of condoms. Condom promotion should be an integral part of health promotion activities to avoid HIV infection rather than being an autonomous activity. With demand growing considerably in recent years, making sufficient condoms available at an affordable price has become a formidable challenge. A variety of approaches to promote condom use include interpersonal communication, entertainment and social marketing; this last strategy has been an increasingly successful approach to promote condoms and make them available.

Health care-seeking behaviour

In addition to health promotion as a strategy for the primary prevention of STI, health care-seeking behaviour to promote early diagnosis and treatment is an important strategy for STI and HIV control. Health care-seeking behaviour is influenced by a large number of factors, cultural and economical as well as knowledge and awareness of STI. Examples of these factors are:

- Ignorance of STI and possible outcomes.
- Absence of signs or symptoms in women.
- Reluctance to discuss sexual matters.

- Fear of a judgemental approach on the part of the health care worker.
- Fear that others will find out.
- Reluctance on the part of the patient to be examined by a health care worker of the opposite sex.
- Lack of knowledge of where to go.
- Lack of confidence in public sector services.
- Unaffordable charges for services.

The importance of health care-seeking behaviour is illustrated in Fig. 12.1.1: a large number of women with STI do not recognize the significance of symptoms or, if recognized, do not come for treatment. Inability to pay is also a major barrier to seeking effective health care, and with economic structural adjustment programmes operating in a large part of the developing world the introduction of fees for medical care must be considered carefully. In the Nairobi STI clinic, for instance, after introduction of fees, attendance dropped by 60% among men and 35% among women. This means that a large proportion of STI patients (of whom 40–60% are HIV-positive) remained untreated or turned to ineffective STI care.

Immunization

While immunization is a highly effective strategy for controlling and even eradicating infectious diseases, the development of STI vaccines that are effective has been very disappointing, except for hepatitis B virus (HBV) infections. HBV vaccines, first plasma-derived and now genetically engineered, are highly protective, and due to a decrease in cost are now more widely available. The strategy to control HBV infection in developing countries is universal vaccination of newborns and infants as part of the national vaccination programme. The availability of combination vaccines, for instance

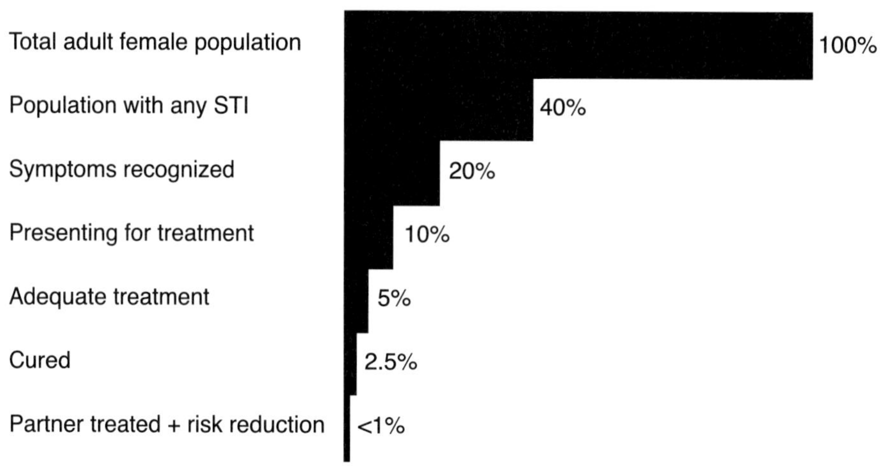

Fig. 12.1.1. Health care-seeking behaviour of women with STI.

HBV combined with diphtheria, tetanus, pertussis and polio, would achieve greater coverage than is actually the case with the HBV vaccine alone. No other STI vaccines are actually available for general use (see Chapter 12.2 for further details).

Ocular prophylaxis at birth

In many developing countries, gonorrhoea rates in pregnant women are high, up to 5–15%. This leads to many babies becoming infected at birth as they pass through the birth canal, the transmission rate from mother to newborn being between 20 and 30%. Thus the incidence rate of gonococcal ophthalmia neonatorum can be as high as 1–5% of all newborns. The factors to be considered are: (i) gonococcal ophthalmia neonatorum is a potentially blinding disease; (ii) effective treatment of the disease in developing countries is often not possible, because the treatment is expensive and the recommended antibiotics (ceftriaxone, spectinomycin or kanamycin) are often not available; and (iii) case-finding of gonorrhoea in pregnant women cannot be implemented as the laboratory infrastructure is not available.

As was shown by Crédé in the 1880s, ocular prophylaxis is highly effective in preventing gonococcal ophthalmia neonatorum, and this intervention should be fully implemented in developing countries. In practice, this means that immediately at birth all newborns should have silver nitrate (1%) eye drops or tetracycline (1%) ointment applied to their eyes. Ocular prophylaxis has only poor protection against chlamydial conjunctivitis in the neonate, but fortunately this is largely a self-limiting disease with no major consequences. At a cost of approximately US$0.05 per newborn, ocular prophylaxis at birth is highly cost effective and should now be a priority intervention for all maternal and child health (MCH) programmes in the developing world.

Patient management

STI care

Comprehensive management of patients with STI remains the cornerstone of an STI control programme. This can be done through the provision of accessible, effective and acceptable services for STI care.

Potential sources of STI care

Patients in most countries have a choice of services from which to seek STI care (Box 12.1.3). In many countries, in particular in urban areas, most STI care is obtained outside the public sector, and this should be considered when planning improved quality services. Due to the crisis in the public health sector (economic and social readjustment programmes), the importance of the private and informal sector is growing rapidly in large parts of the developing world.

Improved STI services need to be sustainable; some additional resources

Box 12.1.3. Potential sources of STI care (WHO/UNAIDS, 1997).

Public/government sector

- First level care at health posts, dispensaries, health centres and general out-patient departments of district hospitals.
- Maternal and child health (MCH) and family planning (FP) clinics.
- Specialized STI or dermatovenereology clinics.

Private sector

- First level care through private physician (general practice, dermatovenereology, urology, gynaecology, etc.)
- Private or non-governmental organizations providing care through health centres, general out-patient department at hospitals, MCH/FP clinics.
- Private STI or dermatovenereology clinics.
- Pharmacists (where they can dispense antibiotics without prescription).

Informal sector

- Traditional healers.
- Unqualified medical practitioners – 'quacks'.
- Pharmacists (where it is illegal to sell antibiotics without prescription).
- Antibiotics vendors.

can be obtained through schemes of cost recovery from the users of STI care, e.g. the Bamako initiative (standard charges for STI services, decentralized revolving funds for drugs or laboratory tests).

General health care services

Primary health care (PHC) facilities have the potential to reach the whole community. They already provide most of the STI care in many areas, and they should be targeted towards increased provision of effective and acceptable STI care. Increasing the STI care package in PHC can meet with resistance from the PHC workers. They may be reluctant to take on more work and responsibilities; this can be overcome by education for PHC workers, training and supervision, and a shift of resources away from specialized services (sophisticated laboratory tests, categorical STI clinics, inefficient testing strategies, hospitalization facilities to the PHC). The STI specialists who fear loss of their position, loss of quality of the services and loss of income, particularly in fee-for-service health systems may also put up resistance; this can be overcome by giving them the responsibility for referral services, training and supervision, and operational research.

Categorical STI clinics

Organizing the delivery of STI services in a developing country largely through specialized STI or dermatovenereology clinics is often unsatisfactory for reasons of high cost, poor accessibility for large parts of the population and poor acceptability, as they may be stigmatizing, particularly for women. However, categorical STI or dermatovenereology clinics have an important role in STI control, firstly in STI service delivery: provision of first line STI care in their geographical catchment areas, for instance a substantial area in a large city; referral care for STI seen at public and private PHC facilities; voluntary HIV testing and counselling; ambulatory care for AIDS patients; comprehensive reproductive health services; and first line care for sex workers and other priority groups. They also have an important role as reference centres for training of health care providers and for performing operational research, e.g. treatment trials, aetiology of STI 'syndromes', evaluation of 'syndromic' management of STI patients, evaluation of different approaches to patient counselling and partner notification, and gonococcal antimicrobial susceptibility monitoring, etc.

Comprehensive patient management

Comprehensive management of STI patients includes:

- correct diagnosis;
- effective treatment and counselling on compliance with treatment instructions;
- counselling on risk reduction including promotion of condoms;
- partner notification and treatment;
- testing for other STI;
- clinical follow-up and referral where appropriate.

Patient management must be effective wherever provided, from the basic to the more sophisticated sources of STI care. National guidelines for effective STI patient management are, therefore, of great importance. They must be adapted to the different levels of care (PHC services using a 'syndromic' approach, pharmacists advising patients on appropriate referral, STI clinic with laboratory support). Most patients rely on a public or private PHC setting for their STI care. The principles for patient management that apply to these settings are:

- The presenting symptoms and signs define the health problem to be solved. Decisions on treatment must be based on the history, physical examination and, if available, simple laboratory tests.
- Routinely performing laboratory tests is useful only if they influence decisions on treatment.
- Correct patient management must often be done within 5 min.
- Choice of treatment should be rational, needing standardized treatment regimens.
- Referral of patients should be exceptional, preferably less than 5% for each health problem.

Referral is a basic element in a stratified health system, but in practice it is often problematical for the STI patients; constraints on referral are lack of time, distance to travel, and financial and sociocultural barriers between peripheral and more sophisticated levels of care.

Diagnosis

Academic medicine puts a major emphasis on an aetiological diagnosis, identifying the causative agent of an STI. This ideal is not only expensive but also impractical, as results of laboratory tests are usually not available during the patient's initial visit. Thus a decision on treatment needs to be made either without the results or at a return visit. This is not feasible in many settings (long distances and costs for travel). So, many patients fail to come back, remain untreated and infectious or go to a private provider. Even if they come back, the period of infectivity and the risk of complications is increased due to delay in therapy. This does not mean that the laboratory is useless for STI care at PHC level; simple tests such as microscopy of Gram-stained urethral smears, wet mounts of vaginal specimens or urine sediment, or leukocyte esterase dip-stick on urine give immediate results and are useful in making treatment decisions.

Based on previous experience and clinical acumen, some health care providers rely solely on a clinical diagnosis. This has been shown to be unreliable even if performed by experienced STI specialists, and misses concurrent infections. A problem-oriented approach, also called syndrome-based approach, provides the STI care provider with a practical tool for improving the diagnostic process.

STI-associated syndromes/problems

Patients with a STI generally present with one or more of the following symptoms:

- urethral discharge;
- genital ulceration;
- inguinal bubo;
- swollen scrotum;
- vaginal discharge;
- lower abdominal pain;
- conjunctivitis in newborns or adults.

The WHO has encouraged the implementation of the syndromic/problem-oriented approach at PHC level as the most cost-effective way of delivery of STI care. The approach met with considerable opposition, the major criticism being that it lowered 'medical standards'. The approach can be highly effective in dealing with urethral discharge in men and genital ulcers in both sexes; flowcharts for vaginal discharge and lower abdominal pain in women are much less satisfactory. A risk assessment has, therefore, been included in some flowcharts on vaginal discharge to increase their validity in differentiating cervicitis from vaginitis.

Following the general acceptance that effective STI care is a major intervention to decrease HIV transmission, the 'syndromic' approach has become a major activity of STI/AIDS programmes. See Chapters 10.1 and 10.2 for flowcharts (also known as algorithms or decision trees) which have been implemented and evaluated. The general principles for the design of STI flowcharts have been outlined. The most important are knowledge of the local aetiology of the STI 'syndromes' including mixed infections, information on the laboratory tests available (sensitivity, specificity, cost, operational value in local routine circumstances) and cost-effectiveness of treatments.

Standardization of STI treatments is essential, and this can be established by treatment trials, knowledge of local antimicrobial susceptibility patterns, information from neighbouring countries or regions, and international guidelines.

The feasibility of specific flowcharts is determined by:

- The infrastructure available for physical examination (examination room with privacy, examination table, specula, gloves and light source, facilities to disinfect specula regularly).
- The level of training of the health care worker (skilled to perform a speculum examination).
- The drugs available at the health care facility.
- Staff time available per patient (clinician, counsellor).
- Presence of laboratory facilities.
- Access to higher levels of care.

Health care-seeking behaviour and cultural perceptions about STI and sexuality will also determine the usefulness of certain flowcharts (e.g. acceptability of a genital examination by a health care worker of the opposite sex).

Treatment

The availability of effective drugs is an essential requirement for effective STI services. Two misconceptions still exist in many settings. Provision of STI drugs is not necessarily very expensive and therefore a bottomless pit: low-cost antibiotics which also are available as generic medications still provide high cure rates for the majority of STI, but gonorrhoea, in most countries, has to be treated with the newer, more expensive drugs, and this should be done in a rational way to delay the emergence of resistant organisms. A two-tier drug policy with the provision of cheaper and less effective drugs at the peripheral health care level and the most effective, and usually more expensive, drugs only at referral level may result in an unacceptably high level of treatment failures, complications and referrals; it also erodes confidence in the STI care services. This policy discredits the public sector and patients may turn to the private and informal sectors and continue to do so for future episodes. Less effective drugs can also lead to a carrier state and continued transmission of the STI to sexual partners. Therefore, drugs used for STI care, in particular also for gonorrhoea, should be at least 95% effective. Criteria for the selection of STI drugs are outlined in Box 12.1.4.

The WHO has produced STI treatment recommendations and regularly updates them; these guidelines encompass specific STI infections as well as the STI-associated 'syndromes'. They have been the basis for national treatment guidelines in many developing countries.

In Indonesia, for instance, ciprofloxacin, ceftriaxone, spectinomycin and thiamphenicol have been shown recently to be still highly effective against gonorrhoea in recommended treatment regimens, but the costs of these regimens vary greatly: ciprofloxacin, 500 mg single oral dose = US$1.85–3.12; ceftriaxone, 250 mg single intramuscular dose = US$12.97; spectinomycin, 2 g single i.m. dose = US$5.88; thiamphenicol, 3.5 g single oral dose = US$3.15. For the treatment of chlamydial infection, doxycycline, 100 mg orally twice a

Box 12.1.4. Preferred characteristics of STI drugs (WHO, 1994b).

- High efficacy.
- Lowest cost.
- Acceptable toxicity and tolerance.
- Microbial resistance is either unlikely to develop or delayed.
- Single-dose regimen.
- Oral administration.
- Not contraindicated for pregnant or lactating women.

day for 7 days, costs US$11.97 as a branded drug but only US$1.26 as the generic drug. Similarly for the treatment of trichomoniasis or bacterial vaginosis, a single oral dose of metronidazole, 2 g costs US$1.98 as a branded drug and US$0.13 as the generic drug.

Drug prices can differ considerably from country to country. It is the responsibility of national or local drug procurement agencies to use techniques that result in low-price procurement of STI drugs (international tenders for generic products, collaboration with non-profit organizations, joint drug procurement, etc.).

Quantifying drug needs is a critical step in the process of STI drug supplies. This quantification needs the merging of three sets of data: (i) a list of drugs used for STI treatment in the country with their unit prices; (ii) average drug quantities needed for treatment of each STI condition; and (iii) an estimate of the incidence of STI or STI-associated 'syndromes' in the country.

An 'historical' example of estimation of STI drug needs and costs for Mozambique is given in Table 12.1.1. The sum of US$137,587 had to cover all STI drugs for 1 year for a population of 1 million at estimates of very high STI incidence. The STI drug provision was supported by a major international donor (European Union – AIDS Task Force) and was an essential element in a considerably strengthened STI programme. While costs for STI drugs are substantial (US$0.13 per inhabitant), this must be weighed against the cost of inadequate treatment (complications, relapse, further transmission, increased HIV transmission).

Acceptable STI care

However accessible and effective services may be, unless patients are prepared to use them, they are valueless. The acceptability of services is likely to be greatest when care is integrated into routine health services. Examples of the constraints on acceptability include:

- Inconvenience of opening times and long waiting periods.
- Poorly maintained and unattractive physical facilities.
- Judgemental staff attitudes.
- Poor staff communication skills.
- Stigmatization of those seeking STI care.
- Failure to relieve symptoms.
- Lack of privacy and (perceived) lack of confidentiality.

Table 12.1.1. Estimated cost of STI drugs needed for 1 million population in Mozambique in 1988.

Drug	Unit price (US$)	Units needed for 1 million population	Total price (US$)
Benzathine penicillin vial 2.4 mega-units	0.35	41,275	14,446
Kanamycin vial 2 g	0.62	122,500	75,950
Spectinomycin vial 2 g	1.61	6,250	10,063
Doxycycline capsule 100 mg	0.03	454,000	13,620
Erythromycin capsule 500 mg	0.077	82,500	6,353
Erythromycin syrup	0.56	2,500	1,400
Metronidazole tablet 250 mg	0.0065	500,000	3,250
Cotrimoxazole tablet 80/400 mg	0.015	427,000	6,405
Nystatin vaginal tablet	0.02	42,000	840
Gentian violet 250 g packs	6.5	40	260
Tetracycline eye ointment	0.5	10,000	5,000
Total			137,587

Early detection

Detection programmes for STI aim at reaching asymptomatic individuals, mainly by two strategies: case-finding and screening of specific population groups.

Case-finding

Case-finding is the testing for STI of individuals seeking health care for reasons other than STI; for instance, STI detection and care can be provided as part of MCH and family planning (FP) services. Women in particular may often and for a protracted time be asymptomatic when infected with STI; they can be reached through MCH and FP services in an acceptable and non-stigmatizing way. Although asymptomatic, they are infectious for their partner, fetus or newborn, and they are at risk of developing severe STI complications.

Testing of women for syphilis at antenatal clinics is a classic example of case-finding. It has been shown to be highly cost effective in preventing congenital syphilis and the other complications of syphilis, if the whole process including testing and treatment of seropositives is monitored carefully.

A demonstration project in Zambia, based on syphilis testing at MCH clinics, showed that syphilis intervention in pregnancy is culturally acceptable and highly cost effective, at a cost of US$0.60 per woman screened (including RPR testing, health education materials and training) and US$12 per adverse pregnancy outcome averted.

Although most developing countries have a programme for maternal syphilis control, the intervention is very often implemented ineffectively. A careful evaluation, too seldomly done, can detect all the flaws in the system and allows remedial action to be taken. Operational research in Nairobi, Kenya showed that less than 15% of pregnant women with syphilis receive adequate treatment through the case-finding programme.

In many areas, FP and MCH attendees have a high prevalence of chlamydial and gonococcal infections, and case-finding would be a cost-effective intervention in preventing transmission and complications.

These case-finding programmes cannot be implemented in many developing countries because of lack of resources: a good laboratory infrastructure is essential (laboratory tests available in sufficient quantity and quality of performance regularly checked), and this support component most often is grossly inadequate.

Mass treatment can be an alternative to case-finding in situations of high prevalence of treatable STI and non-availability or inefficient laboratory testing. Mass treatment of pregnant women (with a high prevalence of gonococcal infections) in Nairobi, with a single dose of ceftriaxone, 250 mg, increased birth weight significantly and decreased portpartum endometritis.

Screening

Screening is testing in individuals who have not directly sought health care. Donors of blood, tissue or semen should be screened for at least HIV, hepatitis B and C, and syphilis. This activity is the responsibility of the blood transfusion services ('provide safe blood'), but collaboration with the STI/AIDS programme is necessary particularly for adequate case management of donors found to be infected, including pre- and post-test counselling if results of tests are communicated, and treatment for syphilis.

Screening for curable STI among 'core groups' such as female prostitutes, the military, etc., and among other groups such as specific occupational groups, is often implemented and is a popular intervention with the lay public and politicians. A particular problem with these activities is the potential for infringement of the individual's rights due to lack of confidentiality and, except for high prevalence groups, these check-ups are not cost effective. Most countries have organized regular STI screening of female prostitute populations. The effectiveness of most of these programmes is questionable due to inaccurate methodologies (Gram-stained cervical or vaginal smears), poor quality of testing, ineffective treatments and low coverage rates. In Indonesia, infection rates in the three largest cities among sex workers ranged from 15 to 31% for gonorrhoea and from 18 to 39% for chlamydial infection; 2-monthly screening by gonorrhoea culture and chlamydia ELISA combined with treatment with azithromycin, 1 g, immediately reduced infection rates to approximatively 50% of their initial level in all three cities. A further reduction probably needs a higher frequency of screening, increased safer sex practices and as wide a coverage as possible of STI services for sex workers, clients and their regular partners. These types of high-quality screening and other STI services are neither sustainable nor generalizable as a routine intervention for such target groups.

HIV testing

HIV testing may be carried out for various purposes: to screen blood donors and blood units; to monitor the epidemic through surveillance of sentinel populations; to test patients with symptoms and signs (diagnostic testing as part of HIV/AIDS patient management); or to perform voluntary testing on healthy persons (early detection).

A single HIV antibody test may not be sufficient to give a reliable result; WHO has elaborated HIV testing strategies using one, two or three different HIV tests depending on the purpose of testing (see above) and the HIV prevalence in the area.

Unless testing is for screening or surveillance purposes and the results cannot be linked in any way to the individual (unlinked anonymous testing), informed consent must be obtained: it means that the individual understands what the test involves, what the result may mean to him or her, and voluntarily accepts testing.

When testing for early detection (screening or case-finding) or diagnostic purposes, individuals should participate in pre-test and post-test counselling sessions, face to face with a qualified counsellor. Confidentiality of HIV test results is an absolute necessity which means that all testing in the laboratory must be done on coded specimens and only the doctor and counsellor should be able to link code numbers with the individual. Much care should be taken to avoid errors in the coding process.

Screening and case-finding for HIV infection should always be organized on a voluntary basis; it is often considered, especially, for individuals with high-risk behaviour. In developing countries, it is not an intervention strategy which should receive high priority for various reasons: its effectiveness depends on the individuals who test HIV positive to adopt consistently safe sex practices; HIV testing is costly and widespread testing is a serious drain on scarce resources for STI/AIDS prevention and control; the other needs for HIV testing, blood safety, surveillance and diagnosis deserve priority; and the accuracy of HIV antibody tests in field conditions is also considerably lower than in reference laboratories and necessitates repeat testing to avoid mislabelling individuals as HIV positive.

Partner notification

Partner notification is a public health activity by which the partners of those with an STI or HIV infection are notified, informed of their exposure and offered medical and counselling services. Notification can be through patient referral, whereby the patient is encouraged to notify his/her partners of their possible infection, or through provider referral whereby health care workers notify a patient's partners (with agreement of the patient). Partner notification should be voluntary and non-coercive, and all information should remain strictly confidential.

Management of sexual partners is based on the disease diagnosed ('syndromic' or aetiological) in the index patient. It is recommended that epidemiological treatment (with the same treatment regimen used as in the index patient) is given to all sexual partners. Different strategies are possible for treatment of partners: (i) immediate epidemiological treatment without any laboratory investigation; (ii) immediate epidemiological treatment, but specimens are obtained for laboratory confirmation of infection; and (iii) delay of treatment until the results of laboratory tests are available.

Partner notification of STI patients or HIV-infected persons offers an important opportunity for identifying persons who are likely to be infected themselves. Further transmission of STI/HIV, re-infection and development of complications can be prevented. Infection in the partners is often asymptomatic, and although important in both sexes this is particularly important for women who are otherwise difficult to reach for early detection.

STI services for core groups

Individuals with multiple sexual partners are particularly vulnerable for acquiring and transmitting STI; members of such 'core' groups play a significant role in maintaining a high reproductive rate of STI and therefore it is logical to target interventions on them. Examples of potentially high-frequency transmitters of STI are given in Box 12.1.5.

Core group members may be reluctant to seek STI care or to reveal their high-risk behaviour. The STI/AIDS programme should seek information on types of core groups in the community, where they can be reached and on their STI health-seeking behaviour. This information allows for interventions tailored to their STI needs and demands. STI services must be improved so that they are acceptable for individuals of core groups, or STI services can be developed specifically for them. Examples of this are 'drop-in' clinics for sex workers, situated inside or close to a red-light area having convenient hours, a non-judgemental approach by staff, and which can also offer family planning

Box 12.1.5. Potential core groups (WHO/UNAIDS, 1997).

- Sex workers, female and male.
- Clients of sex workers belonging to specific groups, e.g.
  - the military
  - long-distance truck drivers
  - tourists – male and female, business people
  - seafarers
  - migrant workers, refugees, displaced persons
  - 'single' men in urban settings.
- Men who have sex with men, e.g.
  - self-identifying homosexual men
  - bisexual and covert homosexual men.
- Injecting drug users and their sexual partners: particularly of importance where there is a high HIV level amongst injecting drug users and where prostitution is used to support a drug habit.

and other services, voluntary testing, legal and social advice, etc. The STI services should be as comprehensive as possible: health promotion and counselling on safer sex including condom use, STI care when symptomatic and screening and treatment where it can be organized effectively.

In Nairobi, Kenya, it was estimated that enhanced STI services, including promotion of condom use and diagnosis and treatment of STI, in a cohort of 1000 sex workers (80% HIV-positive) prevents 6000–10,000 new HIV infections annually in the community; at a cost of US$8–12 per HIV infection averted. Such a targeted intervention is highly cost effective. Results of numbers of infections prevented are even more impressive for a conventional STI with a high transmission rate, such as gonorrhoea.

Mass treatment

Mass treatment, i.e. periodical epidemiological treatment of sex workers, remains highly controversial, but the strategy should be considered under certain circumstances, e.g. high numbers of sex workers, inadequate, insufficient or too costly laboratory facilities, high mobility. Treatments selected could be directed against gonorrhoea and chlamydia (ciprofloxacin plus doxycycline, or azithromycin) or against gonorrhoea and chancroid (spectinomycin, or ceftriaxone).

One of the arguments against mass treatment is the development of antimicrobial resistance. Therapeutic doses must be used for mass treatment. Furthermore, in nearly all settings, sex workers regularly take different types of antibiotics which frequently are totally ineffective because of low dosages and wrong choice of antibiotics.

STI information systems

Surveillance system

A surveillance system is an integral part of the STI/AIDS programme in order to provide the information required for programme decisions, e.g. definition of resources needed, advocacy of support from policy makers, improvement of activities, etc. The main objectives of surveillance are: (i) to estimate the magnitude of the AIDS/STI problem and its determinants; and (ii) to monitor trends in different areas and population groups.

Methods used for surveillance of HIV/AIDS and STI do not differ technically from those used for other infectious diseases. However, due to the severity of the infection and the extreme social and personal implications of being identified as HIV-positive, surveillance issues such as anonymity and confidentiality are of paramount importance.

Surveillance is the routine collection and analysis of data which are needed to take appropriate action. For an STI/AIDS programme, data to be collected are on HIV, AIDS, STI and risk behaviours. Data on the number of patients with STI or AIDS can be generated through a reporting system from the health services. This reporting can cover comprehensively all health units, but more reliable data at much less cost can be obtained through reporting from sentinel sites only. Reporting of cases gives us an estimate of disease incidence.

Another set of data is the number of people infected with HIV or STI in specific populations, which yields prevalence estimates in sentinel populations, e.g. blood donors, STI patients, pregnant women, core groups, etc.

Monitoring and evaluation

Monitoring is the process of assessing how well various programme activities have been implemented, and should be both quantitative (how much is being achieved) and qualitative (how well activities are being carried out). Its purpose is to ensure that work is progressing as planned, and to anticipate or detect implementation problems, e.g. adequacy of supplies, appropriateness of training, performance of service providers, etc.

Supervision is one of the most important methods used in monitoring and to assess performance and outputs in the light of the situation and the resources available. Supervision is a way of ensuring competence through observation, discussion, support and guidance. In practice, supervisory checklists are produced to establish systematically that all items in the plan of action are monitored carefully.

Evaluation is the critical assessment, on as objective a basis as possible, of the degree to which the objectives and the targets of the programme are being attained. Evaluation assembles information from the surveillance system, monitoring and supervision to determine whether the planned outcomes are in fact achieved. This can best be done by setting targets for the different activities of the programme and using an indicator to determine whether the targets have been met.

The WHO has developed and tested a number of prevention indicators (PIs) for evaluating the progress of STI/AIDS programmes (Box 12.1.6). The methods used for the measurement of the PIs are a population survey (PI 1, 3, 4, 5 and 9), a health facility survey (PI 6, 7), an analysis of records (PI 2), and a serosurvey (PI 8, 10).

While monitoring is much more an ongoing activity and the responsibility of the more peripheral levels of programme management, evaluation is done at regular intervals, for instance initially, at mid-term and at the end of programme planning periods, and is the responsibility of the central management.

STI/AIDS programme management

Programme management is the organization and control of available human, material and financial resources to ensure that these are being used in the most effective and efficient manner to achieve the objectives of the programme. A clearly defined management structure is crucial. As far as possible,

Box 12.1.6. List of prevention indicators (PI) (Mertens *et al.*, 1994).

PI 1: Knowledge of prevention practices
No. of people citing at least two acceptable ways of protection from HIV infection
divided by
No. of people aged 15–49 years surveyed.

PI 2: Condom availability (central level)
Total no. of condoms available for distribution during the preceding 12 months
divided by
population aged 15–49 years.

PI 3: Condom availability (peripheral level)
No. of people who can acquire a condom
divided by
population aged 15–49 years.

PI 4: Reported non-regular sex partners
No. of people aged 15–49 years who report having had at least one sex partner other than a regular sex partner(s) in the last 12 months
divided by
no. of people aged 15–49 years who report having been sexually active in the last 12 months.

PI 5: Reported condom use with non-regular sex partner
No. of people aged 15–49 years who report condom use during the last sexual intercourse with a non-regular sex partner
divided by
no. of people aged 15–49 years who report sexual intercourse with a non-regular sex partner in the last 12 months.

PI 6: STI case management
No. of people presenting with STI in health facilities assessed and treated in an appropriate way (according to national standards)
divided by
no. of people presenting with STI in health facilities.

PI 7: STI case management
No. of people presenting with STI in health facilities who received basic advice on condoms and on partner notification
divided by
no. of people presenting with STI in health facilities.

PI 8: STI prevalence, women
No. of pregnant women aged 15–24 years with positive serology for syphilis
divided by
no. of pregnant women aged 15–24 years attending antenatal clinics whose blood was tested for syphilis.

PI 9: STI incidence, men
No. of reported episodes of urethritis in the last 12 months in men aged 15–49 years
divided by
no. of men aged 15–49 years surveyed.

PI 10: HIV prevalence, women
No. of HIV seropositive pregnant women aged 15–24 years
divided by
no. of pregnant women aged 15–24 years attending antenatal clinics whose blood was tested for HIV.

the implementation of programme management should be decentralized.

At district or provincial level, health authorities must define a programme and its components that are in line with national policy; steps to be taken at this level also include a situation analysis, development of a plan of operation and a plan of action, implementation of the activities, monitoring and evaluation. To be successful, STI/AIDS programmes need to be multisectorial, involving the planning, education, community development and other sectors of the district in collaboration with the health sector, and to make a maximum effort to involve non-governmental (NGOs) and community-based organizations.

Nevertheless, a central management structure has major responsibilities to ensure that STI/AIDS control receives the high priority and attention it deserves; the World Bank estimated that in sub-Saharan Africa AIDS and STI ranked fifth among health problems in terms of disability-adjusted life years (DALYs), with 8.8% of DALYs lost, after malaria (10.8%), respiratory infections (10.8%), diarrhoea (10.4%) and vaccine-preventable diseases (9.6%).

Responsibilities at the central level include:

- political advocacy;
- national policy decisions including setting of priorities in the implementation of activities;
- allocation of resources;
- planning and guidance on service delivery and necessary referral systems;
- ensuring sustainability of programme activities;
- developing and monitoring training for all types of health workers involved;
- developing and distributing guidance on programme activities;
- planning of specific activities, e.g. interventions targeted at core groups;
- ensuring that recommended drugs are available: importance of essential drug lists and guidance on cost recovery mechanisms;
- ensuring procurement and availability of condoms of standard quality;
- supervision of coverage and quality of services;
- situational analysis and planning of essential operational research;
- surveillance systems;
- programme evaluation, based on indicators of achievement and after setting realistic targets.

The national programme thus has promotional, technical, planning and coordination roles.

Conclusion

STI/AIDS are significant health problems in the developing world and their importance is still increasing. This means that, in addition to the need for the current control programmes to be sustained, an expansion in programme activities is required. This will only be possible if the programmes deliver 'value for money' through adequate programme management. Therefore, the planning and the implementation of the STI/AIDS programme should comprise a number of steps as part of a systematic approach: a situational assessment, a political commitment, a national AIDS/STI policy, a selection of programme priorities, setting objectives and designing strategies, planning the implementation, development of support components, mobilization of resources, and monitoring and evaluation.

Further reading

Adler, W.M. (1996) Sexually transmitted diseases control in developing countries. *Genitourinary Medicine* 72, 83–88.

Arya, O.P. and Lawson, J.B. (1977) Sexually transmitted diseases in the tropics: epidemiological, diagnostic, therapeutic and control aspects. *Tropical Doctor* 7, 51–56.

Dallabetta, G., Laga, M. and Lamptey, P. (1996) *Control of Sexually Transmitted Diseases. A Handbook for the Design and Management of Programs.* AIDSCAP/Family Health International, USA.

Gerard, C., Sondag-Thull, D., Watson-Williams, E.J. and Fransen, L. (1995) *Safe Blood in Developing Countries. Principles and Organisation.* European Commission, Brussels.

Germain, A., Holmes, K.K., Piot, P. and Wasserheit, J.N. (1992) *Reproductive Tract Infections, Global Impact and Priorities for Women's Reproductive Health.* Plenum Press, New York.

Hayes R., Wawer, M., Gray, R., Whitworth, J., Grosskurth, H., Mabey, D. and HIV/STD Trials Workshop Group (1997) Randomized trials of STD treatment for HIV prevention: report of an international workshop. *Genitourinary Medicine* 73, 432–443.

Lamptey, P. and Piot, P. (1990) *The Handbook for AIDS Prevention in Africa.* Family Health International, Durham, North Carolina.

Lande, R.E. (1993) *Controlling Sexually Transmitted Diseases. Population Report L-No. 9.* Johns Hopkins University, Population Information Programme, Baltimore, Maryland.

Meheus, A., Schulz, K.F. and Cates, W. (1990) Development of prevention and control programs for sexually transmitted diseases in developing countries. In: Holmes, K.K., Mårdh, P.A., Sparling, P.F., Wiesner, P.J. Cates, W., Lemon, S.M. and Stamm, W.E. (eds) *Sexually Transmitted Diseases.* McGraw-Hill, New York, pp. 1041–1046.

Mertens, T., Caraël, M., Sato, P., Cleland, J., Ward, H. and Smith, G.D. (1994) Prevention indicators for evaluating the progress of national AIDS programmes. *AIDS* 8, 1359–1369.

Ng'weshemi, J., Boerma, T., Bennett, J. and Schapink, D. (1997) *HIV Prevention and AIDS Care in Africa: a District Level Approach.* Royal Tropical Institute, Amsterdam.

Wasserheit, J.N., Aral, S.O. and Holmes, K.K. (1991) *Research Issues in Human Behavior and Sexually Transmitted Diseases in the AIDS Era.* American Society for Microbiology, Washington, DC.

World Health Organization Study Group (1991) *Management of Patients with Sexually Transmitted Diseases.* WHO Technical Report Series no. 810, Geneva.

World Health Organization (1994a) *Evaluation of a National AIDS Programme: a Methods Package 1. Prevention of HIV Infection.* WHO, Geneva.

World Health Organization (1994b) *Management of Sexually Transmitted Diseases.* WHO/GPA/TEM/94.1., WHO, Geneva.

World Health Organization (1995) *Condom Promotion for AIDS Prevention.* WHO, Geneva.

World Health Organization/United Nations Programme on HIV/AIDS, WHO/UNAIDS (1997) *Sexually Transmitted Diseases: Policies and Principles for Prevention and Care*, pp. 1–47.

Chapter 12.2
Vaccination against STI, HIV and AIDS

T.F. Schulz
Department of Medical Microbiology and Genitourinary Medicine,
University of Liverpool, Liverpool, UK

Despite extensive efforts to develop effective vaccines against common viral and bacterial STI, clear-cut success has so far only been achieved for hepatitis B. For several other sexually transmitted infectious agents, experimental results are promising enough to expect that an effective vaccine will be technically feasible in the not too distant future. This chapter reviews current knowledge and prospects for the development of effective vaccines.

Vaccines for bacterial STI

Vaccination for the four most important bacterial STI (gonorrhoea, syphilis, chlamydial infection and chancroid) has been considered, but no clinically tested vaccine is yet available. Immunogenic bacterial proteins which elicit protective immune responses have been identified in the case of *Neisseria gonorrhoeae* and *Chlamydia trachomatis*, and represent potential vaccine candidates. Much less detailed knowledge is currently available for *Treponema pallidum* and *Haemophilus ducreyi*.

Gonorrhoea

Clinical experience suggests that infection with *N. gonorrhoeae* can induce a type-specific immunity. Porin (Por) is an abundant membrane protein with multiple membrane-spanning domains that exhibits isolate-specific antigenic epitopes in some surface-exposed domains. Two main Por-based serogroups, Por A and Por B, can be distinguished, and Por may play a role in pathogenesis. Monoclonal and polyclonal antibodies to certain Por antigens are both bactericidal and opsonizing. Recombinant Por-based vaccine candidates have been expressed in *Escherichia coli* and engineered into *Salmonella typhimurium* strains. It is possible that sialylation of lipo-oligosaccharide (LOS) moieties on *N. gonorrhoeae* may interfere with the antibacterial properties of antibodies to Por *in vitro*, and these issues are presently under investigation. *N. gonorrhoeae* pili are important for adherence to host cells and elicit antibodies capable of blocking infection *in vitro*. However, pili can undergo extensive phase and antigenic variation and protective anti-pilin monoclonal antibodies are directed preferentially against highly variable epitopes. Partial protection of human volunteers produced by a Pil vaccine against a homologous strain has been observed in one, but not other trials, and an exclusively Pil-based vaccine is, therefore, unlikely to succeed.

Another set of *N. gonorrhoeae* adherence proteins, termed opacity proteins (Opa), also undergo extensive phase and antigenic variation. Although monoclonal antibodies to some Opas decrease adherence *in vitro*, little experience of their use as vaccines is available at present.

LOS core sugars can elicit antibacterial antibodies, and anti-LOS IgM antibodies occur in individuals who have never been exposed to *N. gonorrhoeae*. This may be due to mimicry of host antigens which could represent an obstacle to the development of high-affinity IgG antibodies to such antigens. In addition, sialylation of these core sugars results in partial masking of LOS core sugars and Por proteins located in close proximity and can interfere with antibody binding to these structures.

Therefore, while several antigens eliciting bactericidal and opsonizing antibodies are known in *N. gonorrhoeae*, natural escape/protection mechanisms may limit their potential as vaccine candidates, and further work is required to identify a combination of *N. gonorrhoeae* proteins which will prove effective in human volunteers.

Chamydia trachomatis infection

The immune response to *C. trachomatis* is known to involve protective antibodies as well as antibodies which may play a role in the pathogenesis of the disease. The presence of antibodies to a 57-kDa heat shock protein, related to the groEL product, correlates with salpingitis, ectopic pregnancy and tubal infertility, and may be predictive of the emergence of some complications in women infected with *C. trachomatis*. A cellular hypersensitivity reaction to this antigen may play a role in the pathogenesis of these conditions and Reiter's syndrome which can complicate genital chlamydial infection. It is thus important to exclude this and other 'immunopathogenic' antigens from any vaccine preparation. The major outer membrane protein (MOMP) elicits neutralizing antibodies which protect against tissue culture infection and may react with different serovars. Neutralizing epitopes are located on surface-exposed, variable loops of this transmembrane protein, and T-helper (T_H) cell epitopes are present in conserved as well as variable domains of MOMP. Synthetic peptides combining epitopes for neutralizing antibodies with T_H epitopes have shown initial promising results in animal experiments, and whole recombinant MOMP is also a possible vaccine candidate. Unlike the gonococcal Por, MOMP does not appear to be protected from antibody attack by blocking antibodies or sialylation of neighbouring structures. Other *C. trachomatis* proteins, such as the recently described 75-kDa outer membrane protein, may also find use as a vaccine component.

Syphilis

Clinical experience, as well as experiments in humans, suggests the development of protective immunity after infection with *T. pallidum*. This develops slowly, and infectious bacteria may persist in the presence of an active immune response. Following early experimentation with the Nichols strain of *T. pallidum*, killed by irradiation or cold storage, the current focus is on recombinant *T. pallidum* proteins. Limited efficacy in animals has been reported for three antigens (TPN19, TPN36/TmpB and endoflagellar protein), but much further work is needed.

Chancroid

Crude extracts of *H. ducreyi*, possibly containing cytotoxins, have been used to elicit antibodies in rabbits, and outer membrane as well as pilin proteins have been identified. Since serial propagation of *H. ducreyi* in one individual has been demonstrated, it is unclear whether protective immunity can develop *in vivo*, and much remains to be learnt regarding the immune response to this organism.

Vaccines for viral STI

Hepatitis B (see also Chapter 6.7)

HBV is the only sexually transmissible virus for which an effective vaccine is available. Following the demonstration, more than 25 years ago, that serum containing HBsAg retained its immunogenic properties after heat inactivation, HBsAg purified from plasma of HBV carriers was shown to be an effective vaccine. Recombinant HBsAg, produced in yeast or mammalian cells, is also highly immunogenic and now licensed as a vaccine.

These vaccines achieve excellent protection against sexually transmitted HBV infection, as shown by two large-scale randomized trials involving adult US homosexual men with protective efficacies of around 90%. Immunogenicity is reduced in individuals who are immunosuppressed as a result of HIV infection or after transplantation. In addition, there are a small number of immunocompetent non-responders and this may in part be determined genetically.

Whereas sexual transmission among adults accounts for a significant proportion of HBV infections in Western countries (the other main route of transmission being parenteral), perinatal transmission is common in some Asian countries, and horizontal infection in childhood predominant in many African countries. Large-scale studies in China and the USA have shown that HBsAg vaccination is also effective in newborns and provides significant protection against perinatal infection when given in combination with hepatitis B immunoglobulin. Similarly, studies in populations in which horizontal childhood transmission is common (West Africa, Alaska) have all reported protective efficacies in excess of 85% and, in some studies, higher than 95%.

Thus, HBsAg vaccination, when carried out on a large scale (such as in Gambia, Hong Kong and Taiwan), has the potential to change the epidemiology of HBV infection profoundly. Indeed, introduction of universal HBV vaccination in Taiwan in 1984 had, by 1994, halved the incidence of childhood hepatocellular carcinoma.

Herpes simplex virus type 2 (HSV-2) infection

Prevalence rates for infection with HSV-2 have been increasing over the last decades, and a vaccine could therefore play an important part in controlling this STI. A series of animal experiments suggests that this might be feasible, but trials in humans are still limited. In mice and guinea pigs, recombinant vaccine preparations containing HSV-2 glycoprotein D, and occasionally glycoprotein B, have been shown to induce a good antibody and T-cell response and to prevent against subsequent challenge with HSV-2. DNA vaccination, using a plasmid which expressed HSV-2 glycoprotein D under the control of the cytomegalovirus promoter, also achieved partial protection of guinea pigs against subsequent viral challenge.

Recombinant vaccine preparation containing glycoproteins B and/or D were well tolerated by HSV-2 seronegative human volunteers, and induced neutralizing antibodies as well as an HSV-2-specific T-cell response. Efficacy studies are therefore warranted.

Immunization of patients with documented genital herpes to reduce the number of clinical episodes (immunotherapy) has also been attempted. During such studies, some limited benefit was observed with vaccine preparations containing either recombinant glycoprotein D or whole inactivated HSV.

Human papillomavirus (HPV) infection

Over 70 different types of HPV have been defined on the basis of DNA sequence homology. Certain high risk HPV types, such as 16, 18, 33, 35, are associated with malignant cervical neoplasia, whereas HPV6 and HPV11 are associated with genital warts and recurrent respiratory papillomatosis. Both capsid and regulatory viral proteins are recognized by the immune system. The papillomavirus capsids consist of major (L1) and minor (L2) capsid proteins, and both contain type-specific and group-specific antigens. Group-specific antigens appear to be hidden inside the capsid complex and become exposed after denaturing native proteins or in antigen preparations based on incorrectly folded recombinant or synthetic proteins. Neutralizing antibodies can be directed against both L1 and L2 proteins. Type-specific antibodies may be directed against conformational epitopes which are only exposed on correctly folded native or recombinant viral capsids. Expression of recombinant L1 and L2, or L1 alone, in mammalian or insect cells results in the formation of 'viral-like particles' (VLPs) which can be used to measure type-specific antibodies and to elicit neutralizing antibodies. VLPs of cottontail rabbit papillomavirus (CRPV), produced in yeast, protect rabbits against challenge with CRPV, and a similar result has been achieved by immunizing rabbits with plasmid DNA encoding the CRPV L1 protein. VLPs of human papillomaviruses have also been generated and represent promising candidates for prophylactic vaccines in humans. Presently available data based on genome detection by PCR suggest that infection with high-risk HPV types is very rare in women who report no previous sexual activity. This would suggest that a vaccine against high-risk HPVs, if available, would have to be used in children or adolescents to provide sufficient protection.

The transforming proteins E6 and E7 of 'high risk' HPV types are almost always expressed in HPV-associated cancers and involved in cellular transformation by interacting respectively, with the p53 tumour suppressor protein, and the retinoblastoma tumour suppressor protein, pRB. E6 and E7 are recognized by the immune system, and vaccination conceivably could induce a regression of established tumours. In animal experiments, vaccination with an HPV16 E7 peptide induces cell-mediated cytotoxic T-cell immunity and protects against challenge with a HPV16-transformed cell line. Efforts currently are being made to enhance the presentation of these antigens and increase the intensity of the immune response.

HIV infection

Despite extensive efforts over the last decade, no effective vaccine against HIV is presently available. Subunit vaccines, replication-competent recombinant vaccinia virus or canarypox virus expressing individual HIV components, synthetic HIV peptides, or a combination of these approaches have all failed to protect reliably in animal experiments, or, where tested, in man. In some primate models, partial protection, or a reduction in virus load, has been achieved. In the macaque model, infection with a molecularly attenuated simian immunodeficiency virus (SIVmac), does, however, protect against challenge with wild-type SIVmac.

Results achieved so far with HIV-1 vaccines

Many subunit preparations (i.e. purified or recombinant viral proteins) of both HIV and some SIVs are potent immunogens and can induce high titres of specific antibodies and T-cell proliferative responses. Recombinant vaccinia or canarypox viruses induce specific cytotoxic T-cell activity. Some also induce antibodies capable of neutralizing tissue-culture adapted HIV, but not, or much less well, 'primary' freshly isolated strains of HIV which are more representative of HIV variants circulating *in vivo*. Antibodies with neutralizing potential for primary HIV-1 strains are, however, present (at low titre) in HIV-infected individuals. Therefore, it seems as if the presently available vaccine preparations are inefficient at inducing antibodies capable of neutralizing primary HIV-1 strains. However, it is also not known whether neutralization of primary strains *in vitro* is really a good correlate of protective immunity against HIV *in vivo*.

Similarly, the strong T-cell response, including the cytotoxic T-cell response, induced by at least some vaccine preparations (mainly recombinant 'live' vaccinia or canarypox viruses), only rarely achieves complete protection in challenge experiments in macaques and did not reduce the number of newly infected volunteers in a phase I/II vaccine trial. It is nonetheless thought that an effective T-cell response can prevent infection with HIV-1, as there are several examples of multiply exposed seronegative individuals with a strong T-cell cytotoxic response to HIV-1.

However, effective resistance to infection with a pathogenic SIVmac can be induced by infecting macaques with attenuated SIV variants, from which the auxiliary '*nef*' gene, alone or in combination with other auxiliary genes, have been removed by molecular techniques. These 'attenuated' SIV variants replicate *in vivo* only at low levels, do not cause any disease in adult macaques, and protect against challenge with pathogenic SIV strains. This resistance builds up slowly. Although both neutralizing antibodies and T-cell immunity are induced in these animals, it is not clear whether they are responsible for the resistance to pathogenic virus. Other possibilities are HIV inhibitory cytokines which have been reported to be released from activated T-cells and include MIP-1α, RANTES and other, as yet unidentified factors. Nevertheless, neonatal macaques develop disease when inoculated with these attenuated SIV strains. This, and the concern that integrated HIV proviruses might rarely be involved in the development of tumours, makes it very unlikely that attenuated HIV vaccines of this kind will be used in humans.

Variability of HIV

If an effective HIV vaccine could be designed, its marked variability may pose additional difficulties. HIV-1 (and HIV-2) occurs in several genomic variants, called 'clades' or 'subtypes'. So far eight different subtypes (A–H) are known and these are grouped together as type M viruses. One even more distinct group of HIV-1 isolates, type O, is sufficiently distinct from 'type M' viruses to be missed by some serological assays.

While some antibodies, including some with neutralizing potential, will show specificity for certain subtypes, it is not clear whether, as was thought initially, vaccines will have to be tailored to the subtypes prevalent in individual geographic areas. In fact, neutralization of primary HIV-1 isolates *in vitro* does not seem to correlate with genomic subtype. As neutralization of primary HIV strains may, however, not be a good correlate of *in vivo* protection, this question is still unresolved.

'Preventive' vs. 'therapeutic' vaccination

The use of vaccines to reduce HIV-1 replication in an already infected individual ('therapeutic' vaccination) has been proposed as an alternative to the complete prevention of HIV-1 infection which appears to be difficult to achieve. However, it is not known at present whether this is technically feasible or would provide any clinical benefit. Because of the progress made in the last 3 years with antiviral therapy for HIV, and the appreciation of the extremely rapid turnover of HIV-1 *in vivo* (which provides the basis for its capacity to adapt rapidly to antibodies, cytotoxic T lymphocytes, antiviral drugs and target cells), 'therapeutic vaccination' appears a less attractive option.

Index

Numbers in **bold** indicate main references.

1

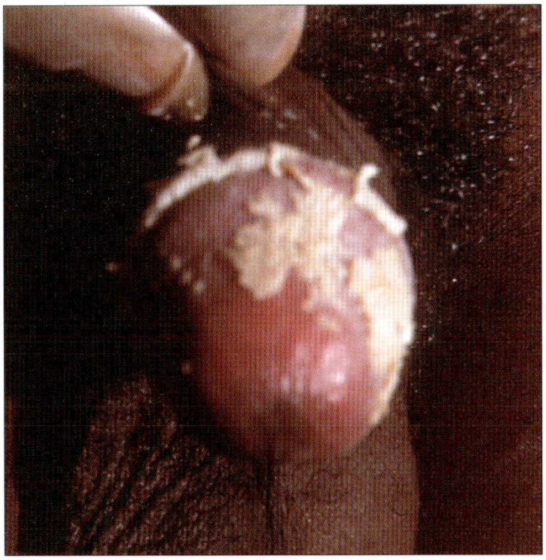

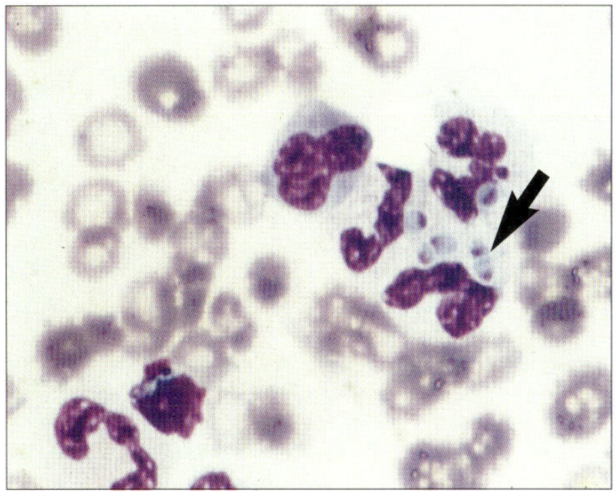

2

3

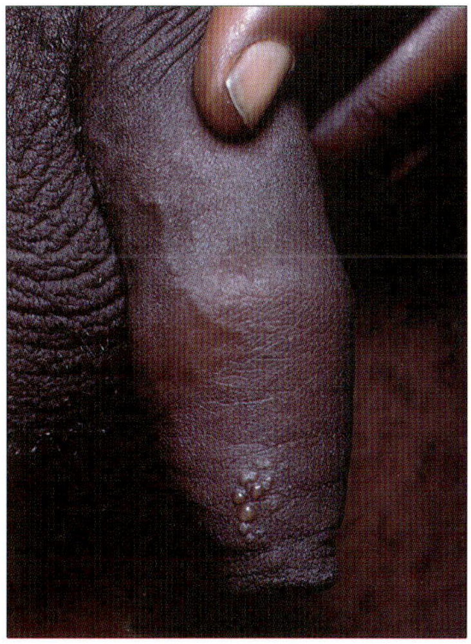

4

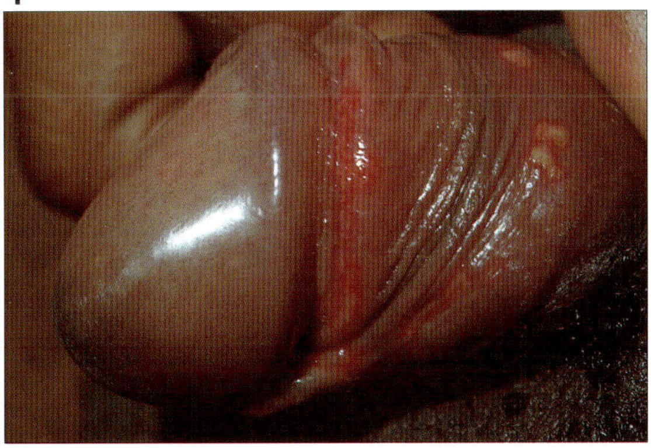

5

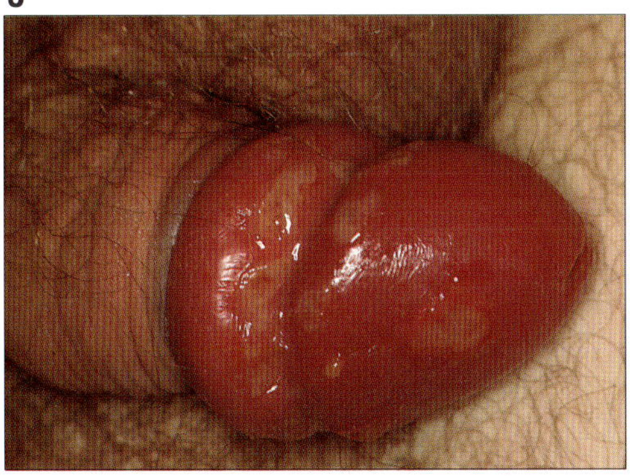

6

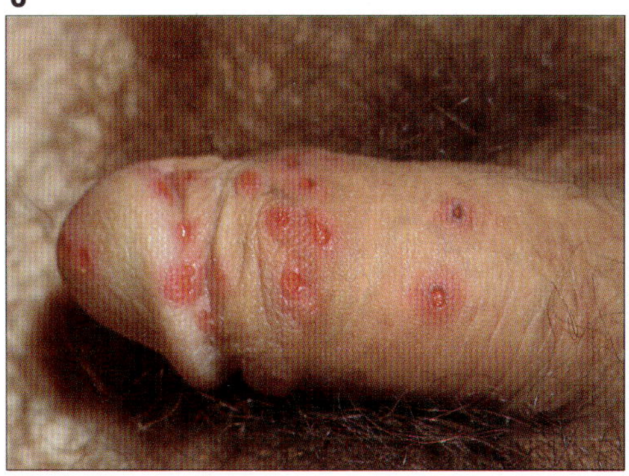

Plate 1. Smegma.
Plate 2. Penicilliosis: intracellular *P. marneffei* elliptical yeast cells with central septation (arrowed).
Plate 3. Genital herpes: a group of herpetic vesicles of the prepuce.
Plate 4. Genital herpes: severe primary HSV infection of the penis with extensive ulceration and surrounding erythema.
Plate 5. Genital herpes: severe primary HSV infection with vesicles, ulcerations and penile oedema.
Plate 6. Genital herpes: multiple ulcers on the penile shaft and glans.

7

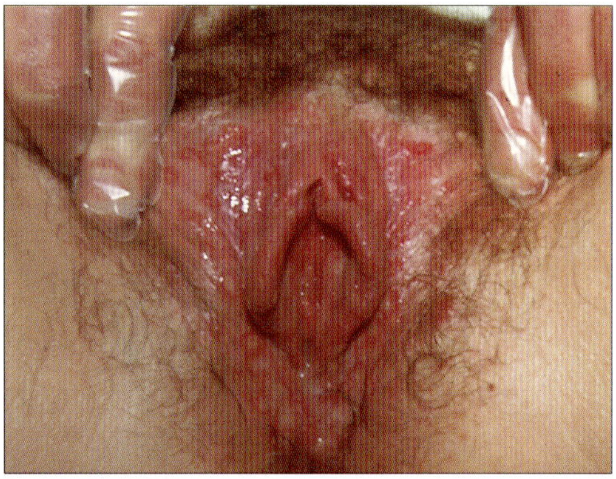

8

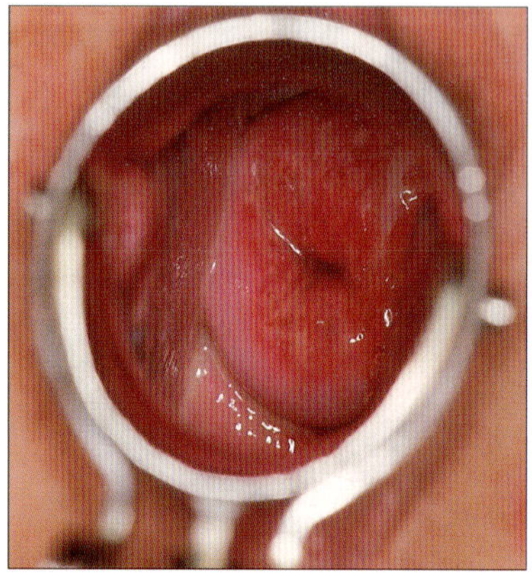

9

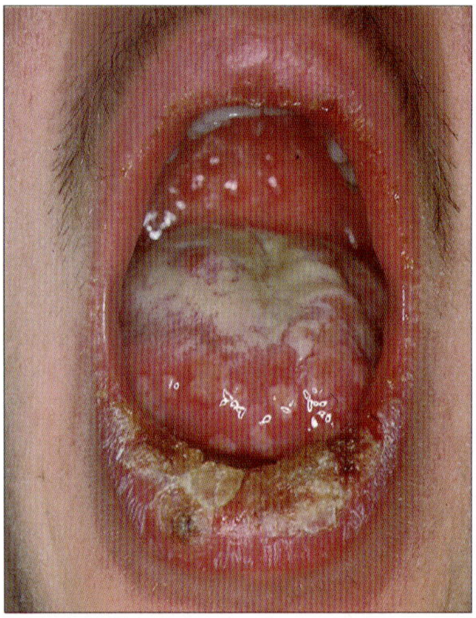

10

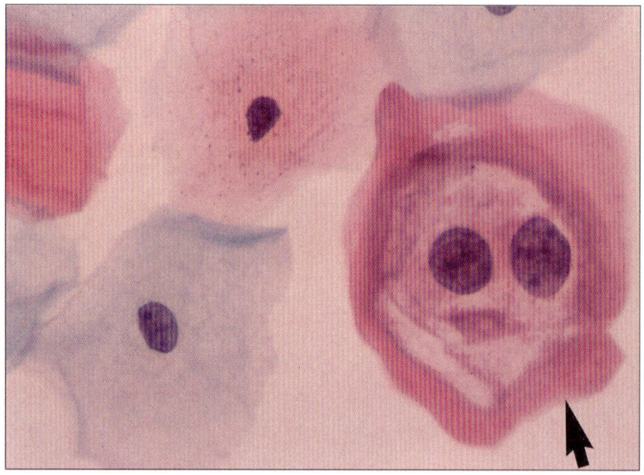

11

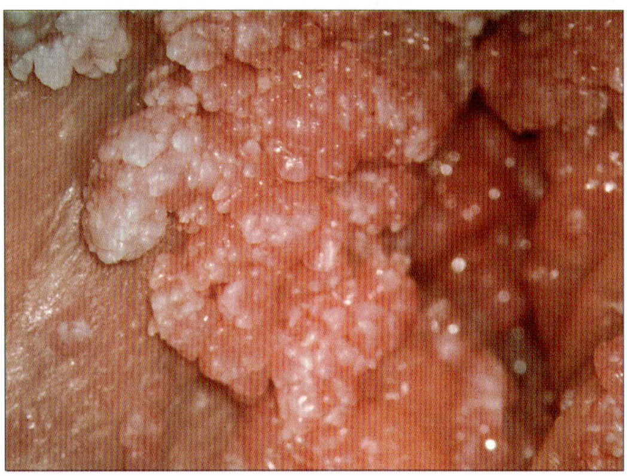

12

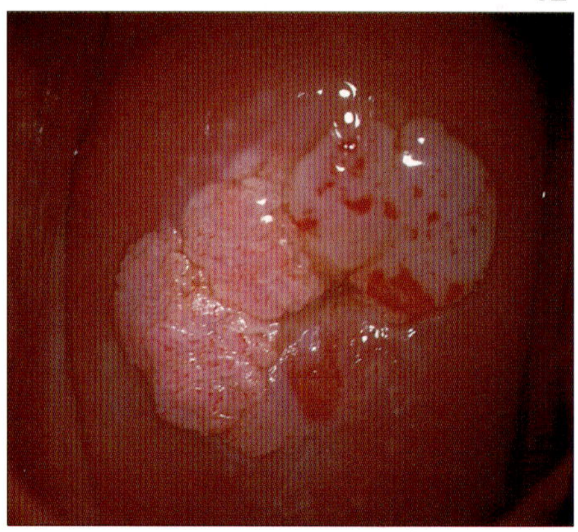

Plate 7. Genital herpes: severe primary HSV infection with extensive ulceration of the vulva (in addition, the vaginal swabs were positive for *T. vaginalis* and *Candida* spp.).

Plate 8. Genital herpes: multiple lesions on the ectocervix.

Plate 9. Extragenital herpes: severe primary HSV infection with extensive vesicles and ulceration of the lips and mouth; the lesions on the lips have crusted.

Plate 10. HPV infection: a cell showing binucleation, koilocytosis and mild dyskaryosis (arrowed).

Plate 11. HPV infection: vulval condylomata acuminata.

Plate 12. HPV infection: cervical condylomas showing capillary patterns.

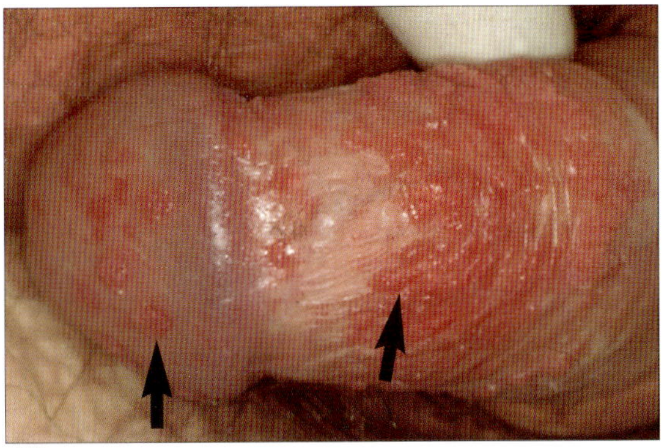

13

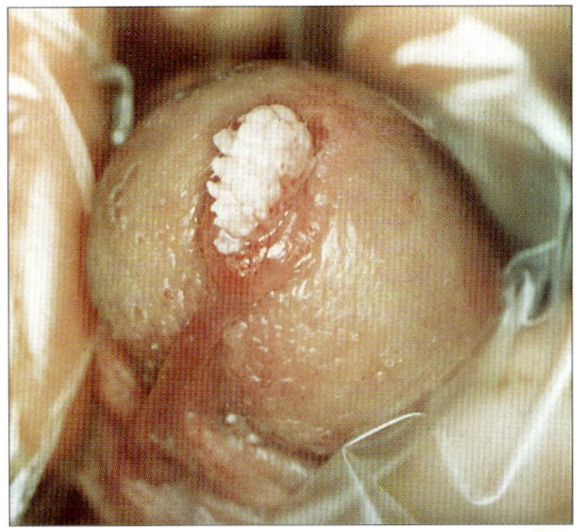

14

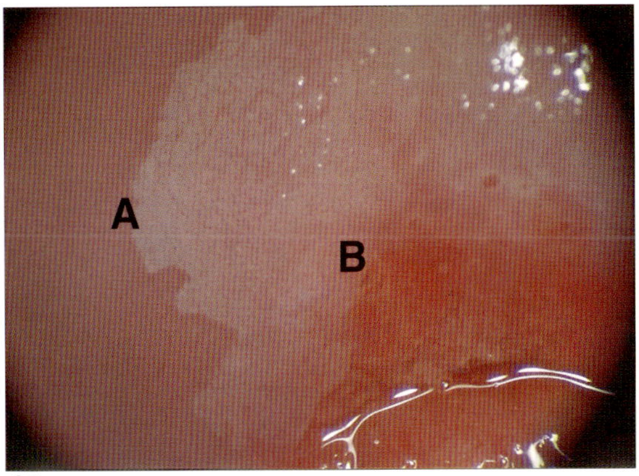

15

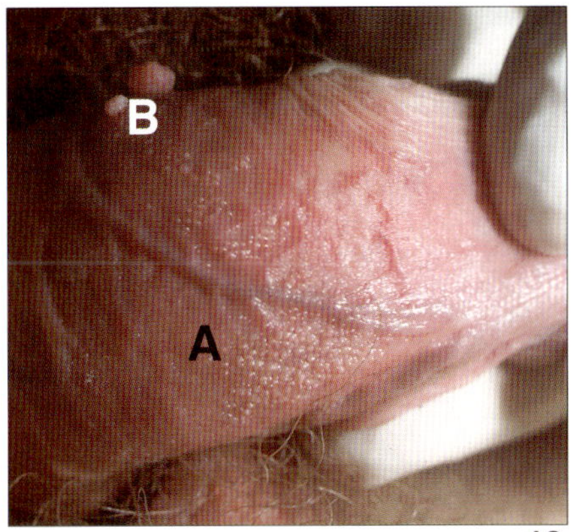

16

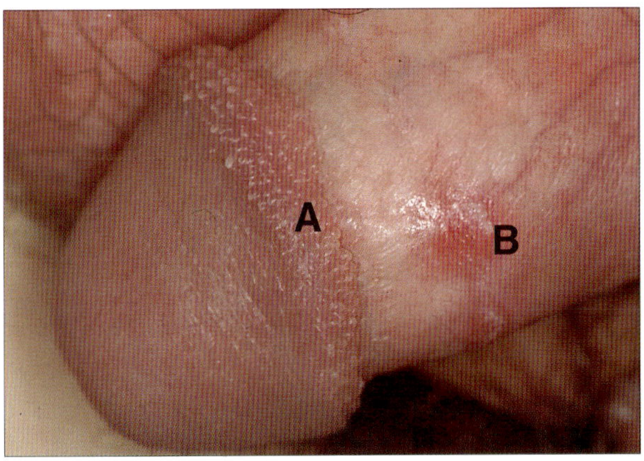

17

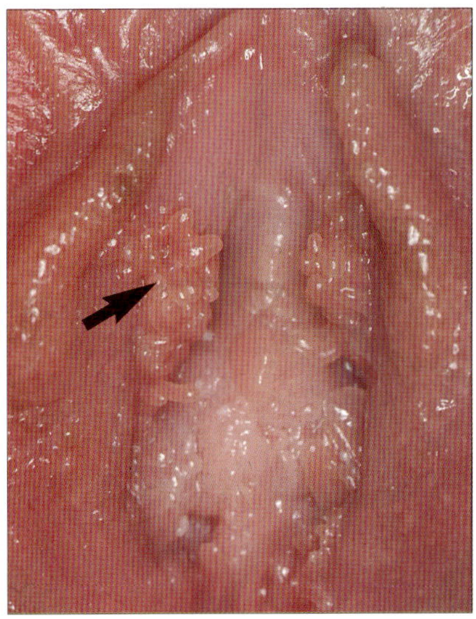

18

Plate 13. HPV infection: penile warts.
Plate 14. HPV infection: meatal warts.
Plate 15. HPV infection: colposcopic appearance of subclinical infection and CIN on application of 5% acetic acid to the cervix showing flat condyloma (A) and CIN3 (B).
Plate 16. Penis: Fordyce's spots (A) and warts (B).
Plate 17. Penis: coronal papillae (A) and warts (B).
Plate 18. Vulva: vestibular papillae.

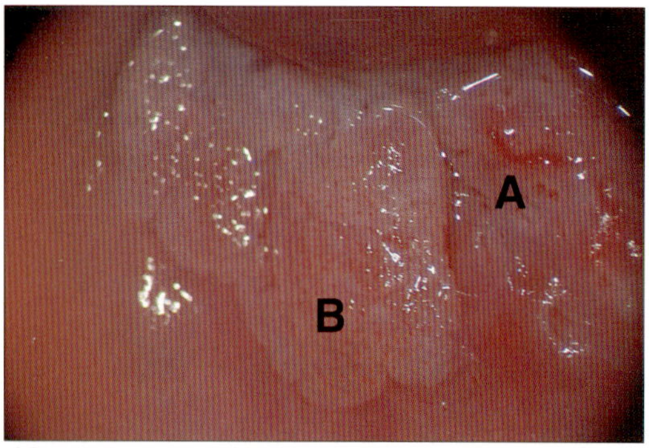

19

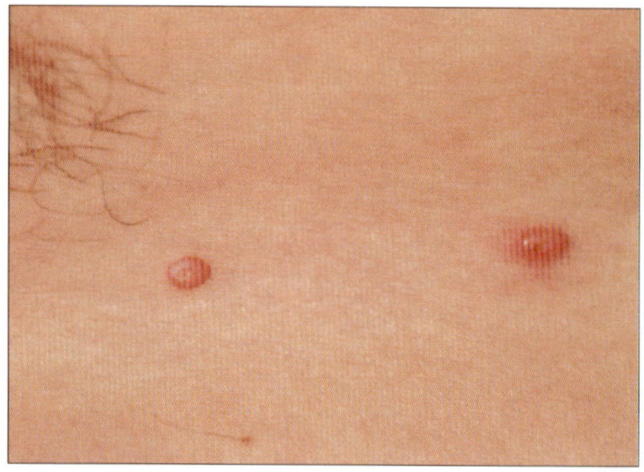

20

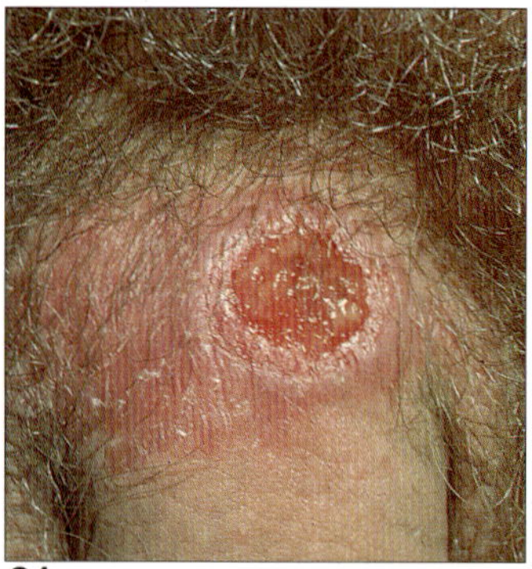

21

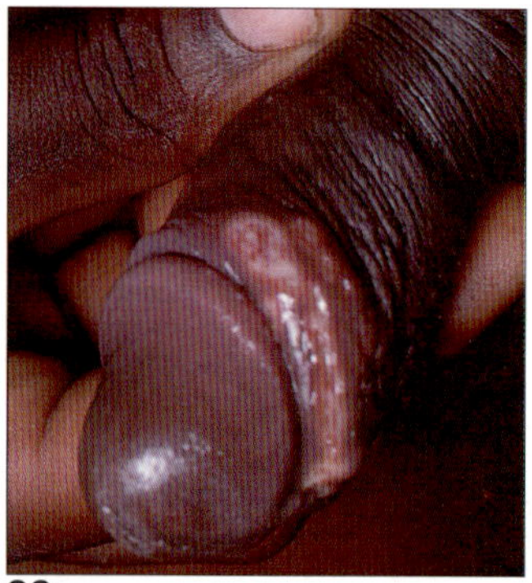

22

24

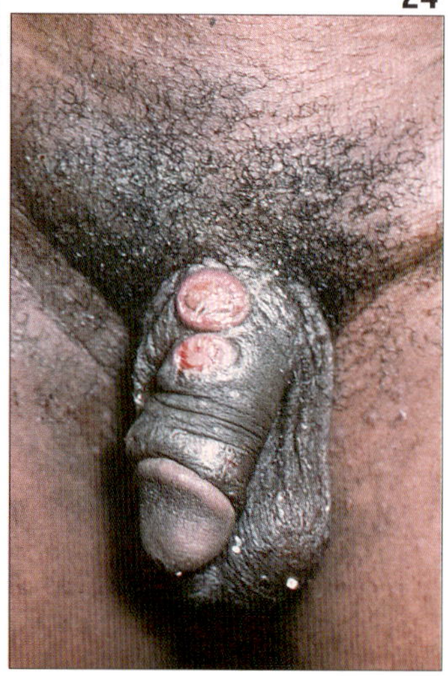

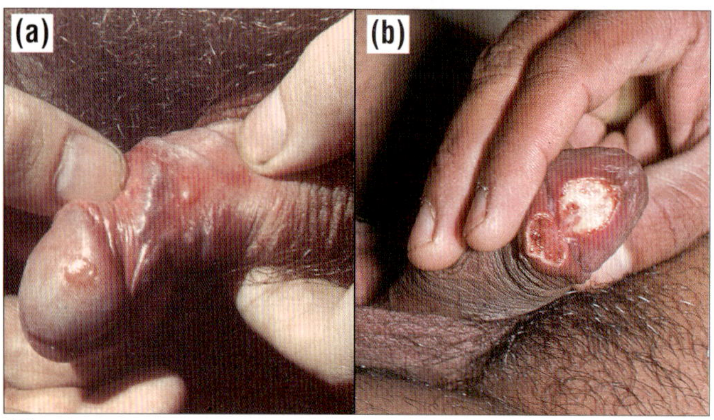

23

Plate 19. HPV infection: colposcopic appearance of the cervix showing frank carcinoma (A) and condylomata acuminata (B).

Plate 20. *Molluscum contagiosum*: dome-shaped papules with central depression on the upper thigh (there were also lesions on the vulva).

Plate 21. Primary syphilis: a typical lesion, single, well-defined, clear ulcer surface. (This patient claimed to have used a condom which did not protect the root of the penis, resulting in the so-called 'condom ulcer'.)

Plate 22. Primary syphilis: an ulcerated chancre (which was painful and tender as a result of secondary infection).

Plate 23. Primary syphilis: (a) small papular kissing lesions and (b) large kissing chancres on the glans penis and reflex prepuce.

Plate 24. Primary syphilis: indurated multiple chancres of the penile shaft and inguinal lymphadenopathy.

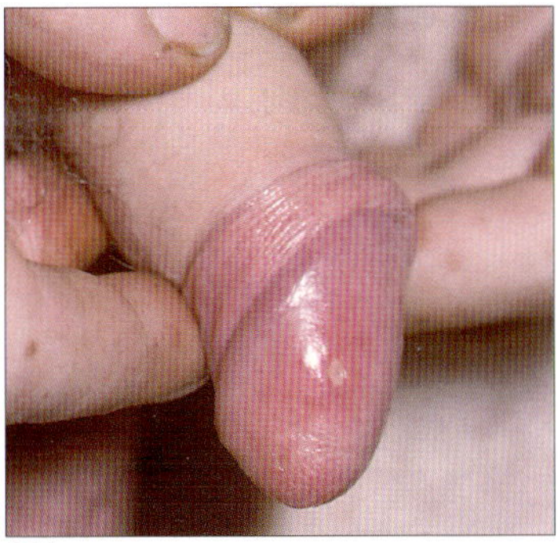

25

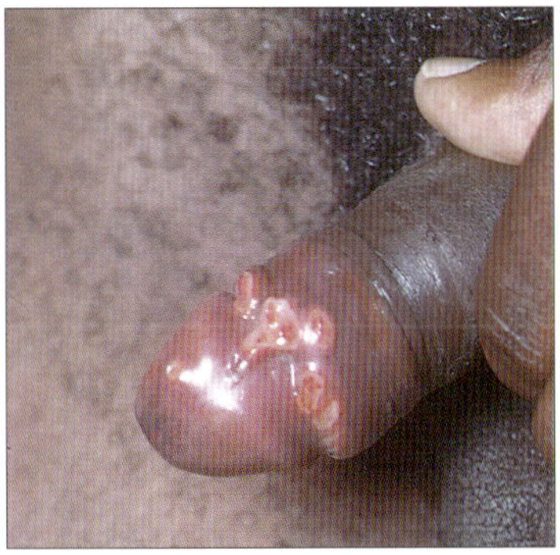

26

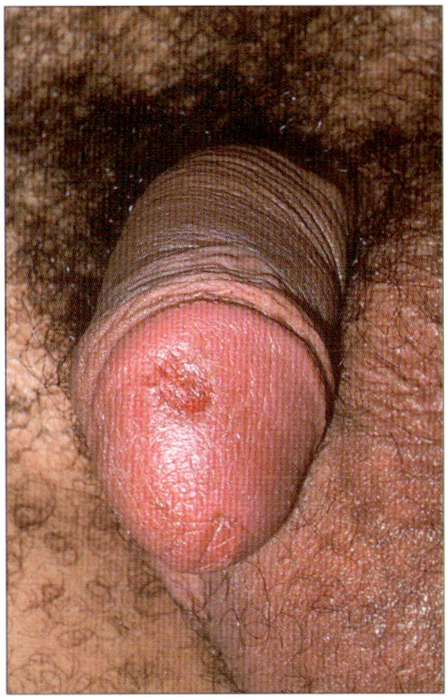

27

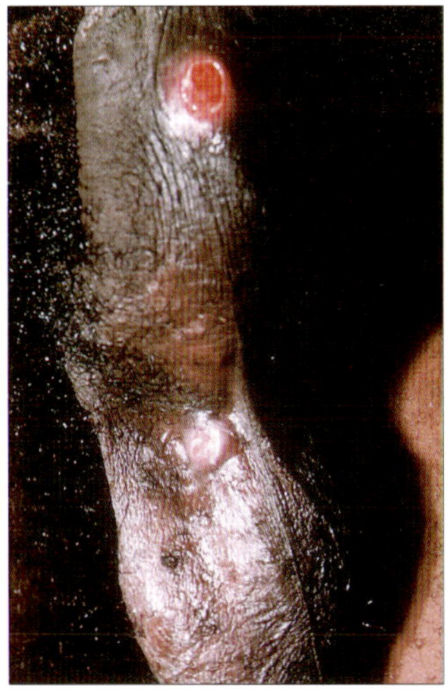

28

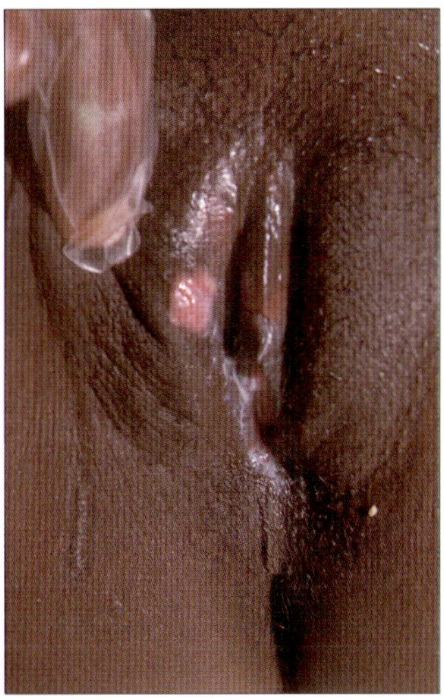

29

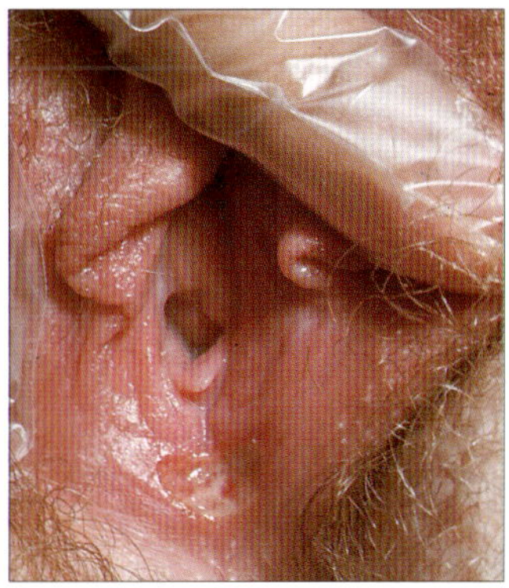

30

Plate 25. Mixed infection (seronegative primary syphilis, chancroid and herpes): a small, tender indurated ulcer of the glans penis (darkfield examination for *T. pallidum* (Fig. 7.1.2), and cultures for *H. ducreyi* and herpes simplex virus were positive).

Plate 26. Mixed infection (primary syphilis and chancroid): multiple and painful syphilitic and chancroidal lesions (some indurated) of the coronal sulcus and fraenum.

Plate 27. Primary syphilis: a small, shallow, non-indurated lesion of the glans penis.

Plate 28. Primary syphilis: a circular scabbed lesion of the penile shaft (initially a kissing chancre; the other part visible on the top area of the scrotum has almost healed).

Plate 29. Primary syphilis: kissing chancres of the labia; the one on the left side has almost healed.

Plate 30. Primary syphilis: chancre of the fourchette.

31

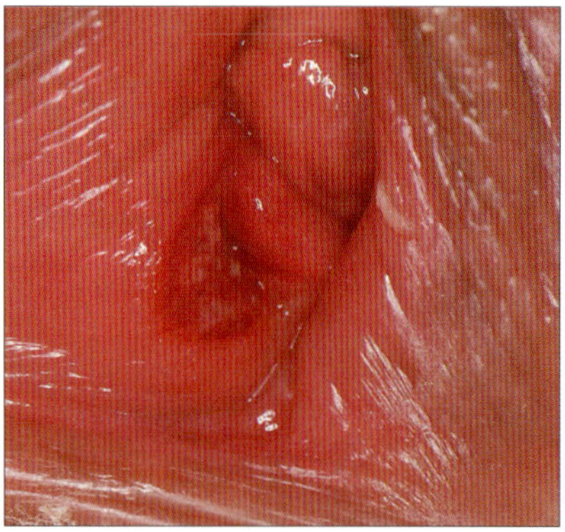

32

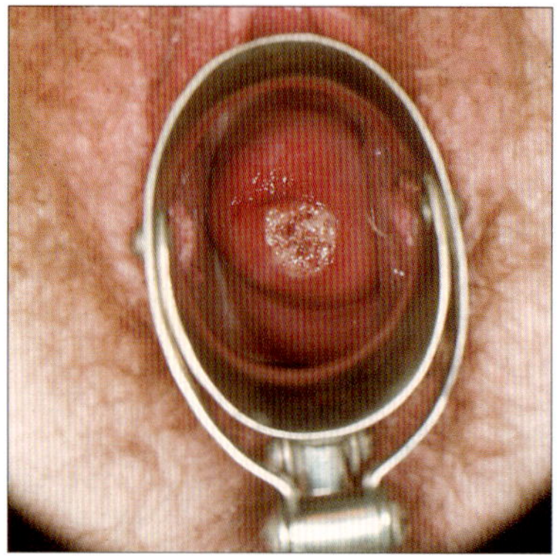

33

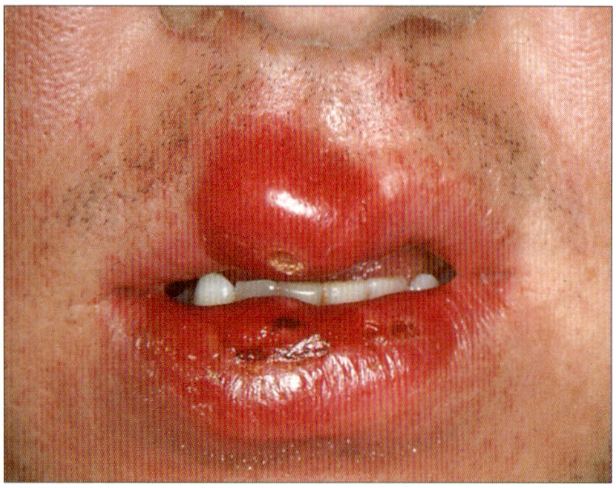

34

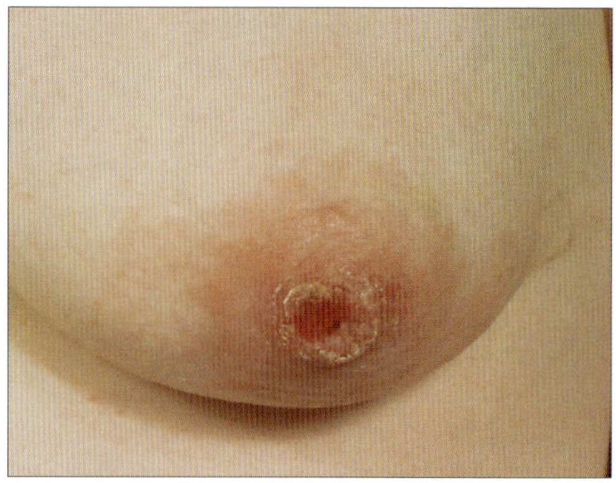

35

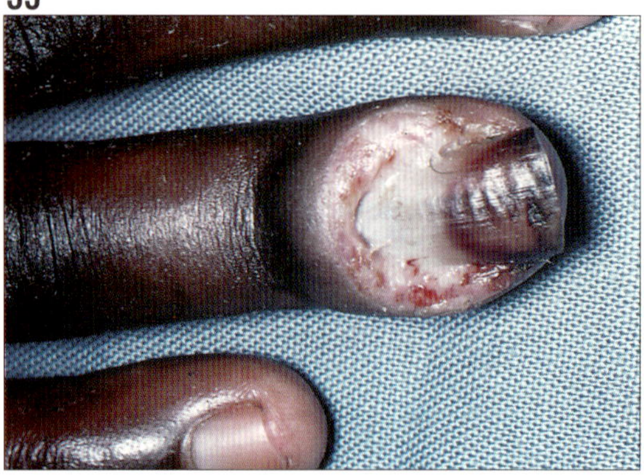

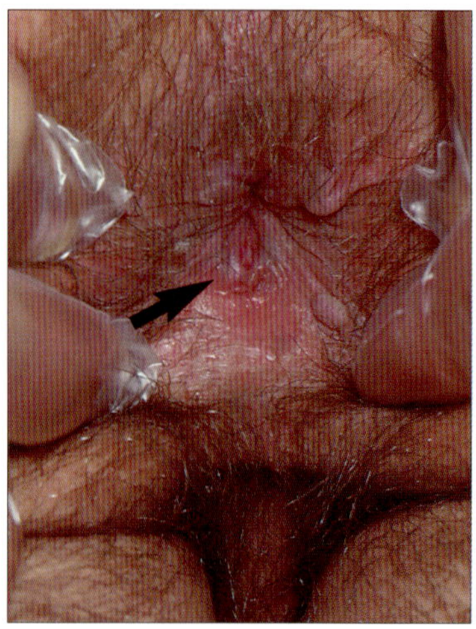

36

Plate 31. Primary syphilis: chancre of the vagina.
Plate 32. Primary syphilis: chancre of the cervix.
Plate 33. Primary syphilis: chancres of the lips (there is marked oedema and the lower lip lesion is scabbed).
Plate 34. Primary syphilis: chancre of the nipple.
Plate 35. Primary syphilis: digital chancre presenting as a non-suppurative whitlow.
Plate 36. Primary syphilis mixed with warts: anal chancre (arrowed) and perianal warts.

37

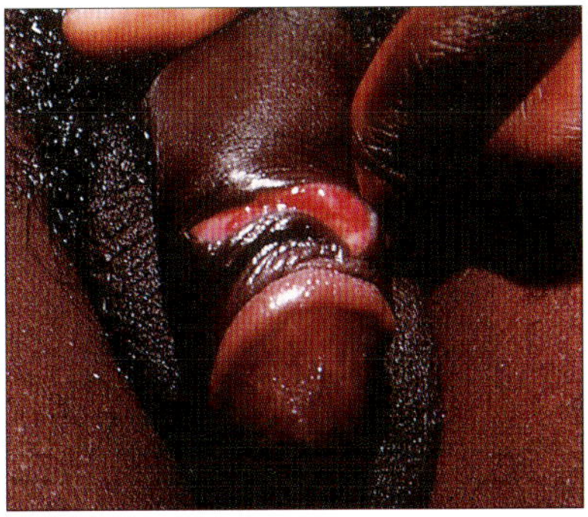

38

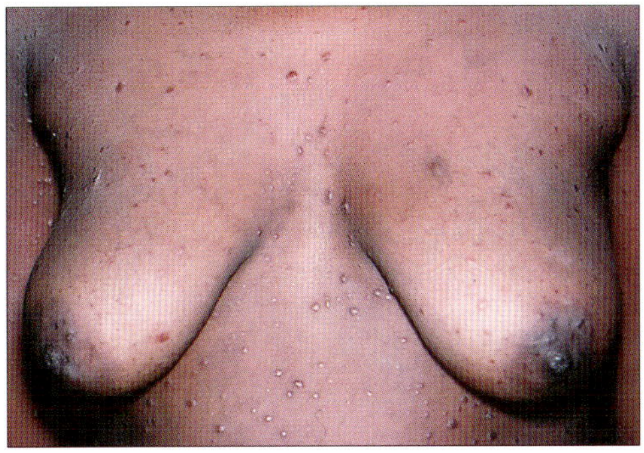

39

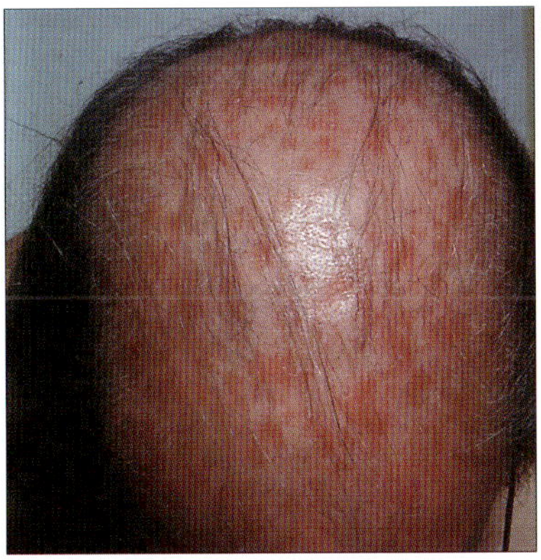

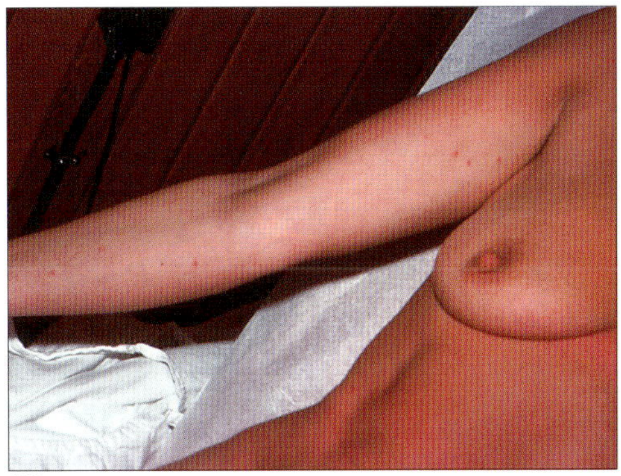

40

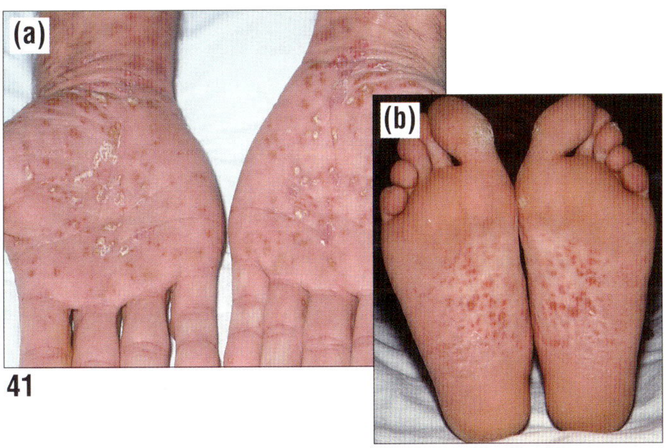

41

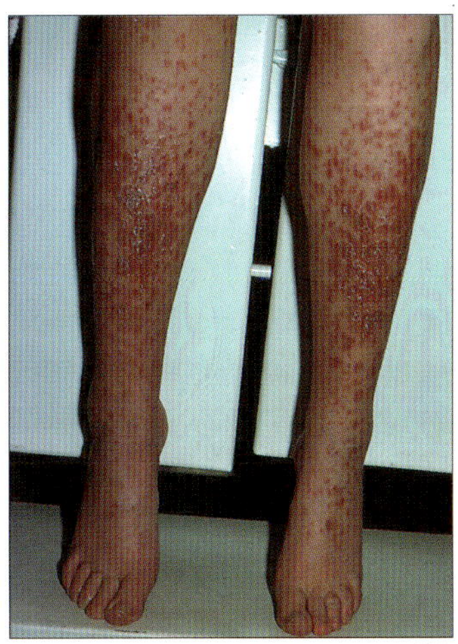

42

Plate 37. Genital trauma: traumatic ulcer of the penis (closely resembling Plate 22 (primary syphilis) and Plate 80 (chancroid)).
Plate 38. Secondary syphilis: profuse, symmetrical maculopapular rash of the trunk (the patient had a generalized rash covering the body).
Plate 39. Secondary syphilis: profuse papular rash of the scalp (this patient also had a generalized rash).
Plate 40. Secondary syphilis: generalized but scanty roseolar rash on the arm and trunk.
Plate 41. Secondary syphilis: lesions on (a) palms and (b) soles.
Plate 42. Secondary syphilis: psoriasiform syphilide.

43

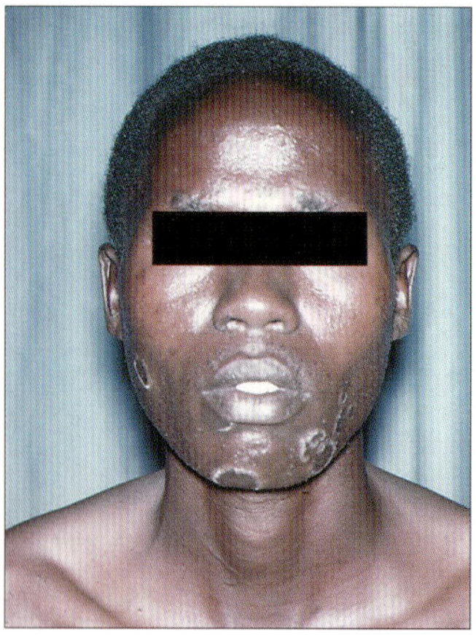

44

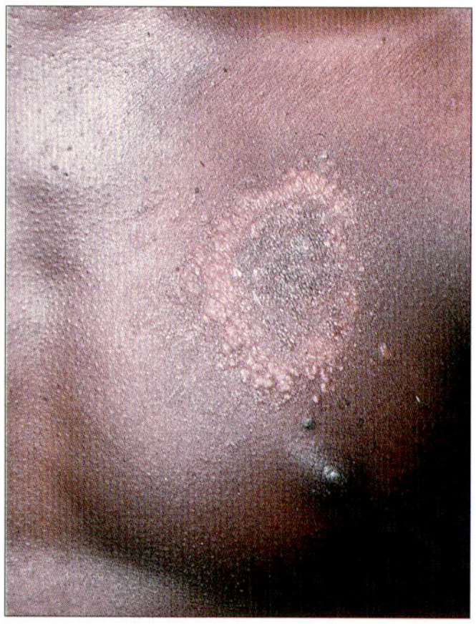

45

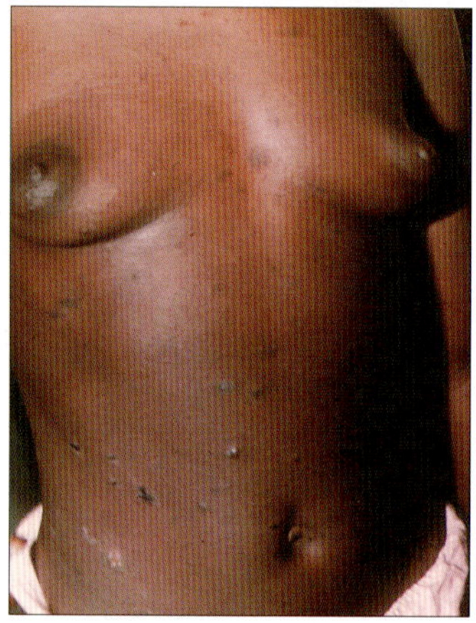

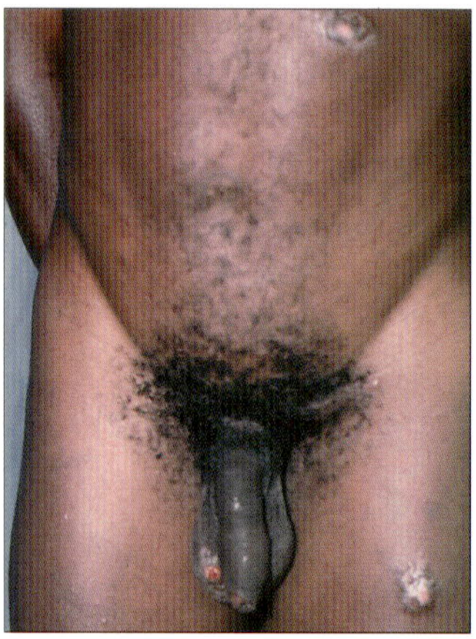

46

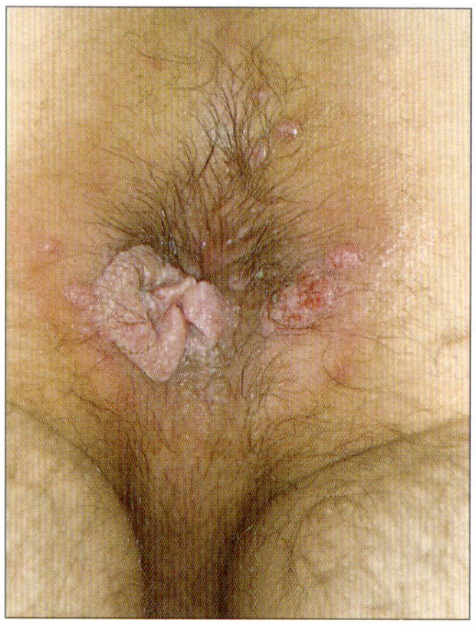

47

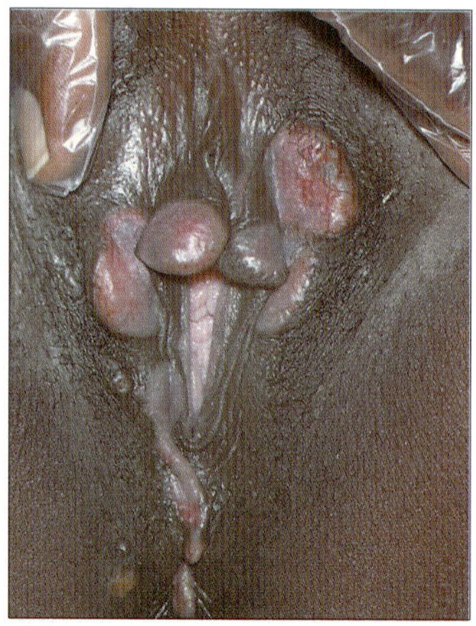

48

Plate 43. Secondary syphilis: annular lesions on the face.
Plate 44. Secondary syphilis: corymbose syphilide.
Plate 45. Secondary syphilis: sparse acneiform rash.
Plate 46. Secondary syphilis: rupial syphilide.
Plate 47. Secondary syphilis: perianal condylomata lata.
Plate 48. Secondary syphilis: vulvar condylomata lata (same patient as in Plate 50).

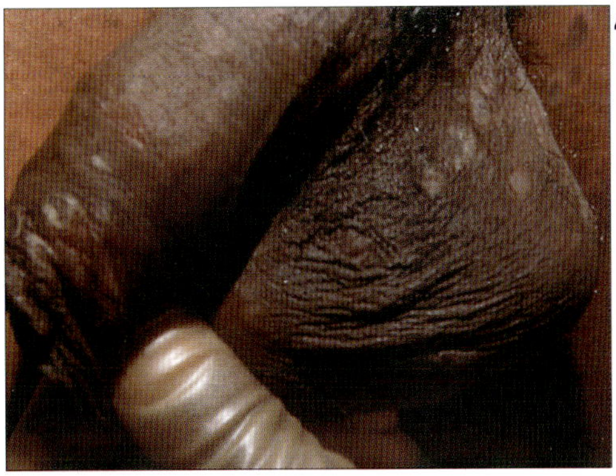
49

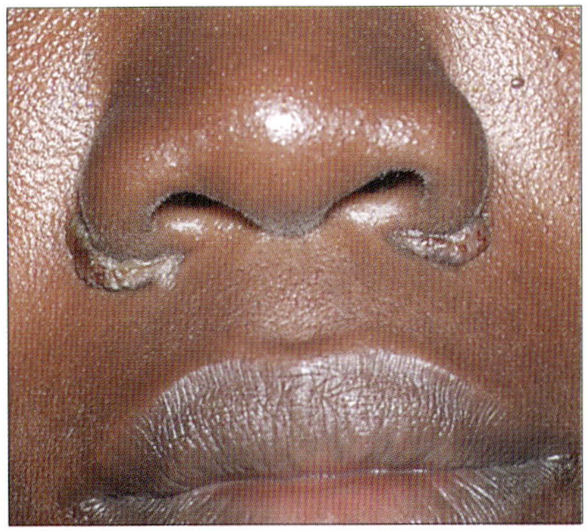
50

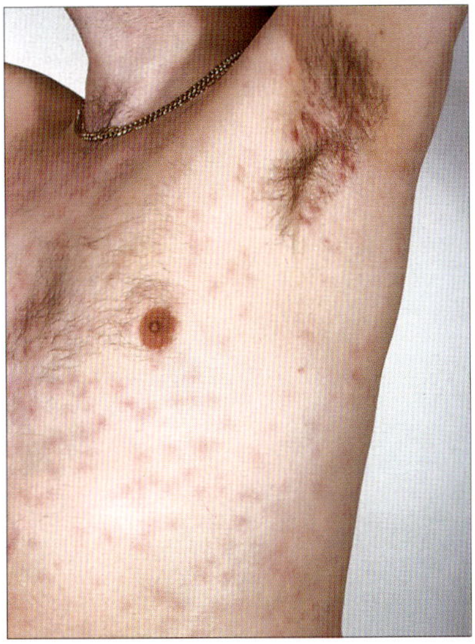
51

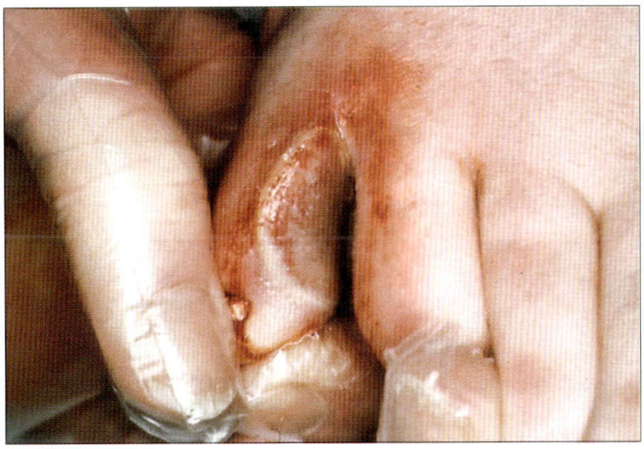
52

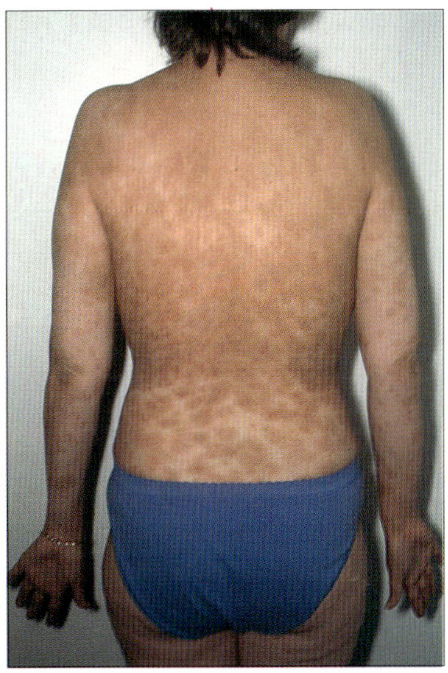
54

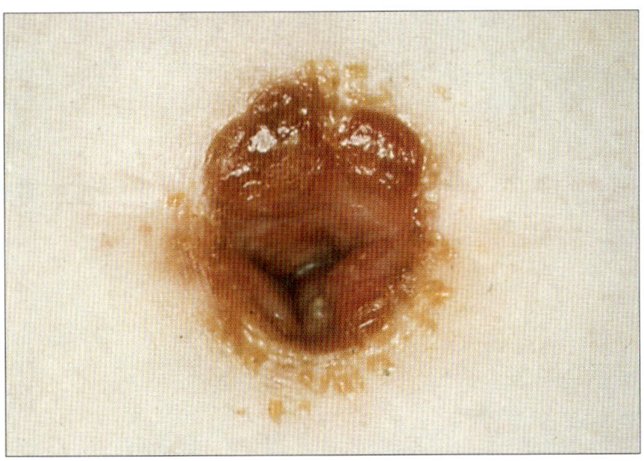
53

Plate 49. Secondary syphilis: condylomata lata on scrotum.
Plate 50. Secondary syphilis: nasolabial condylomata lata (same patient as in Plate 48).
Plate 51. Secondary syphilis: condylomata lata of axilla and generalized rash of the trunk.
Plate 52. Secondary syphilis: condylomata lata between the toes.
Plate 53. Secondary syphilis: condylomata lata of umbilicus.
Plate 54. Secondary syphilis: post-treatment hyperpigmentation following the resolution of skin lesions.

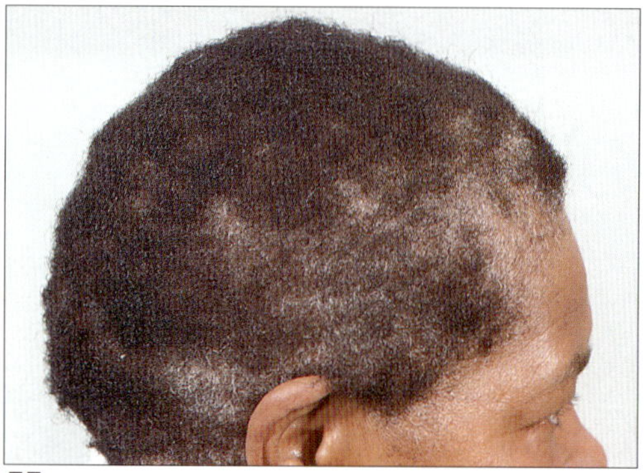

55

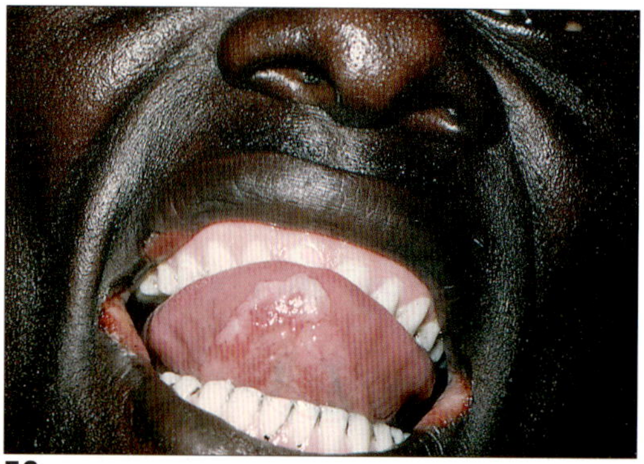

56

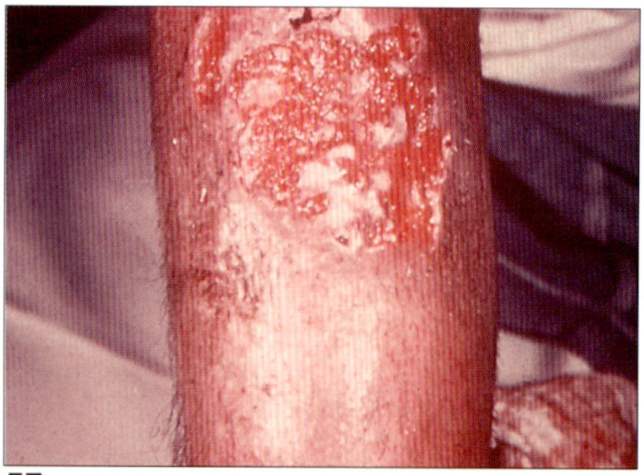

57

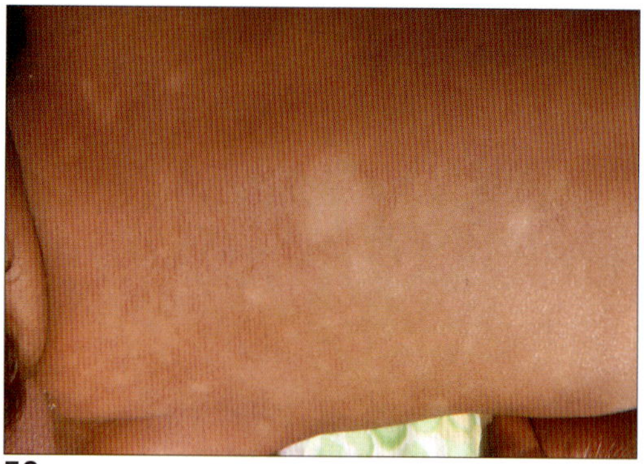

58

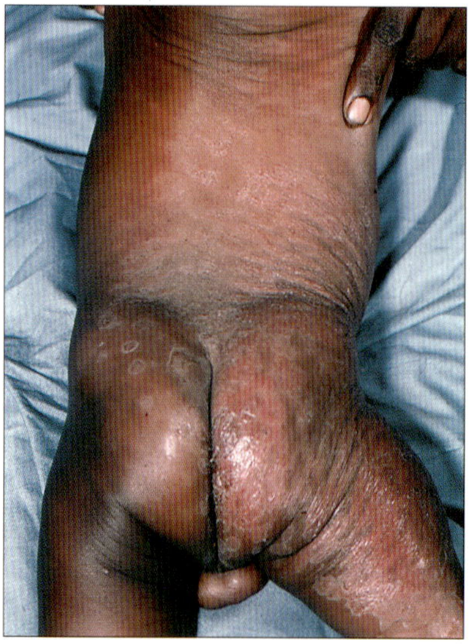

59

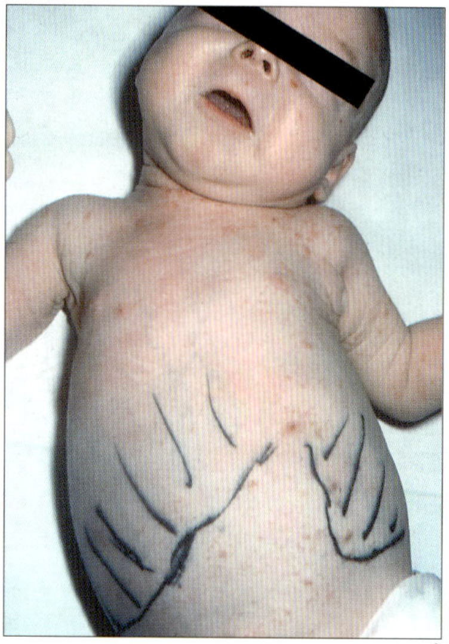

60

Plate 55. Secondary syphilis: alopecia.
Plate 56. Secondary syphilis: mucous patch under the tongue.
Plate 57. Benign late syphilis: nodulo-ulcerative lesion of the leg.
Plate 58. Early congenital syphilis: generalized macular rash.
Plate 59. Early congenital syphilis: generalized papulo-squamous rash.
Plate 60. Early congenital syphilis: generalized rash and hepatosplenomegaly. (Courtesy of Dr D.C. Davidson.)

61

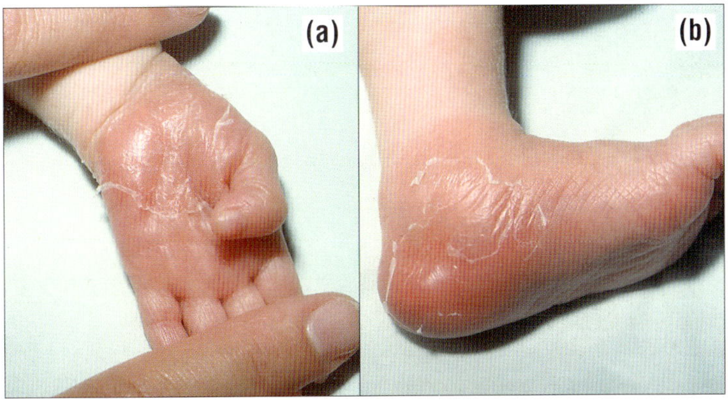

62

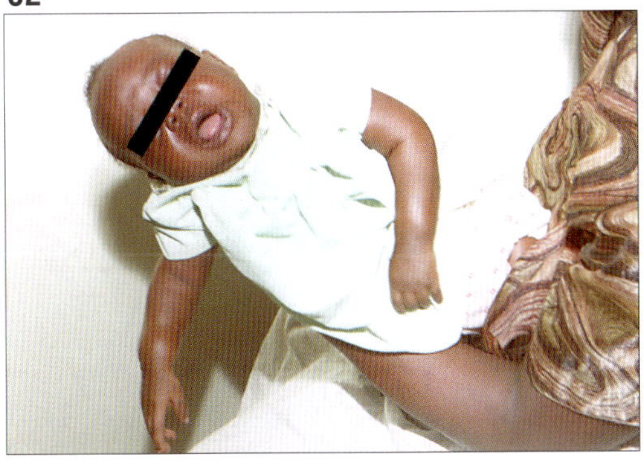

63

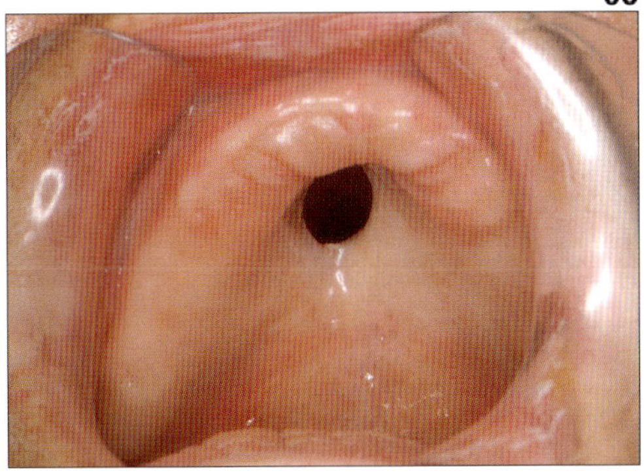

64

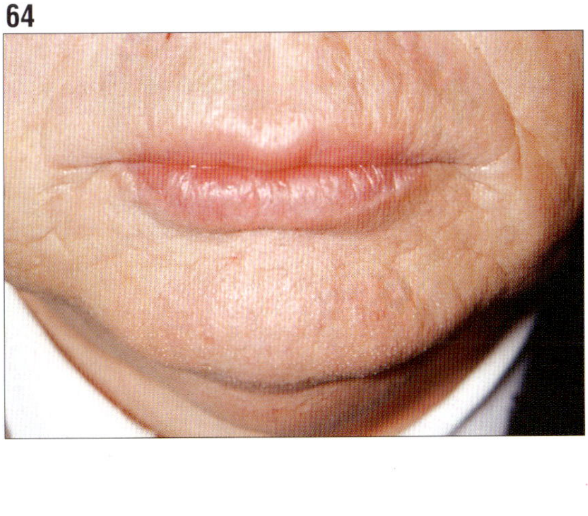

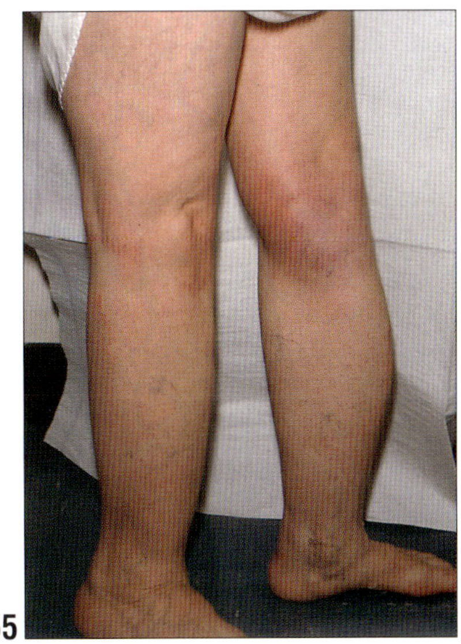

65

Plate 61. Early congenital syphilis: desquamating erythema of (a) palms and (b) soles.

Plate 62. Early congenital syphilis: swellings of the lower ends of forearm bones due to osteochondritis.

Plate 63. Late congenital syphilis: perforation of the hard palate.

Plate 64. Congenital syphilis: radiating scars at the corners of the mouth (rhagades) subsequent to healing of the early lesions.

Plate 65. Late congenital syphilis: anterior bowing of the leg due to 'sabre' tibia.

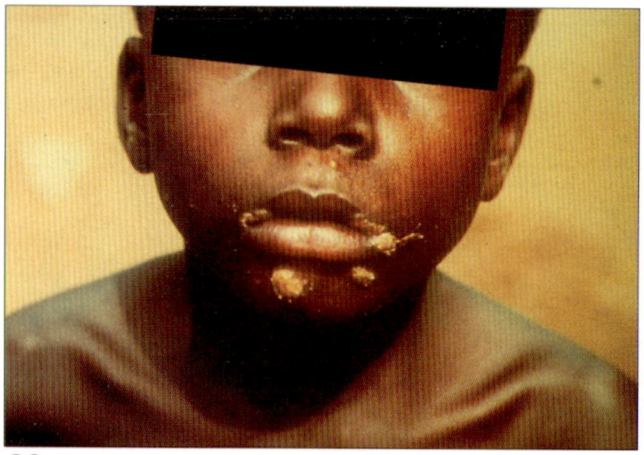

66

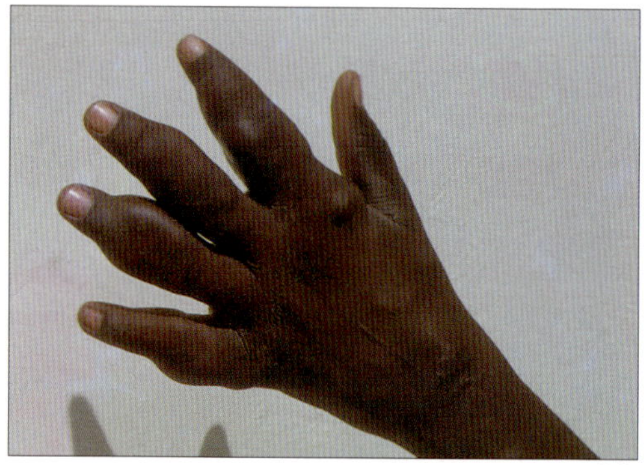

69

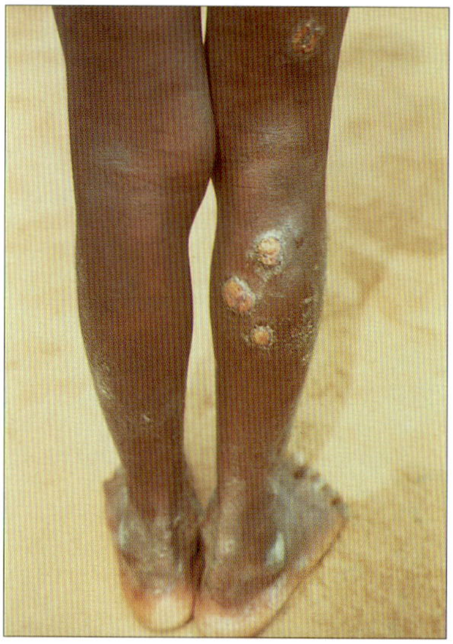

67

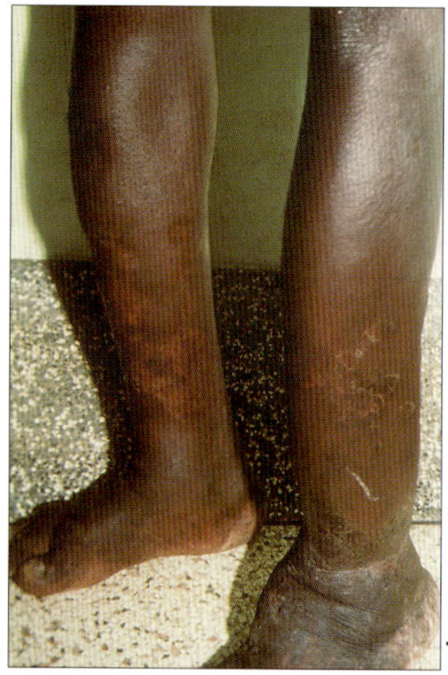

70

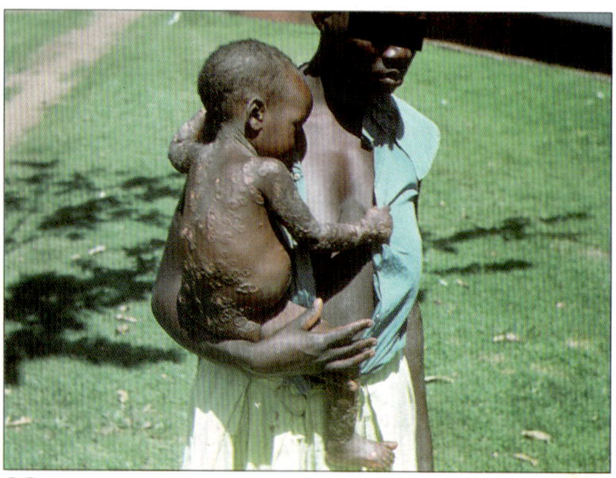

68

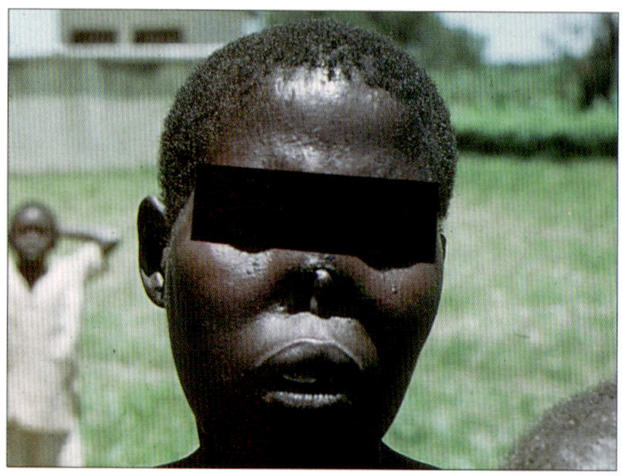

71

Plate 66. Early yaws: mucocutaneous and papillomatous lesions on the face. (Courtesy of Dr P. Perine.)

Plate 67. Early yaws: ulceropapillomatous lesions on the leg. (Courtesy of WHO, Geneva.)

Plate 68. Early yaws: disseminated secondary lesions.

Plate 69. Early yaws: polydactylitis.

Plate 70. Yaws: anterior bowing of the leg due to osteoperiostitis of the tibia ('sabre' tibia).

Plate 71. Yaws (early or late): goundou.

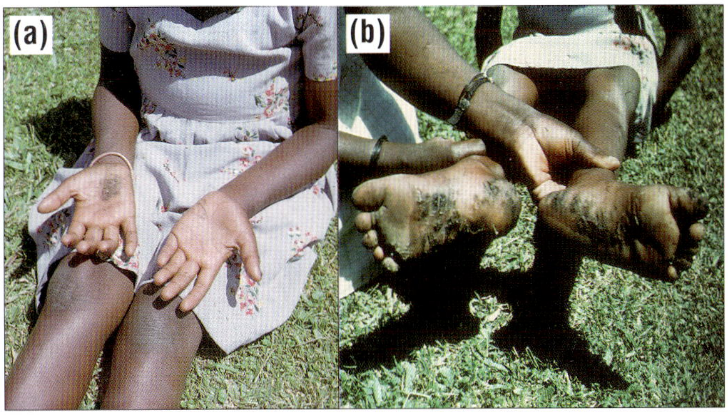

72

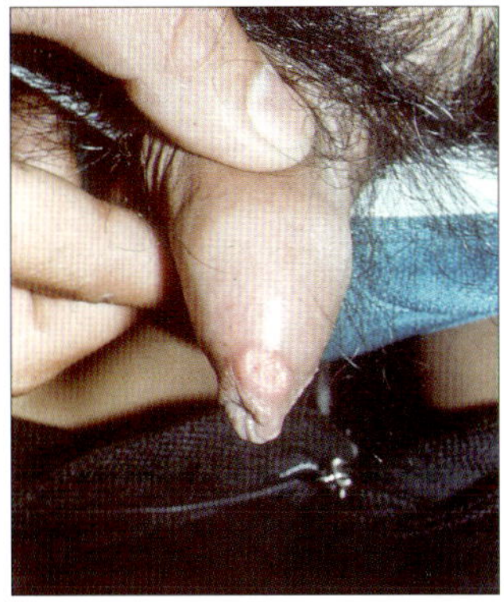
73

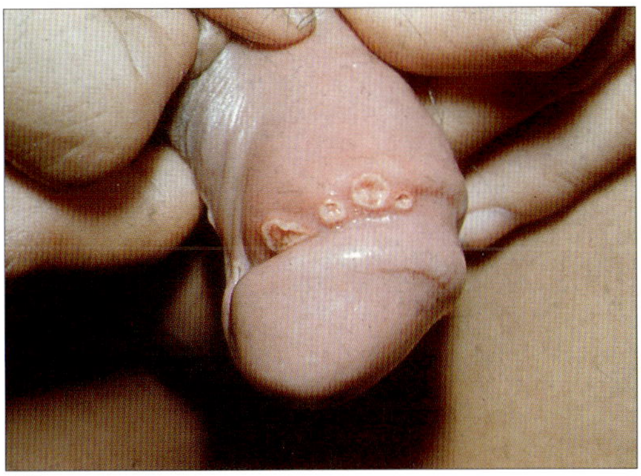
74

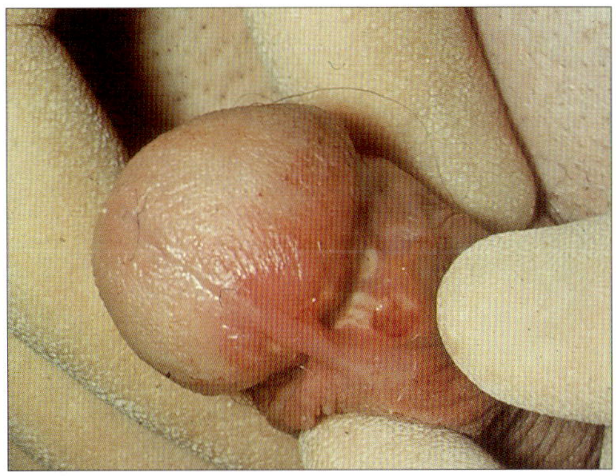
75

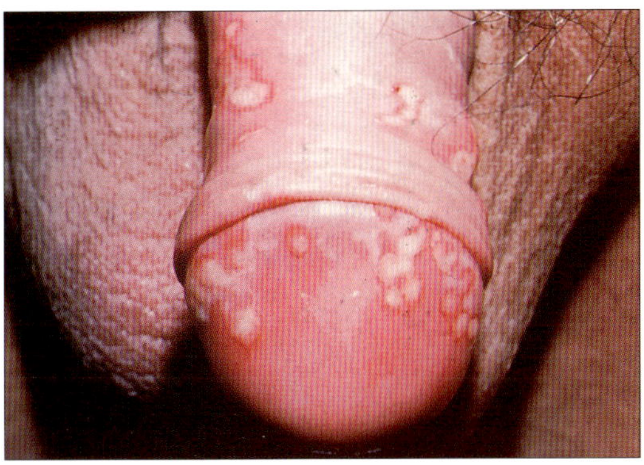
76

77
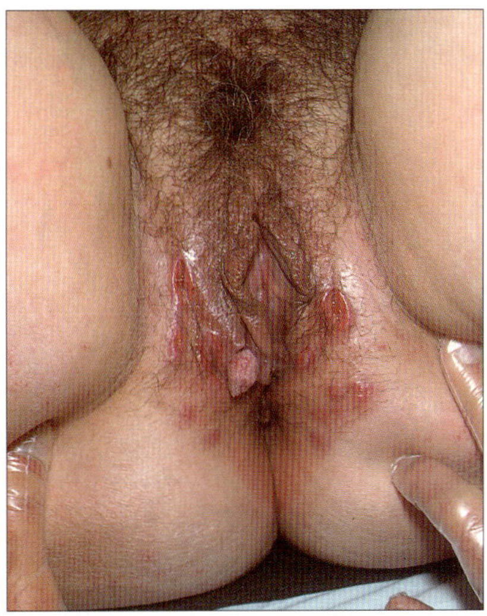

Plate 72. Yaws: (a) palmar and (b) plantar hyperkeratosis in the same patient.
Plate 73. Chancroid: a single well-defined lesion of the prepuce. (Courtesy of the late Dr V.S. Rajan.) This lesion cannot be differentiated clinically from syphilitic chancre.
Plate 74. Chancroid: multiple ulcers at coronal sulcus. Note undermined ragged edges.
Plate 75. Chancroid: lesions of the fraenum.
Plate 76. Chancroid: multiple superficial ulcers of the glans penis and shaft. These lesions are impossible to differentiate clinically from genital herpes.
Plate 77. Chancroid (mixed with warts): multiple ulcers and warts on the vulva.

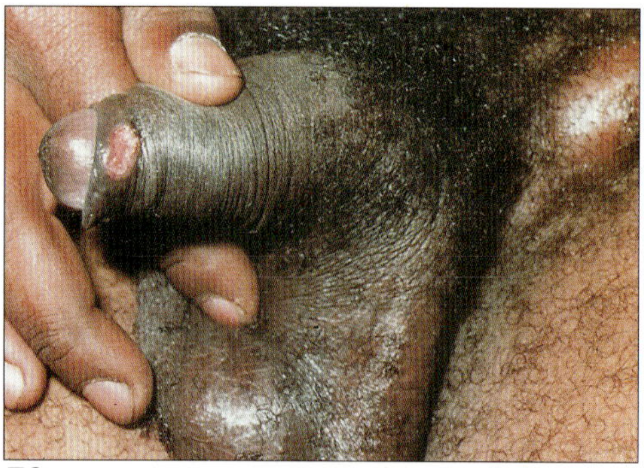

78

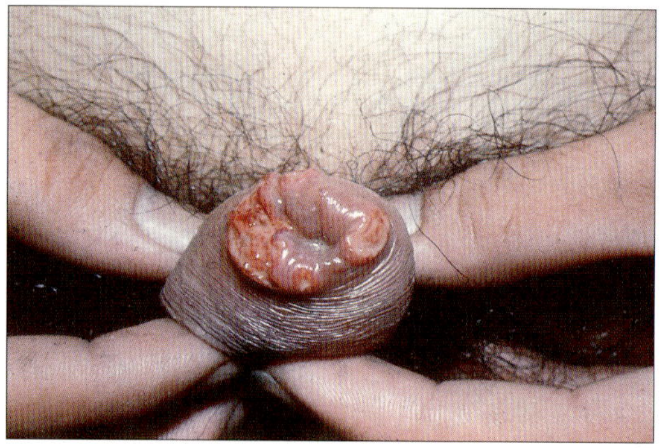

79

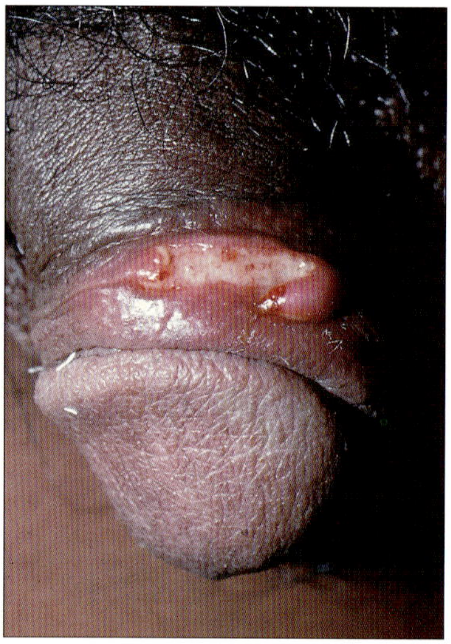

80

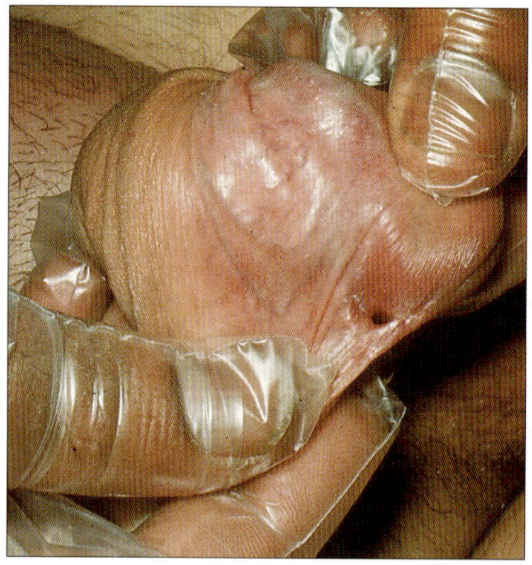

81

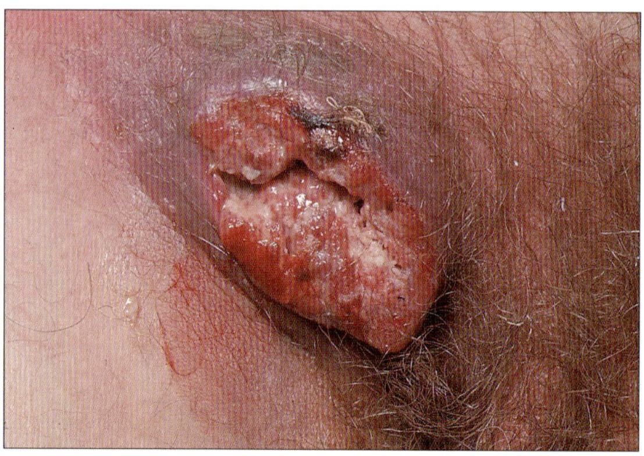

82

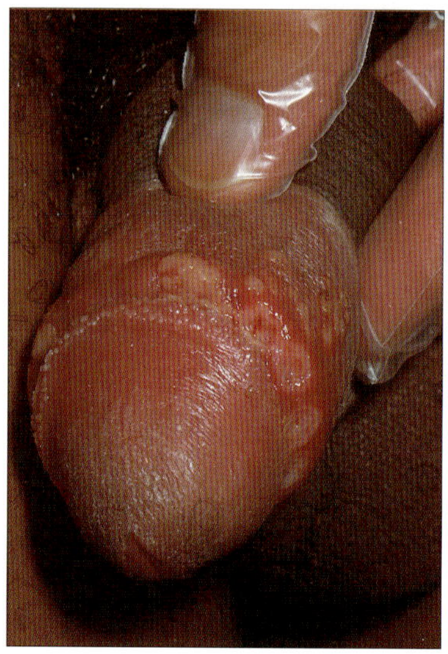

83

Plate 78. Chancroid: ulcer on the penis, and bubo.
Plate 79. Chancroid: phagedenic ulcers at preputial opening.
Plate 80. Chancroid: phagedenic, oedematous ulcer of the prepuce. Note the resemblance with Plate 22 of ulcerated chancre and Plate 37 of traumatic ulcer.
Plate 81. Chancroid: fraenal perforation as a sequel to resolution of the lesions shown in Plate 75.
Plate 82. Chancroid: ulcerated bubo.
Plate 83. Chancroid (mixed with herpes): multiple ulcers and vesicles on coronal sulcus and prepuce.

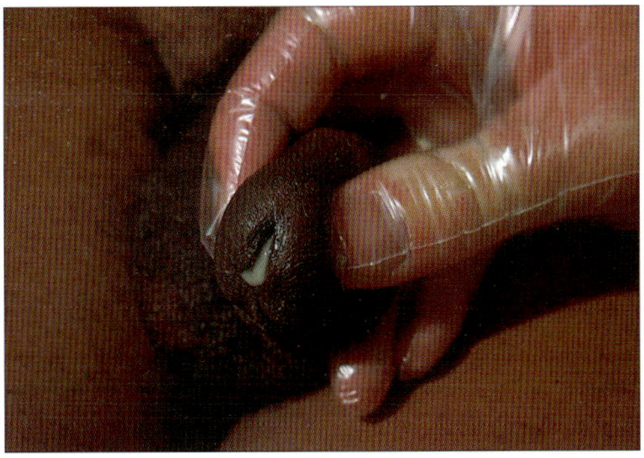

84

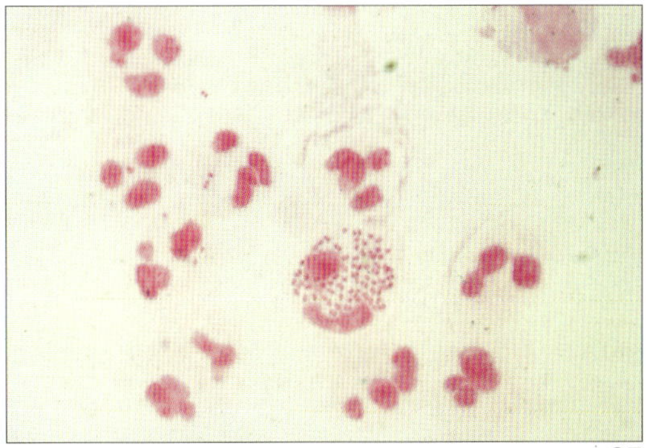

85

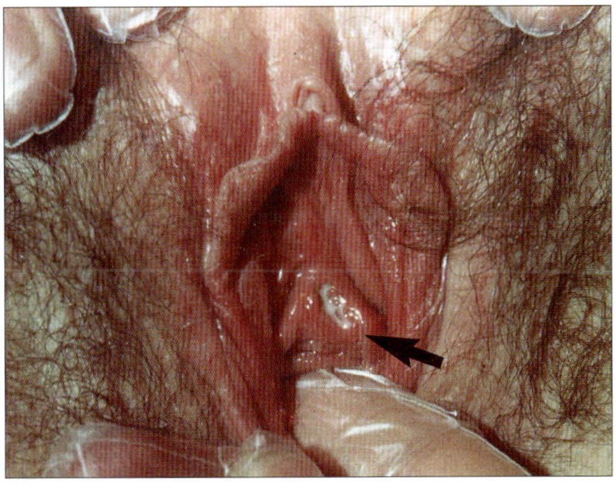

86

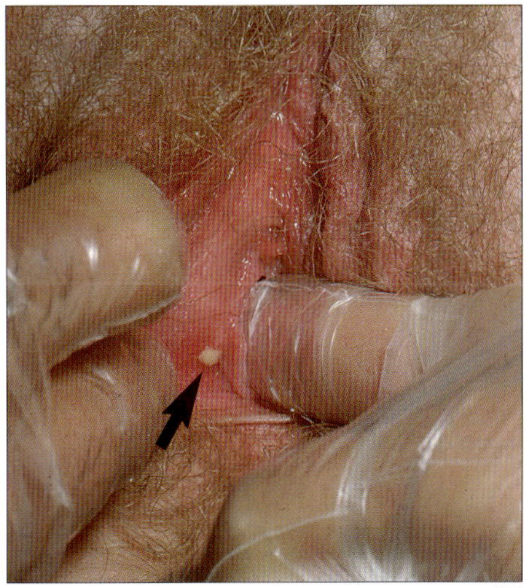

87

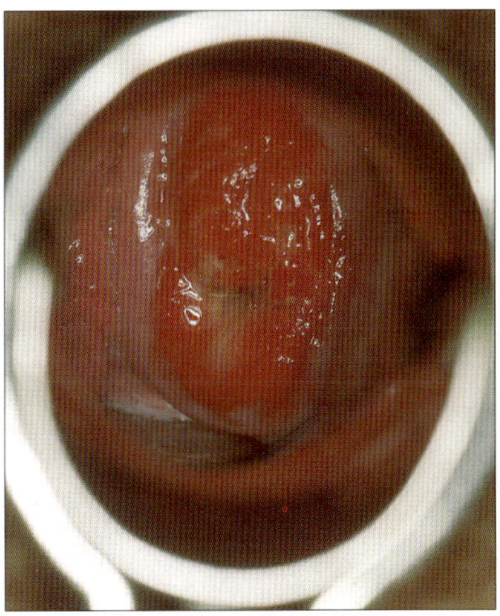

88

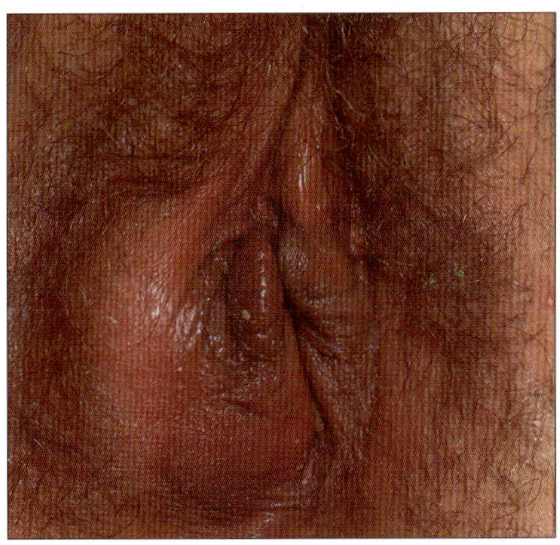

89

Plate 84. Gonorrhoea: purulent urethral discharge in male.

Plate 85. Gonorrhoea: Gram-stained smear of urethral exudate from a man with gonorrhoea, showing polymorphonuclear leukocytes and Gram-negative intracellular diplococci.

Plate 86. Gonorrhoea: mucopurulent urethral discharge in female.

Plate 87. Gonorrhoea: a bead of pus at the duct opening of the right Bartholin's gland.

Plate 88. Gonorrhoea (mixed with chlamydial infection): note oedematous cervical ectopy and scanty, thin mucopurulent discharge exuding from the cervix.

Plate 89. Gonorrhoea: Bartholin's gland abscess.

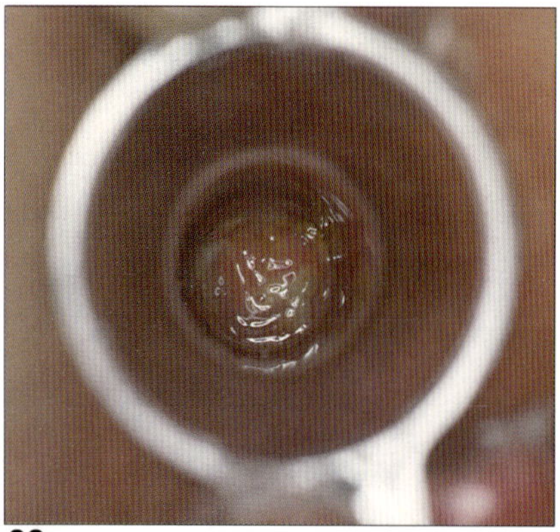

90

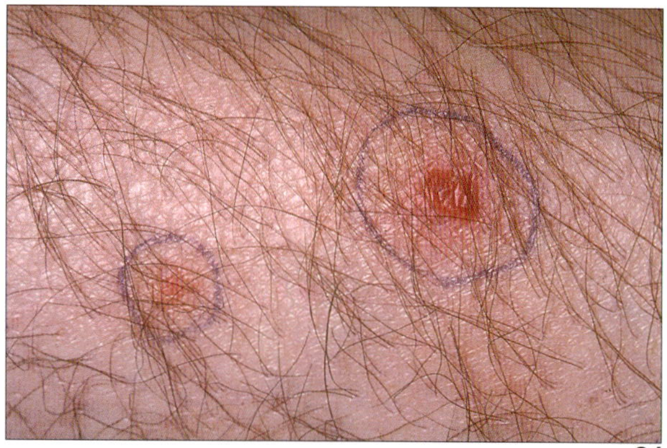

91

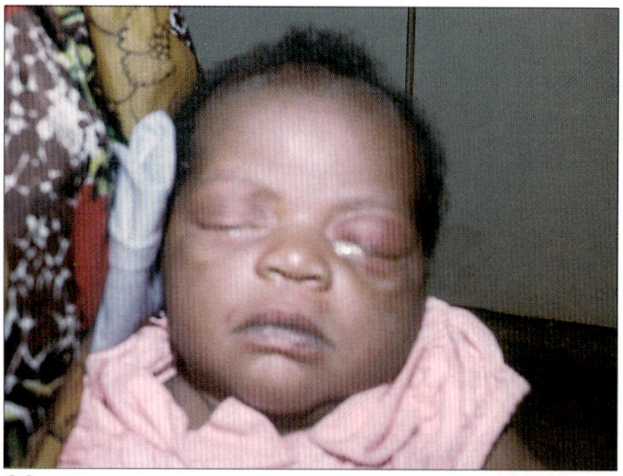

92

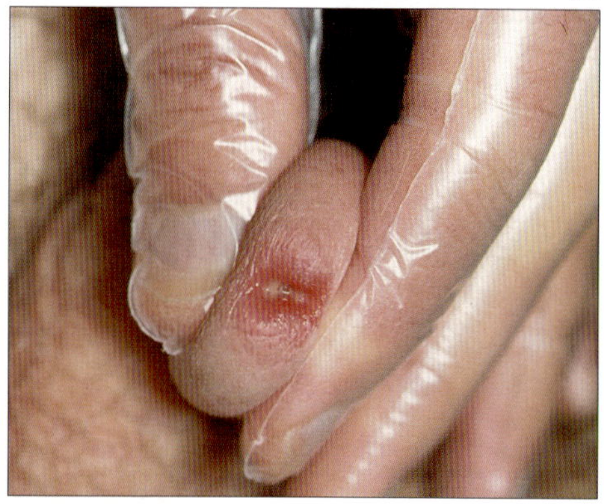

93

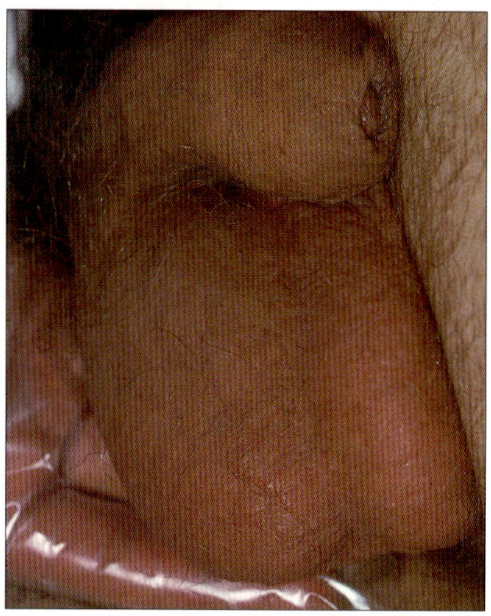

94

Plate 90. Gonorrhoea: mucopurulent exudate on rectal mucosa.

Plate 91. Disseminated gonorrhoea: skin lesions of the leg.

Plate 92. Gonococcal ophthalmia neonatorum: note purulent exudate and oedema of the lids.

Plate 93. Non-gonococcal urethritis: scanty mucopurulent urethral discharge in a male patient which was demonstrated only by massaging the urethra after the patient had held urine for over 4 h. Note also meatal erythema. Within 2 weeks the patient developed Reiter's syndrome (see Plate 99).

Plate 94. Epididymoorchitis: the young man presented with a painful right-sided scrotal swelling. *C. trachomatis* and *U. urealyticum* (the significance of the latter is uncertain) were isolated from his urethral swabs.

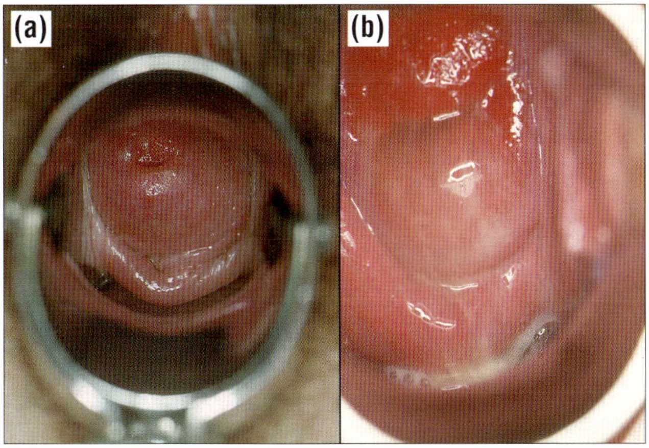

95

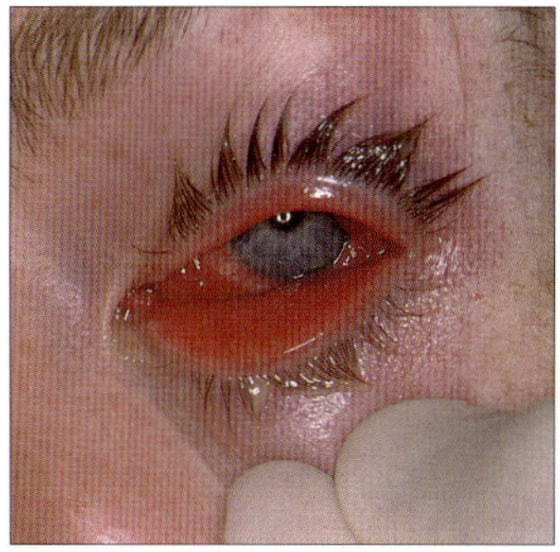

96

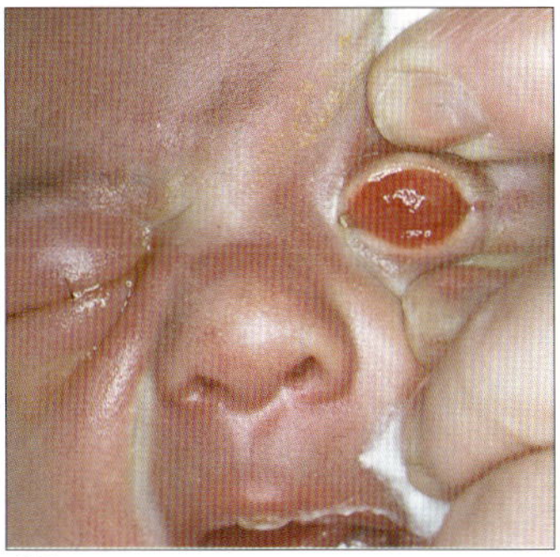

97

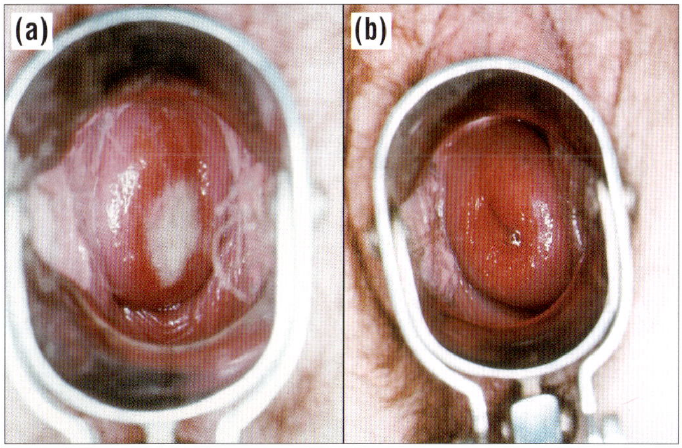

98

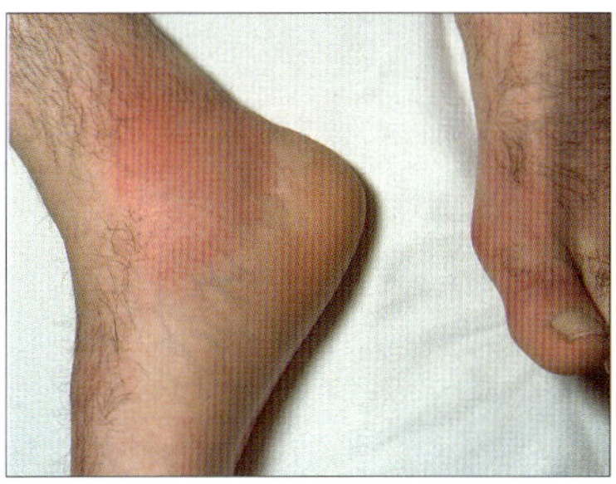

99

Plate 95. Chlamydial infection of the cervix. (a) Macroscopically normal cervix; (b) macroscopic cervicitis. Note oedema and congestion of the cervix, and a thin mucopurulent discharge cascading from the cervix.

Plate 96. Chlamydial conjunctivitis in an adult male. The patient first presented at an eye clinic; he did not have urethritis and urethral swab for chlamydia was negative. His asymptomatic female partner was subsequently found to have chlamydial infection of the cervix.

Plate 97. Chlamydial ophthalmia neonatorum. Note oedema of the lids, conjunctivitis and scanty mucopurulent discharge. (Courtesy of Dr E. Rees.)

Plate 98. Chlamydial infection of the cervix. Mucopurulent cervicitis (a) before treatment and (b) 6 weeks after treatment with tetracycline. (Courtesy of Dr E. Rees.)

Plate 99. Reiter's syndrome: arthritis of the ankle and metatarsophalangeal joint of the big toe (same patient as Plate 93).

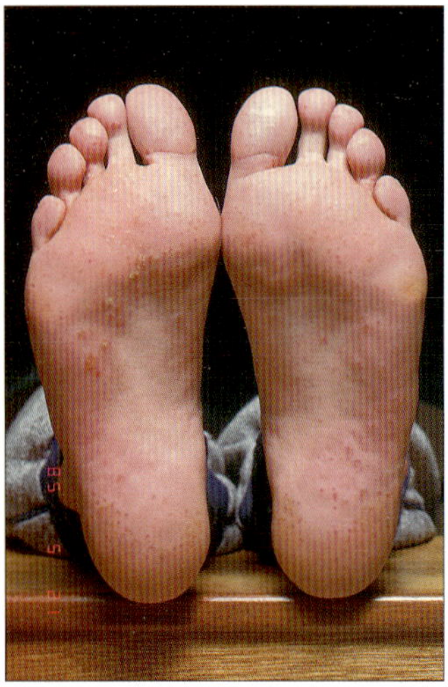

100

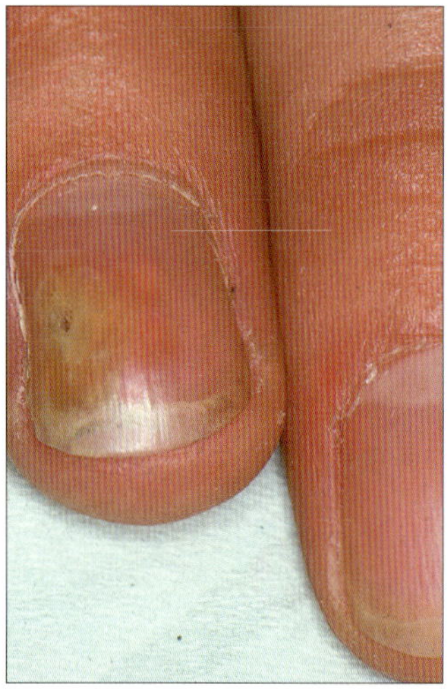

101

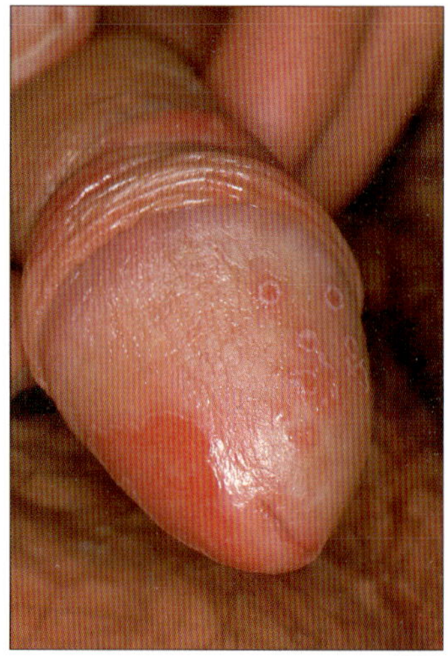

102

103

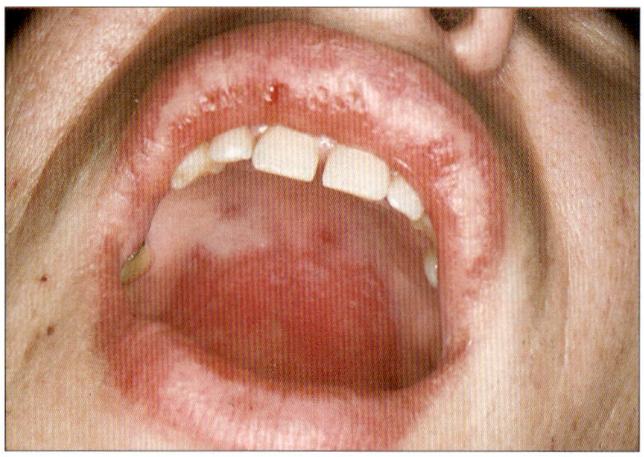

104

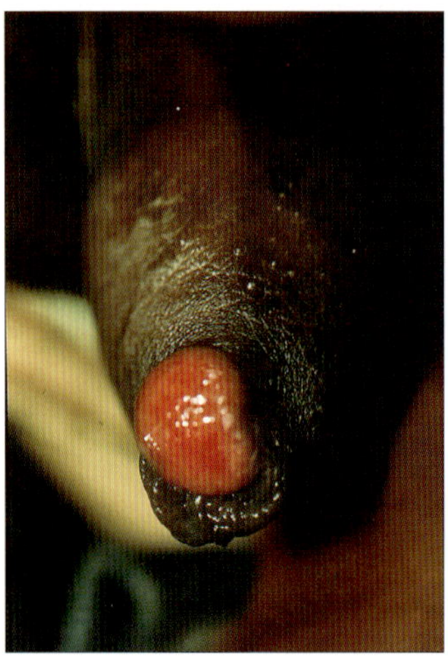

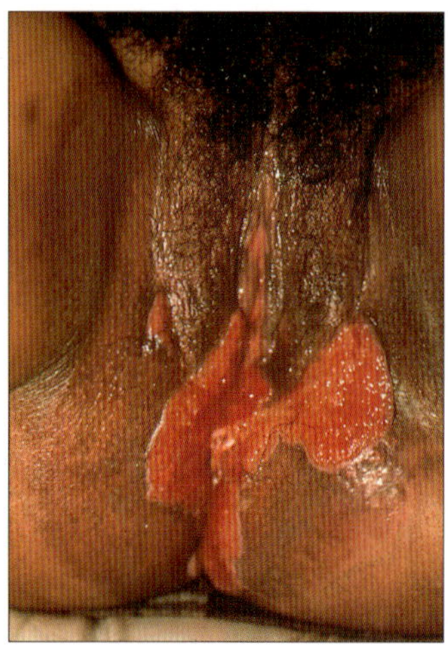

105

Plate 100. Reiter's syndrome: keratodermia blenorrhagica.
Plate 101. Reiter's syndrome: lesion of the nail.
Plate 102. Reiter's syndrome: balanitis circinata (same patient as in Plate 101).
Plate 103. Reiter's syndrome: lesions on the palate.
Plate 104. Donovanosis: early hypertrophic-type lesion of the penis.
Plate 105. Donovanosis: advanced lesion of the vulva displaying serpiginous outline. This patient was the sexual partner of the male illustrated in Plate 104.

106

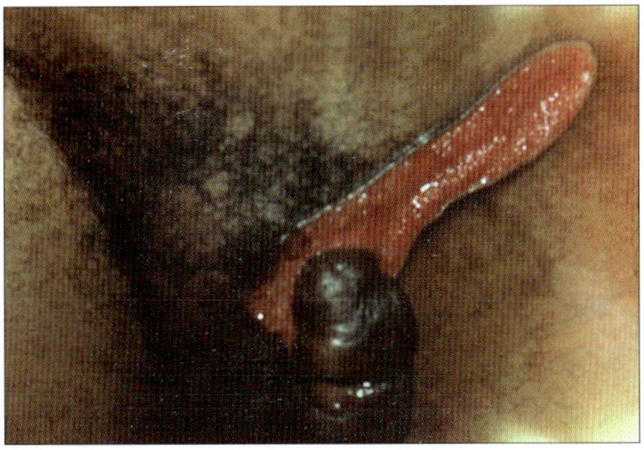

107

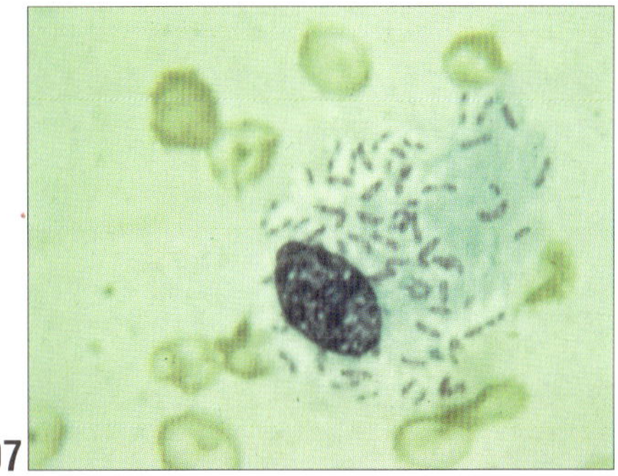

108

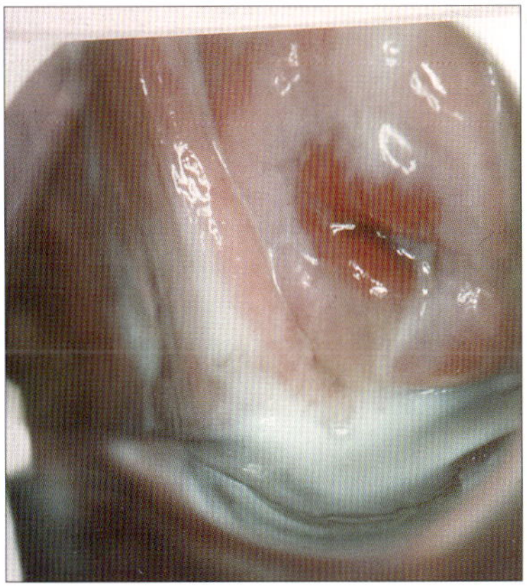

109

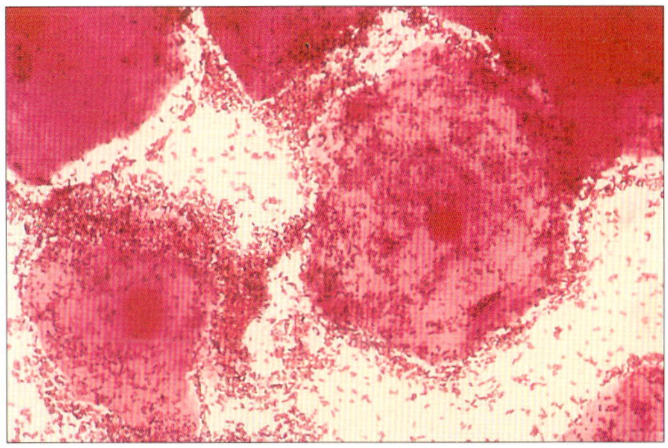

110

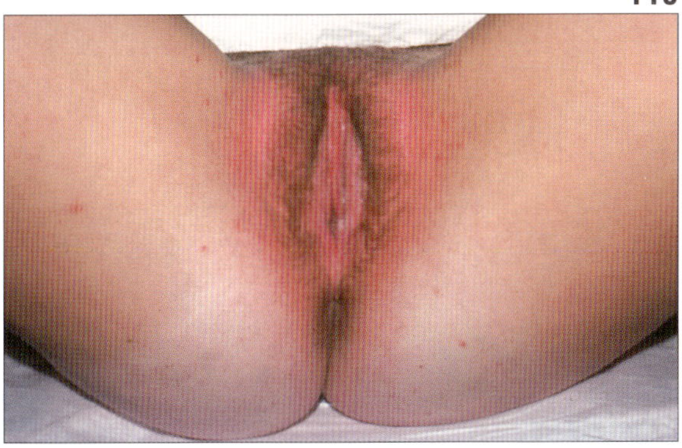

111

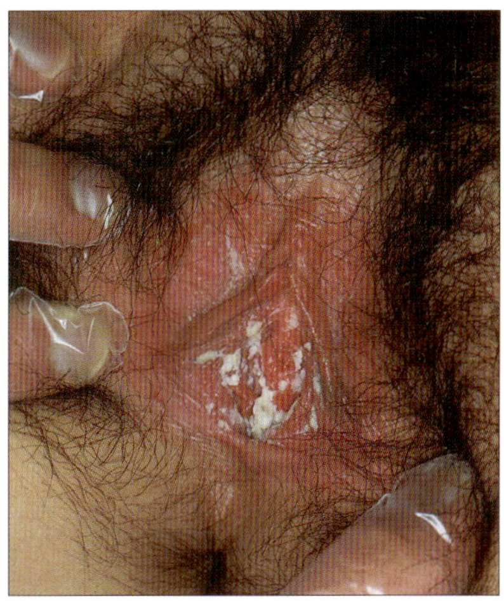

Plate 106. Donovanosis: extensive inguinal ulceration (hence the term 'granuloma inguinale' for this disease) encircling the base of the penis. The lesion, if left unchecked, may result in penile autoamputation.

Plate 107. Donovanosis: crush preparation from a genital ulcer showing Donovan bodies in a mononuclear cell (Giemsa, ×1000).

Plate 108. Bacterial vaginosis: note greyish-white homogeneous discharge. The patient experienced recurrent episodes.

Plate 109. Bacterial vaginosis: Gram-stained smear of vaginal specimen from the patient in Plate 108 showing two clue cells, absence of lactobacilli and a large number of Gram-negative/Gram-variable coccobacilli.

Plate 110. Candidiasis: severe vulvitis – note dry congestion of the vulva. This patient had been using oral contraceptive and taking tetracycline for acne vulgaris for 4 months.

Plate 111. Candidiasis: severe vulvovaginitis with curd-like or cheesy exudate.

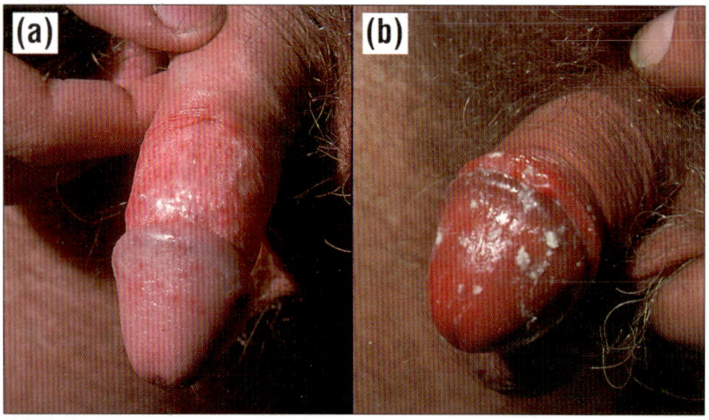

112

113

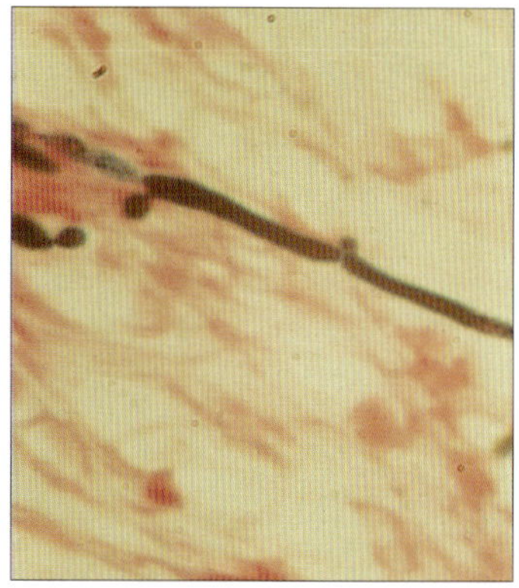

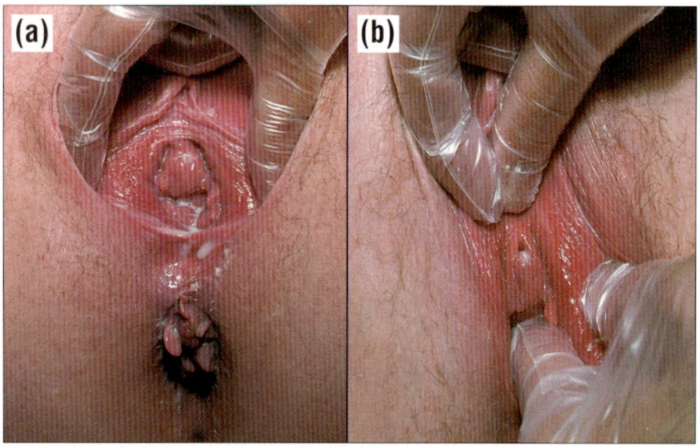

114

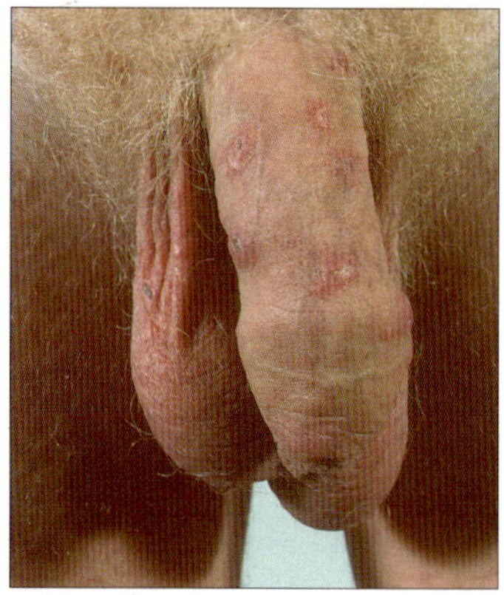

116

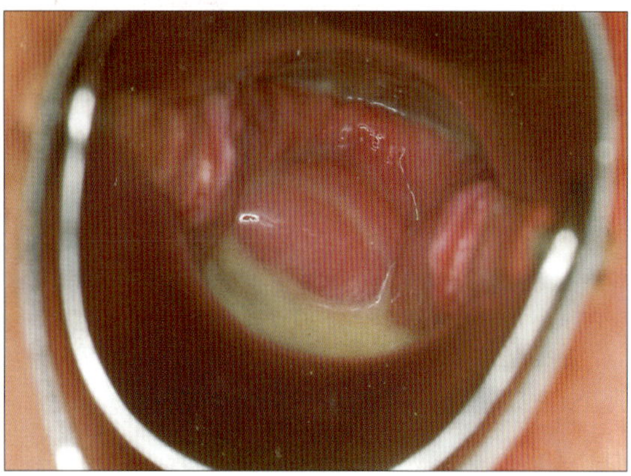

115

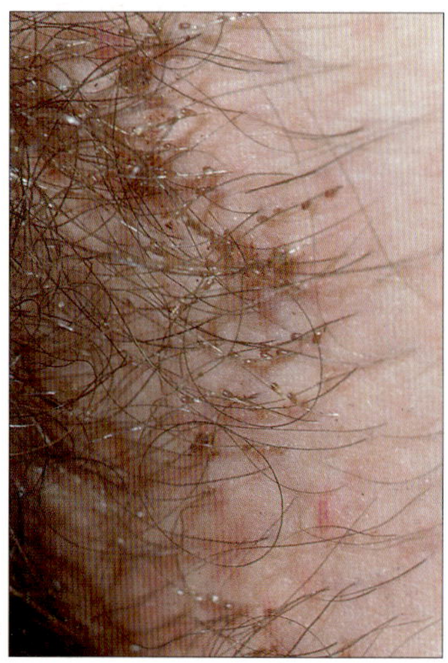

117

Plate 112. Candidiasis. (a) Micropapular balanitis; (b) severe balanoposthitis in a patient with undiagnosed diabetes mellitus.

Plate 113. *Candida albicans*: pseudohyphae and yeast-like spores in a Gram-stained vaginal smear.

Plate 114. Trichomoniasis. (a) Vaginal discharge running out on to the vulva; (b) urethral discharge in the same patient.

Plate 115. Trichomoniasis: copious purulent discharge in the vagina.

Plate 116. Scabies.

Plate 117. Pubic lice and nits.

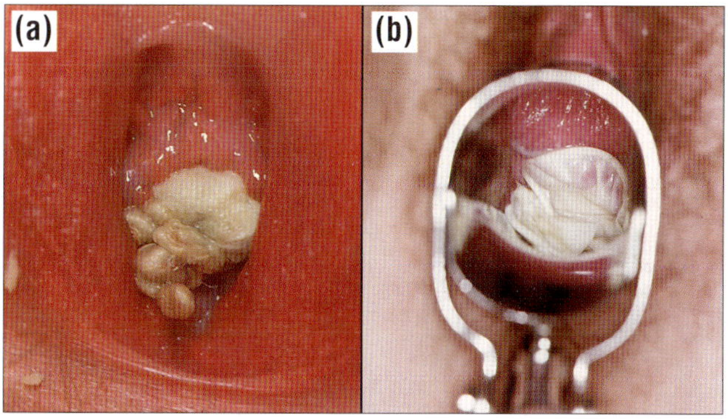

118

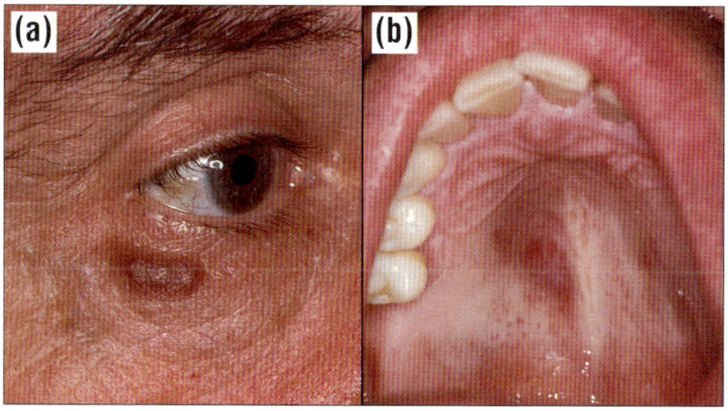

119

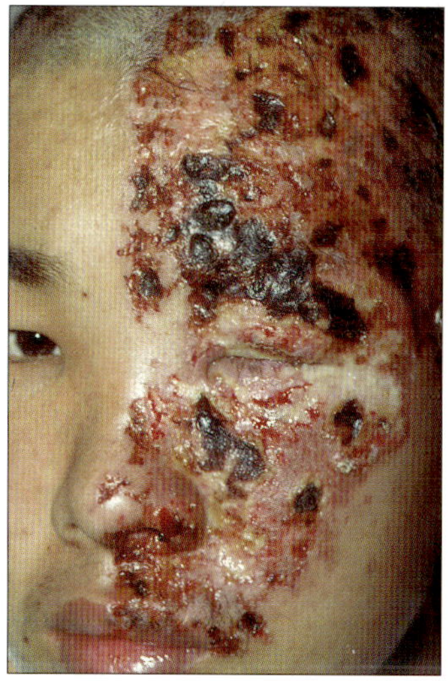

121

120

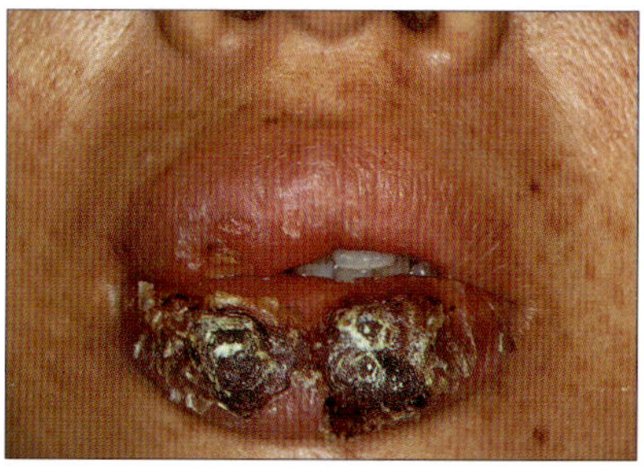

122

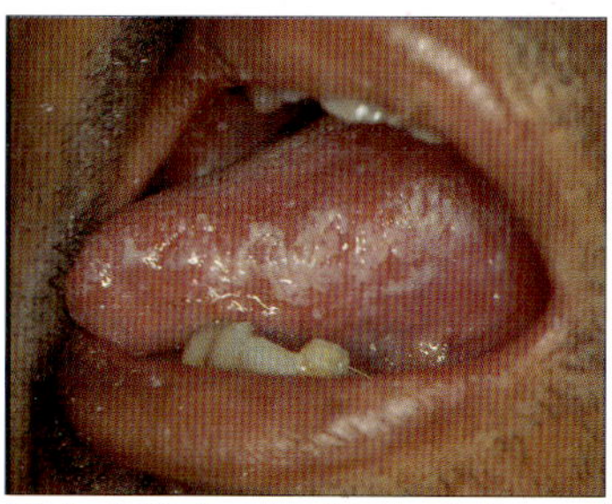

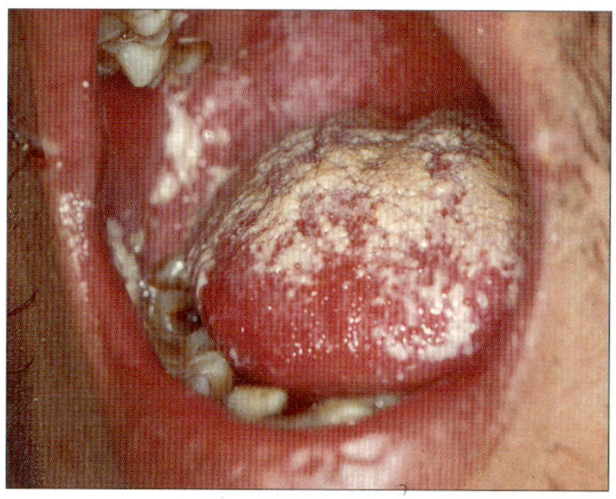

123

Plate 118. Foreign bodies in the vagina. (a) A retained tampon, and (b) a condom. Both these patients presented with smelly vaginal discharge.

Plate 119. Kaposi's sarcoma in a patient with AIDS. Purplish lesions of (a) the face, and (b) the palate.

Plate 120. Persistent necrotic ulceration due to herpes simplex virus infection in an HIV-infected patient.

Plate 121. Necrotizing ulceration of herpes zoster involving ophthalmic and maxillary branches of the trigeminal nerve in a patient with HIV infection.

Plate 122. Oral hairy leukoplakia.

Plate 123. Oral candidiasis in a patient with HIV infection.

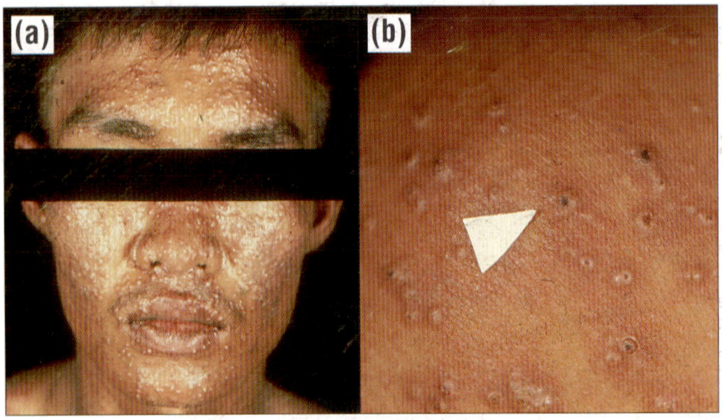

124

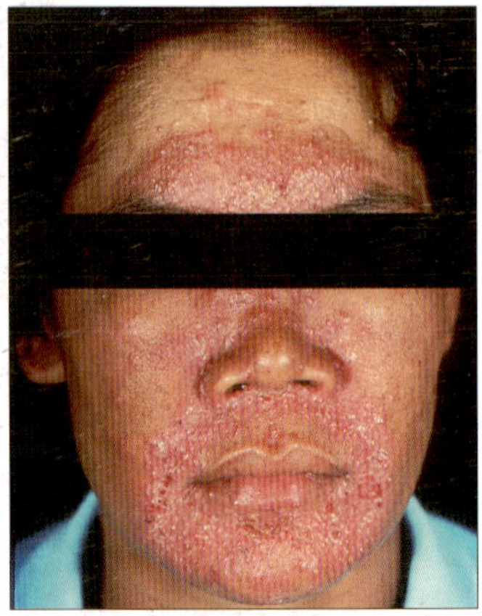

125

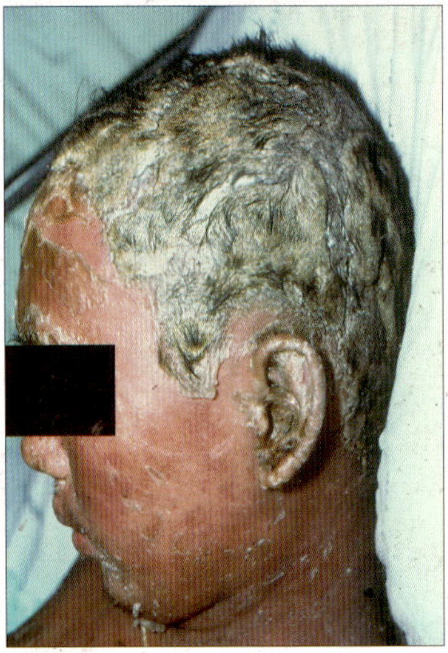

126

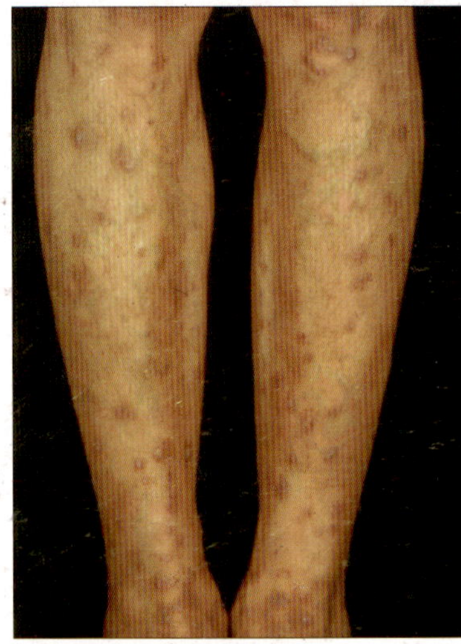

127

128

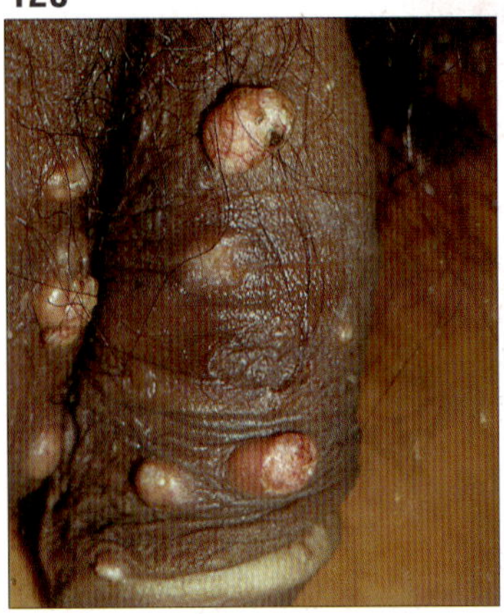

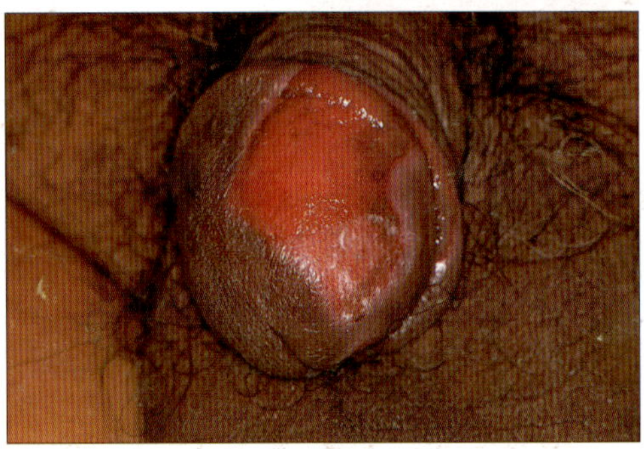

129

Plate 124. *P. marneffei* infection in AIDS. (a) Diffuse papular eruption, and (b) papules with umbilicated necrotic centre.

Plate 125. Severe seborrhoeic dermatitis in a patient with AIDS.

Plate 126. Severe psoriasis in a patient with AIDS.

Plate 127. Diffuse excoriated papules and nodules of pruritic papular eruption in a patient with HIV infection.

Plate 128. Giant lesions of molluscum contagiosum in a patient with AIDS.

Plate 129. Fixed drug eruption due to cotrimoxazole.

130

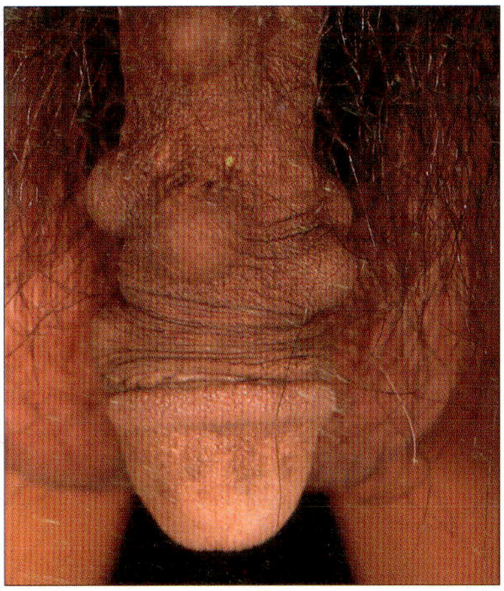

131

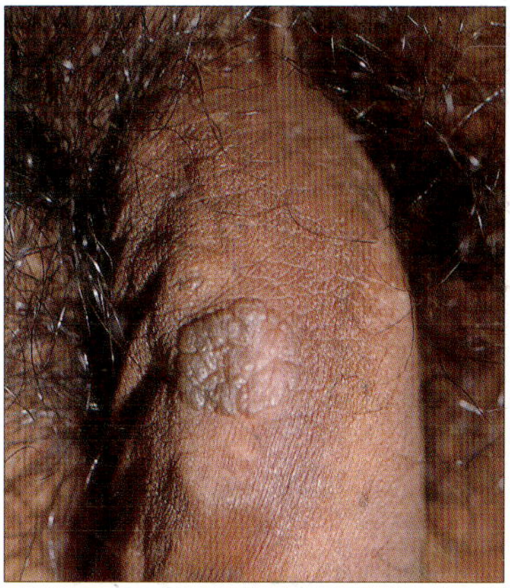

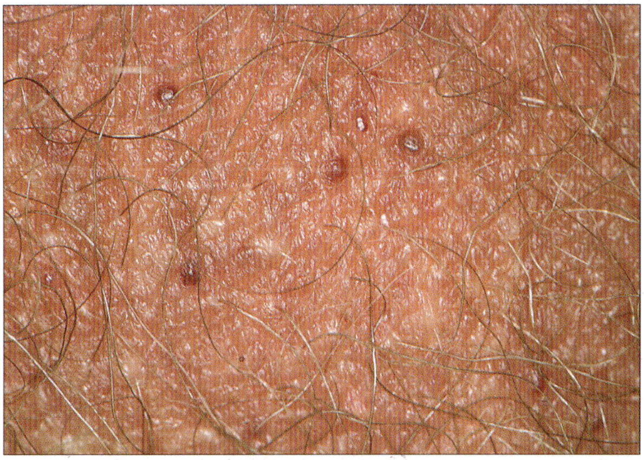

132

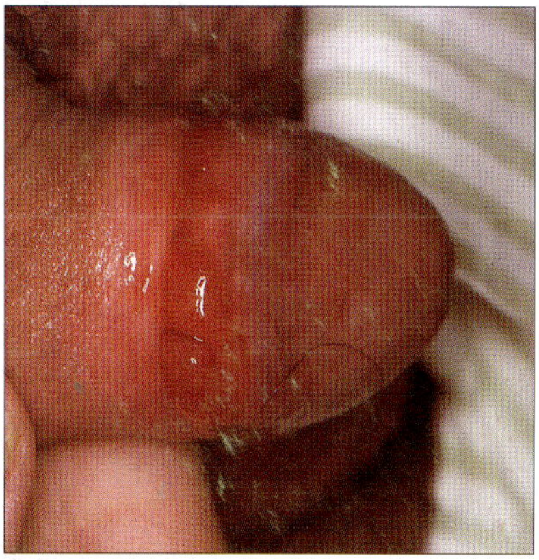

133

134

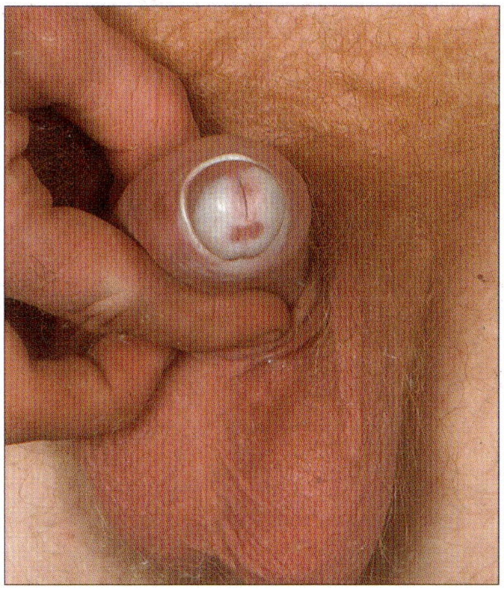

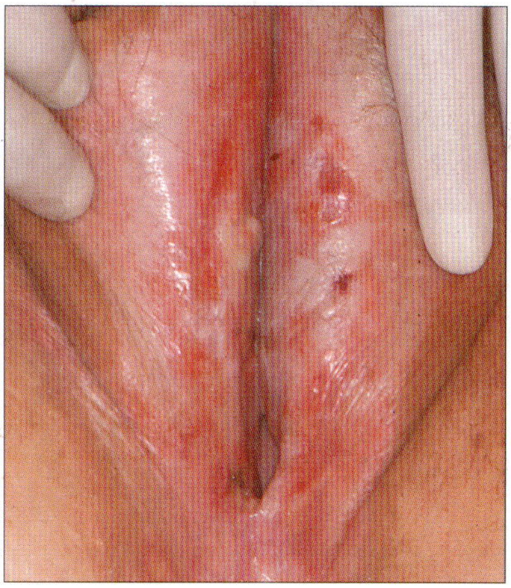

135

Plate 130. Artificial penile nodules.
Plate 131. Seborrhoeic keratosis.
Plate 132. Angiokeratomas of Fordyce.
Plate 133. Balanoposthitis of Zoon.
Plate 134. Balanitis xerotica obliterans; note also meatal stenosis.
Plate 135. Lichen sclerosus et atrophicus of the vulva. (Courtesy of Dr C. O'Mahony.)

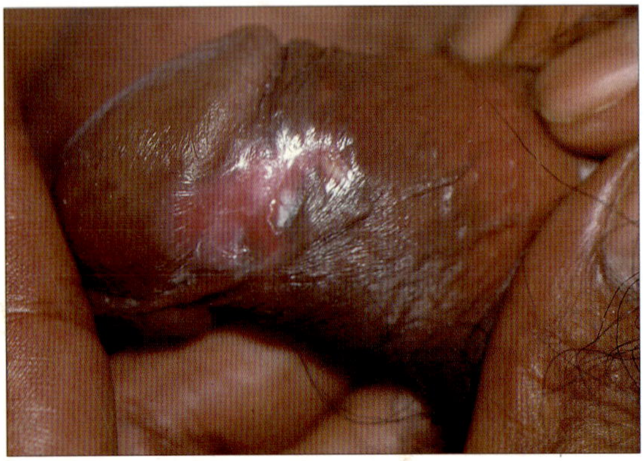

136

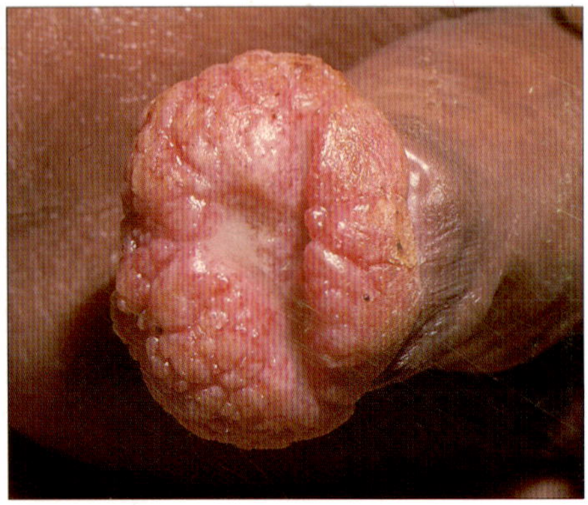

137

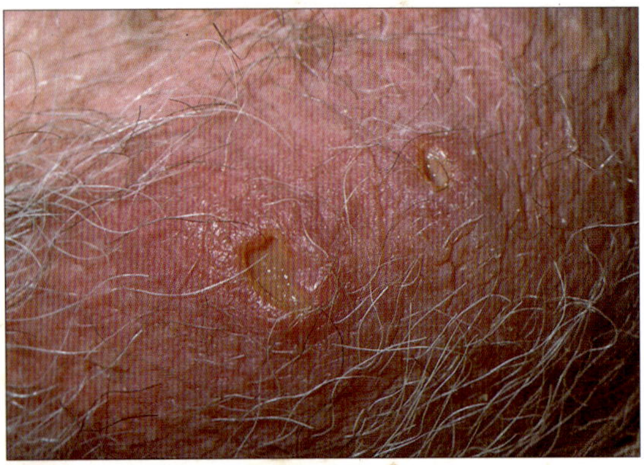

138

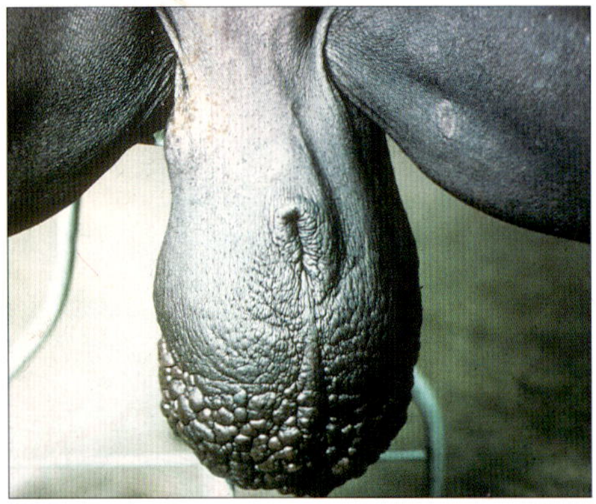

139

140

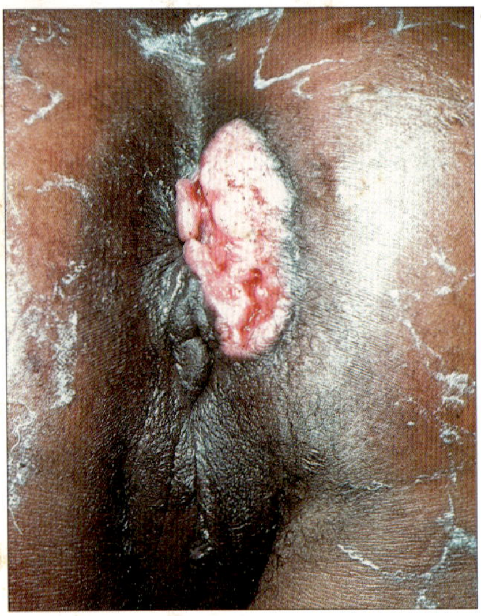

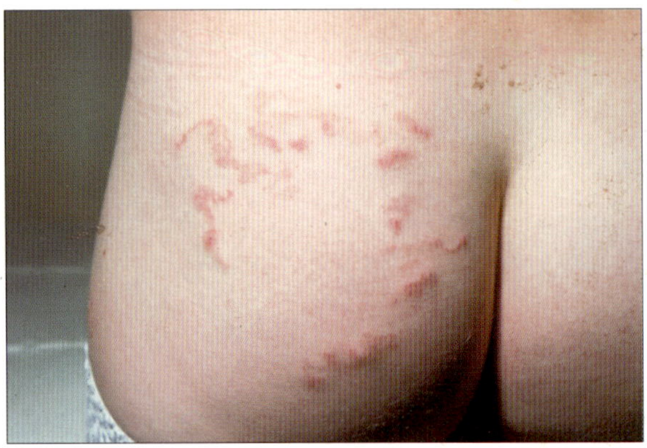

141

Plate 136. Erythroplasia of Queyrat.

Plate 137. Squamous cell carcinoma of the penis.

Plate 138. Behçet's syndrome: ulcers on the scrotum. The patient also had oral ulceration.

Plate 139. Scrotal elephantiasis as a sequel to chronic *Filaria bancrofti* infection.

Plate 140. Perianal ulceration due to *Entamoeba histolytica* in a patient with neglected amoebic dysentery.

Plate 141. Larva migrans of the buttock after a holiday in Zanzibar.